Anaesthesia
for Veterinary Nurses

Edited by

Elizabeth Welsh

Blackwell
Science

© 2003 Blackwell Science Ltd, a Blackwell
Publishing Company
Editorial Offices:
9600 Garsington Road, Oxford OX4 2DQ, UK
    Tel: +44 (0)1865 776868
Blackwell Science, Inc., 350 Main Street,
Malden, MA 02148-5020, USA
    Tel: +1 781 388 8250
Iowa State Press, a Blackwell Publishing
Company, 2121 State Avenue, Ames, Iowa
50014-8300, USA
    Tel: +1 515 292 0140
Blackwell Publishing Asia Pty Ltd,
550 Swanston Street, Carlton South,
Victoria 3053, Australia
    Tel: +61 (0)3 9347 0300
Blackwell Verlag, Kurfürstendamm 57,
10707 Berlin, Germany
    Tel: +49 (0)30 32 79 060

First published 2003 by Blackwell Science Ltd

Library of Congress
Cataloging-in-Publication Data
Anaesthesia for veterinary nurses / edited by
Elizabeth Welsh.
    p. cm.
Includes bibliographical references (p.   ).
  ISBN 0-632-05061-6 (pbk.)
  1. Veterinary anesthesia. I. Welsh, Elizabeth.

SF914.A48 2003
636.089′796--dc21

                              2002155057

ISBN 0-632-05061-6

A catalogue record for this title is available
from the British Library

Set in 10/13 pt Sabon
by Sparks Computer Solutions Ltd, Oxford
http://www.sparks.co.uk
Printed and bound in Great Britain by
TJ International, Padstow

For further information on
Blackwell Publishing, visit our website:
www.blackwellpublishing.com

Contents

Contributors

Kirstin Beard VN, DipAVN(Surg)
University of Edinburgh Hospital for Small Animals, Easter Bush Veterinary
  Centre, Roslin, Midlothian EG25 9RG

Louise Clark BVMS, CertVA, MRCVS
University of Edinburgh Hospital for Small Animals, Easter Bush Veterinary
  Centre, Roslin, Midlothian EG25 9RG

Joan Duncan BVMS, PhD, CertVR, MRCVS
Idexx Laboratories, Grange House, Sandbeck Way, Wetherby LS22 4DN

Derek Flaherty BVMS, DipECVA, DVA, MRCVS
University of Glasgow Veterinary School, Bearsden Road, Bearsden, Glasgow
  G61 1QH

Mary Fraser BVMS, PhD, CBiol, MIBiol, CertVD, MRCVS
No 9 Edderston Ridge Crescent, Peebles EH45 9ND

Simon Girling BVMS, CBiol, MIBiol, CertZooMed, MRCVS
171 Mayfield Road, Edinburgh EH9 3AZ

Janis Hamilton VN, DipAVN(Surg)
University of Glasgow Veterinary School, Bearsden Road, Bearsden, Glasgow
  G61 1QH

Craig Johnson BVSc, PhD, DVA, DipECVA, MRCA, MRCVS
Comparative Physiology and Anatomy, Institute of Veterinary, Animal and
  Biomedical Sciences, Massey University, Private Bag 11-222, Palmerston
  North, New Zealand

Janice MacGillivray VN, DipAVN(Surg)
PDSA, 211 Hawkhill, Dundee DD1 5LA

Joan Freeman VN, DipAVN(Surg)
University of Edinburgh Hospital for Small Animals, Easter Bush Veterinary
  Centre, Roslin, Midlothian EG25 9RG

Elizabeth Welsh BVMS, PhD, CertVA, CertSAS, MRCVS
University of Edinburgh Hospital for Small Animals, Easter Bush Veterinary
  Centre, Roslin, Midlothian EG25 9RG

Preface

In every small animal veterinary surgery, on every day, pet owners entrust their animals into our care. Many of these pets are sedated or anaesthetised and veterinary nurse trainees and listed veterinary nurses play a central role in this process. They are often the people who admit the patient to the clinic, are central to the care of the patient before, during and after anaesthesia, and will frequently discharge the patient into the care of its owner at the end of the day. Thus, it is vitally important that veterinary nurses at all stages of their career are familiar with the physiological, pharmacological and physical principles that underpin clinical anaesthesia.

This is the first book in the UK on the principles and practice of anaesthesia that has been aimed specifically at veterinary nurses. It has been written to help both veterinary nurse trainees and listed veterinary nurses, not only in their studies but also in navigating the daily challenges of anaesthesia more confidently. Throughout, we have aimed to provide the necessary information for this purpose at the right level and in the right detail, and, to reflect the increasing importance of small mammals, birds and reptiles in small animal practice, separate chapters have been dedicated to them.

Acknowledgements

I would like to thank all my colleagues who contributed to this book. I would like especially to mention the veterinary nurses who readily agreed to contribute to the content. The staff at Blackwell Publishing have been patient and supportive, and to them also I express my thanks.

The Role of the Veterinary Nurse in Anaesthesia

Joan Freeman

Veterinary surgeons must work within the legal constraints of the Veterinary Surgeons Act (1966). They must also abide by the rules of conduct for veterinary surgeons ('Guide to Professional Conduct') set up by the Royal College of Veterinary Surgeons (RCVS), the professional body in the United Kingdom. Veterinary surgeons can be found negligent and guilty of malpractice, not only as a consequence of their own actions but also for the injurious actions of an employee, including veterinary nurses and student veterinary nurses. Therefore, veterinary nurses are not entitled to undertake either medical treatment or minor surgery independently. Nevertheless, veterinary nurses have a duty to safeguard the health and welfare of animals under veterinary care and, as anaesthesia is a critical procedure, the need for knowledge and an understanding of the procedures involved in anaesthesia cannot be overestimated.

LEGISLATION GOVERNING VETERINARY NURSES

Student veterinary nurses who pass both Part II and Part III examinations for the veterinary nursing qualification in the United Kingdom and fulfil the practical training requirements at an approved training practice are entitled to have their names entered on a list of veterinary nurses maintained by the RCVS and to describe themselves as listed veterinary nurses.

The Veterinary Surgeons Act (1966) states that only a veterinary surgeon may practise veterinary surgery. Exceptions to this rule apply solely to listed veterinary nurses, and are covered under the 1991 amendment to Schedule 3 of the Act.

The exceptions are:

- Veterinary nurses (or any member of the public) may administer first aid in an emergency as an interim measure until a veterinary surgeon's assistance can be obtained.
- A listed veterinary nurse may administer 'any medical treatment or any minor surgery (not involving entry into a body cavity) to a companion animal' under veterinary direction.

The animal undergoing medical treatment or minor surgery must be under the care of the veterinary surgeon and he or she must be the employer of the veterinary nurse.

The Act does not define 'any medical treatment or any minor surgery' but leaves it to the individual veterinary surgeon to interpret, using their professional judgement. Thus veterinary nurses should only carry out procedures which they feel competent to perform under the direction of a veterinary surgeon, and the veterinary surgeon should be available to respond if any problems arise. Recent changes to the Veterinary Surgeons Act 1966 (Schedule 3 amendment) Order 2002 now entitles listed veterinary nurses to perform nursing duties on all species of animal, not just companion animals, and in addition allows student veterinary nurses to perform Schedule 3 tasks during their training, provided they are under the direct, continuous and personal supervision of either a listed veterinary nurse (Fig. 1.1) or veterinary surgeon.

Currently there are moves towards a system of self-regulation within the veterinary nursing profession. In such a system the privilege of being listed

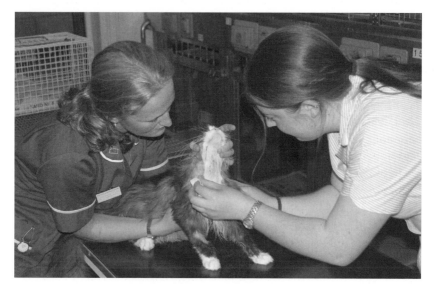

Fig. 1.1 A listed veterinary nurse supervising a veterinary nurse trainee during a clinical procedure.

would entail the veterinary nurse accepting both responsibility and account-ability for their actions. Consequently, it is reasonable to expect listed veterinary nurses to maintain their professional knowledge and competence, for example, through attendance at continuing professional development courses and conferences, and reading veterinary and veterinary nursing journals, and equally to acknowledge their limitations and if relevant make these known to their employer.

Veterinary nurses receive training in many procedures and should be competent to carry out the following under the 1991 amendment to Schedule 3 of the Veterinary Surgeons Act (1966):

- Administer medication (other than controlled drugs and biological products) orally, by inhalation, or by subcutaneous, intramuscular or intravenous injection.
- Administer other treatments such as fluid therapy, intravenous and urethral catheterisation; administer enemas; application of dressings and external casts; assisting with operations and cutaneous suturing.
- Prepare animals for anaesthesia and assist with the administration and termination of anaesthesia.
- Collect samples of blood, urine, faeces, skin and hair.
- Take radiographs.

The veterinary surgeon is responsible for the induction and maintenance of anaesthesia and the management to full recovery of animals under their care. The veterinary surgeon alone should assess the fitness of the animal for anaesthesia, select and plan pre-anaesthetic medication and a suitable anaesthetic regime, and administer the anaesthetic if the induction dose is either incremental or to effect. In addition, the veterinary surgeon should administer controlled drugs such as pethidine and morphine. However, provided the veterinary surgeon is physically present and immediately available, a listed veterinary nurse may:

- administer the selected pre-anaesthetic medication;
- administer non-incremental anaesthetic agents;
- monitor clinical signs;
- maintain an anaesthetic record;
- maintain anaesthesia under the direct instruction of the supervising veterinary surgeon.

DEFINITIONS IN ANAESTHESIA

Many different terms are used in anaesthesia and it is important to be familiar with those listed in Table 1.1.

Table 1.1 Terms used in anaesthesia.

Term	Definition
Anaesthesia	The elimination of sensation by controlled, reversible depression of the nervous system
Analeptic	Central nervous system stimulant, e.g. doxapram
Analgesia	A diminished or abolished perception of pain
General anaesthesia	The elimination of sensation by controlled, reversible depression of the central nervous system. Animals under general anaesthesia have reduced sensitivity and motor responses to external noxious stimuli
Hypnosis	Drug-induced sleep. Originally hypnosis was considered a component of anaesthesia along with muscle relaxation and analgesia, however human patients administered hypnotics could recall events when apparently in a state of anaesthesia
Local anaesthesia	The elimination of sensation from a body part by depression of sensory and/or motor neurons in the peripheral nervous system or spinal cord
Narcosis	Drug-induced sedation or stupor
Neuroleptanalgesia and neuroleptanaesthesia	Neuroleptanalgesia is a state of analgesia and indifference to the surroundings and manipulation following administration of a tranquilliser or sedative with an opioid. The effects are dose dependent and high doses can induce unconsciousness (neuroleptanaesthesia), permitting surgery
Pain	An unpleasant sensory or emotional experience associated with actual or potential tissue damage
Pre-emptive analgesia	Administering analgesic drugs before tissue injury to decrease post-operative pain
Sedative–sedation Tranquilliser–tranquillisation Neuroleptic Ataractic	These terms are used interchangeably in veterinary medicine. The terms refer to drugs that calm the patient, reduce anxiety and promote sleep. However, they do not induce sleep as hynotics do, and although animals are more calm and easier to handle they may still be roused

PRINCIPLES OF ANAESTHESIA

The purposes of anaesthesia are:

• To permit surgical or medical procedures to be performed on animals. The Protection of Animals (Anaesthetics) Acts 1954 and 1964 state that:
  'carrying out of any operation with or without the use of instruments, involving interference with the sensitive tissues or the bone structure of an animal, shall constitute an offence unless an an-

aesthetic is used in such a way as to prevent any pain to the animal during the operation'.
- To control pain.
- To restrain difficult patients. Patients may need to be restrained for radiography, bandage or cast application, etc.
- To facilitate examination by immobilising the patient. Anaesthesia and sedation allow difficult animals to be restrained and handled, reducing the risk of injury to both staff and patients.
- To control status epilepticus in animals. Diazepam and phenobarbitone may be injected to control status epilepticus. Low doses of propofol administered by continuous infusion have also been used for this purpose.
- To perform euthanasia. Euthanasia in dogs and cats is performed using concentrated anaesthetic agents.

Types of anaesthesia

General anaesthesia is the most commonly used type of anaesthesia in small animals. However it is important for veterinary nurses to understand and be familiar with local and regional anaesthetic techniques.

General anaesthesia

General anaesthesia is the elimination of sensation by controlled, reversible depression of the central nervous system. Animals under general anaesthesia have reduced sensitivity and motor responses to external noxious stimuli.

The ideal general anaesthetic would produce these effects without depression of the respiratory or cardiovascular systems, provide good muscle relaxation, and be readily available, economical, non-irritant, stable, non-toxic and not depend on metabolism for clearance from the body. Unfortunately, such an agent is not available, but a balanced anaesthetic technique can be employed using more than one drug to achieve the desired effects of narcosis, muscle relaxation and analgesia. This approach has the added advantage that the dose of each individual agent used may be reduced and consequently the side effects of each agent also tend to be reduced.

General anaesthetic agents may be administered by injection, inhalation or a combination of both techniques. The subcutaneous, intramuscular or intravenous routes may be used to administer injectable anaesthetics. The safe use of injectable agents depends on the calculated dose being based on the accurate weight of the animal. Propofol and thiopentone are commonly used intravenous agents; ketamine and alphaxalone–alphadalone (Saffan®) are intramuscular agents. In addition ketamine may be administered subcutaneously. Inhalational anaesthetic agents may be either volatile agents or gases and administered in an induction chamber, by mask or by tracheal intubation. Halothane, isoflurane and nitrous oxide are commonly used in small animals.

Local anaesthesia

Local anaesthesia is the elimination of sensation from a body part by depression of sensory and/or motor neurons in the peripheral nervous system or spinal cord. Local anaesthetic drugs (e.g. lignocaine) and opioids (e.g. morphine) are commonly used in this way (see chapter 6).

Both general and local anaesthesia have advantages and disadvantages and a number of factors will influence the type of anaesthesia used.

(1) The state of health of the animal: An animal with systemic disease or presented for emergency surgery will be compromised and a different anaesthetic regime may be required to that for a young healthy animal undergoing an elective procedure.
(2) Pre-anaesthetic preparation: Animals presented for emergency procedures are unlikely to have been fasted for an appropriate length of time prior to anaesthesia.
(3) Species, breed, temperament and age of the animal: Certain anaesthetic agents may be contra-indicated in certain species e.g. Saffan® in dogs.
(4) The duration of the procedure to be performed.
(5) The complexity of the procedure to be performed.
(6) The experience of the surgeon will influence the duration of the procedure and trauma to tissues.
(7) A well-equipped and staffed veterinary hospital may be better able to deal with a general anaesthetic crises.

Anaesthetic period

Veterinary nurses are involved from the time of admission of the patient to the veterinary clinic until discharge of the animal back to the owner's care.

The anaesthetic period can be divided into five phases, with different nursing responsibilities and patient risks associated with each phase. The surgical team is responsible for the welfare of the patient at all stages and it is important that they work as a team. Communication between team members is important to minimise both the risks to the patient and the duration of the anaesthetic. All members of the team must be familiar with the surgical procedure. The anaesthetic area and theatre should be prepared and equipment which may be required checked and available for use. Members of the team should also be familiar with possible intra- and postoperative complications and the appropriate action to be taken should they occur.

(1) *Preoperative period*: The animal is examined and an anaesthetic protocol devised by the veterinary surgeon to minimise the risk to the individual animal. The animal's health, the type of procedure, the ability and experience

of both the anaesthetist and the surgeon are all factors that should be considered. The area for induction and maintenance of anaesthesia must be clean and prepared. All equipment should be checked for faults, and drugs and ancillary equipment should be set up for use.

(2) *Pre-anaesthetic period*: Pre-anaesthetic medication is given as part of a balanced anaesthesia protocol. Sedatives and analgesics are used to reduce anxiety, relieve discomfort, enable a smooth induction and reduce the requirement for high doses of anaesthetic induction and maintenance agents. The animal should be allowed to remain undisturbed following administration of the pre-anaesthetic agents, although close observation during this period is recommended.

(3) *Induction period*: Anaesthesia should be induced in a calm and quiet environment. Placement of an intravenous catheter allows for ease of administration of intravenous agents and prevents the risk of extravascular injection of irritant drugs. To ensure a smooth transition from induction to maintenance, appropriate endotracheal tubes, anaesthetic breathing system and ancillary equipment must be prepared for use. Suitable intravenous fluids should be administered during anaesthesia.

(4) *Maintenance period*: Unconsciousness is maintained with inhalational or injectable agents. This allows the planned procedure to be performed. A properly trained person should be dedicated to monitor anaesthesia. Unqualified staff should not be expected to monitor anaesthesia. An anaesthetic record should be kept for every patient. Monitoring needs to be systematic and regular, with intervals of no more than 5 minutes recommended. This enables trends and potential problems to be identified.

(5) *Recovery period*: Administration of anaesthetic drugs ceases and the animal is allowed to regain consciousness. Monitoring should continue until the patient is fully recovered.

THE NURSE'S ROLE DURING THE ANAESTHETIC PERIOD

- To ensure that the animal is prepared for anaesthesia according to the instructions of the veterinary surgeon.
- To observe the patient following administration of the pre-anaesthetic medication.
- To ensure that the necessary equipment is prepared.
- To assist the veterinary surgeon.
- To monitor both the patient and equipment during the anaesthetic period.
- To observe the patient during the postoperative period.
- To administer treatments as directed by the veterinary surgeon.

Consent for anaesthesia

Initial communication with the client is very important, and often for elective procedures the veterinary nurse is the initial contact. In addition to being a legal requirement, completion of an anaesthetic consent form is also an opportunity for the nurse to introduce himself or herself to the client.

The nurse needs to maintain a professional friendliness and be approachable. It is important that the client understands the risks associated with all anaesthetics and surgical procedures. The nurse can explain to the client how the practice aims to minimise these risks. In addition, they can reassure the client by informing them that their pet will receive a full physical examination prior to administration of the anaesthetic, and that the practice will contact the client should further diagnostic tests be required, for example, blood tests or radiographs. The nurse can explain to the client that modern anaesthetics are safer than those used in the past and that their pet will receive pre-anaesthetic medication, which will help both by calming the animal and by reducing the total amount of anaesthetic required. It is also important to reassure the client that trained veterinary nurses or supervised trainees will monitor their pet throughout the procedure and during recovery.

Details required on the anaesthetic consent form may include:

- The date.
- The client's name and address.
- Contact telephone number.
- The animal's identification.
- The surgical or diagnostic procedure to be performed, including identification of lesion(s) for removal if appropriate.
- Known allergies.
- Current medication.
- A brief summary of the risks relating to anaesthesia.
- The client's signature.
- Extra information may be recorded, such as an estimate of the cost of the procedure, any items left with the animal, dietary requirements, and so on.

HEALTH AND SAFETY ASPECTS OF ANAESTHESIA

Health and safety legislation ensures that the workplace is a safe environment in which to work. A number of regulations are enforced to minimise the risk of exposure to hazardous substances and accidents within the workplace.

The Health and Safety at Work Act (1974)

This act states that the employer is responsible for providing safe systems of work and adequately maintained equipment, and for ensuring that all substances are handled, stored and transported in a safe manner. Safe systems of

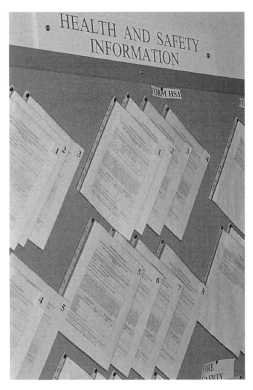

Fig. 1.2 Health and safety documentation prominently displayed within a veterinary hospital.

work should be written as standard operating procedures (SOPs) and be displayed in the appropriate areas of the workplace (Fig. 1.2).

The Control of Substances Hazardous to Health (COSHH) (1988)
COSHH assessments involve written SOPs, assessing hazards and risks for all potential hazards within a veterinary practice. All staff should be able to identify hazards, know the route of exposure and the specific first aid should an accident occur.

Misuse of Drugs Act (1971) and Misuse of Drugs Regulations (1986)
In the United Kingdom the use of drugs is controlled by the Misuse of Drugs Act (1971) and the Misuse of Drugs Regulations (1986). The 1971 Act divides drugs into three classes depending on the degree of harm attributable to each drug. Class A drugs (or class B injectable agents) are deemed to be the most harmful and class C drugs the least. The 1986 Regulations divide controlled drugs into five schedules that determine the nature of the control.

The 1986 Regulations cover a wide range of drugs, of which only a few are in regular use in veterinary practice. Schedule 1 drugs, for example, LSD, are stringently controlled and are not used in veterinary practice. Schedule 2 drugs include morphine, pethidine, fentanyl (Hypnorm®), alfentanil, methadone and etorphine (Immobilon®). Codeine and other weaker opiates and opioids are also Schedule 2 drugs. An opiate is a drug derived from the opium poppy while an opioid refers to drugs that bind to opioid receptors and may be synthetic, semi-synthetic or natural. Separate records must be kept for all Schedule 2 drugs obtained and supplied in a controlled drugs register. These drugs can only be signed out by a veterinary surgeon and the date, animal identification details, volume and route of administration must be recorded. The controlled drug register should be checked on a regular basis and thefts of controlled drugs must be reported to the police. Schedule 2 drugs must be kept in a locked receptacle, which can only be opened by authorised personnel (Fig.1.3). Expired stocks must be destroyed in the presence of witnesses (principal of the practice and/or the police) and both parties involved must sign the register.

Schedule 3 drugs are subject to prescription and requisition requirements, but do not need to be recorded in the controlled drugs register. However, buprenorphine is required to be kept in a locked receptacle. It is recommended that other drugs in this schedule such as the barbiturates (thiopentone, pentobarbitone, phenobarbitone) and pentazocine should also be kept in a locked cupboard.

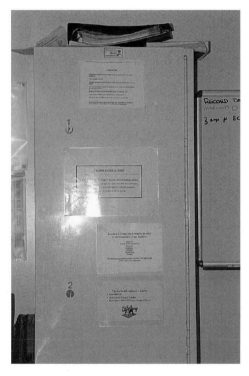

Fig. 1.3 A locked, fixed receptacle for storing controlled drugs. Keys should never be left in the lock of controlled drug cabinets.

The remaining two Schedules include the benzodiazepines (Schedule 4) and preparations containing opiates or opioids (Schedule 5).

Specific hazards
Compressed gas cylinders
Anaesthetic gas cylinders contain gas at high pressure and will explode if mishandled. Gas cylinders should be securely stored in a cool, dry area away from direct sunlight. Size F cylinders and larger should be stored vertically by means of a chain or strap. Size E cylinders and smaller may be stored horizontally. Racks used to store cylinders must be appropriate for the size of cylinder. Cylinders should only be moved using the appropriate size and type of trolley. Cylinders should be handled with care and not knocked violently or allowed to fall. Valves and any associated equipment must never be lubricated and must be kept free from oil and grease.

Both oxygen and nitrous oxide are non-flammable but strongly support combustion. They are highly dangerous due to the risk of spontaneous combustion when in contact with oils, greases, tarry substances and many plastics.

Exposure to volatile anaesthetic agents
Atmospheric pollution and exposure to waste gases must be kept to a minimum. Long-term exposure to waste anaesthetic gases has been linked to congenital abnormalities in children of anaesthesia personnel, spontaneous abortions, and liver and kidney damage. Inhalation of expired anaesthetic gases can result in fatigue, headaches, irritability and nausea. In 1996 the British Government Services Advisory Committee published its recommendations, *Anaesthetic Agents: Controlling Exposure Under the Control of Substances Hazardous to Health Regulations 1994*, in which standards for occupational exposure were issued. The occupational exposure standards (OES) (see box) are for an 8-hour time-weighted average reference period for trace levels of waste anaesthetic gases.

> OCCUPATIONAL EXPOSURE STANDARDS
> 100 ppm for nitrous oxide
> 50 ppm for enflurane and isoflurane
> 10 ppm for halothane
> 20 ppm for sevoflurane. The Health and Safety Executive currently has not set an official OES for sevoflurane but an employee exposure limit of 20 ppm is proposed (Abbott, personal communication).

These values are well below the levels at which any significant adverse effects occur in animals, and represent levels at which there is no evidence to suggest human health would be affected. Personal dose meters may be worn to measure exposure to anaesthetic gases. A separate dose meter is required for each anaesthetic agent to be monitored. These should be worn near the face to measure the amount of inspired waste gas. The dose meter should be worn for a minimum of 1.5 hours, but it will give a more realistic reading if worn over a longer period. At least two members of the surgical team should be monitored on two occasions for the gases to which they may be exposed. When analysed, an 8-hour weighted average is calculated and a certificate issued.

Sources of exposure

The main ways in which personnel are exposed to anaesthetic gases involve the technique used to administer the anaesthetic and the equipment used.

Anaesthetic techniques

- Turning on gases before the animal is connected.
- Failure to turn off gases at the end of the anaesthetic.
- Use of uncuffed or too small a diameter endotracheal tubes.
- Use of masks or chambers for induction.
- Flushing of the breathing system.

Anaesthetic machine, breathing system and scavenging system

- Leaks in hoses or anaesthetic machine.
- Type of breathing system used, and ability to scavenge.
- Refilling the anaesthetic vaporiser.
- Inadequate scavenging system.

Precautions

Anaesthetic vaporisers should be removed to a fume hood or a well-ventilated area for refilling. It is important not to tilt the vaporiser when carrying it. 'Key-indexed' filling systems are associated with less spillage than 'funnel-fill' vaporisers, however, gloves should be worn. The 'key-indexed' system is agent specific and will prevent accidental filling of a vaporiser with the incorrect agent. Vaporisers should be filled at the end of the working day, when prolonged exposure to spilled anaesthetic agent is minimised.

In the event of accidental spillage or breakage of a bottle of liquid volatile anaesthetic, immediately evacuate all personnel from the area. Increase the ventilation by opening windows or turning on exhaust fans. Use an absorbent material such as cat litter to control the spill. This can be collected in a plastic bag and removed to a safe area.

Soda lime

Wet soda lime is very caustic. Staff should wear a face mask and latex gloves when handling soda lime in circle breathing systems.

Safety of personnel

The safety of personnel should not be compromised. Veterinary nurses should wear slip-proof shoes, and 'wet floor' signs should be displayed when necessary to reduce the risk of personal injury from slips and falls. Staff should never run inside the hospital.

Care should be taken when lifting patients, supplies and equipment. Trolleys or hoists should be used wherever possible and assistance should be sought with heavy items.

The risk of bites and scratches can be minimised by using suitable physical restraint, muzzles, dogcatchers and crush cages. Fingers should not be placed in an animal's mouth either during intubation or during recovery. It is important to learn the proper restraint positions for different species and focus attention on the animal's reactions.

Sharp objects such as needles and scalpel blades should be disposed of immediately after use in a designated 'sharps' container. All drugs drawn up for injection should be labelled and dated. If dangerous drugs are used the needle should not be removed and both the syringe and needle should be disposed of intact in the sharps container.

To prevent the risk of self-administration or 'needle-stick' injuries, the following guidelines should be observed:

- Unguarded needles should never be left lying about.
- Needles should not be recapped but disposed of directly into a sharps container.
- Do not place needle caps in the mouth for removal, as some drugs may be rapidly absorbed through the mucous membranes.
- Do not carry needles and syringes in pockets.
- Never insert fingers into or open a used sharps container.

Guidelines on the safe use of multidose bottles or vials in anaesthesia, and the use of glass ampoules in anaesthesia, are to be found at the end of chapter 6 (Figs 6.5 and 6.6).

MORTALITY

Anaesthesia in fit and healthy small animals is a safe procedure and should pose little risk to the animal.

Mortality in small animals appears to be unnecessarily high when compared to man. In a study conducted in healthy dogs and cats in the UK it was estimated that 1 in 679 animals died primarily as a result of anaesthesia (Clarke & Hall 1990), while in man 1 in 10 000 patients died purely as a result of the anaesthetic (Lunn & Mushin 1982).

Many of the animal deaths occurred when the animal was not under close observation. However, deaths were reported to be due to failure of the oxygen supply, overdose of anaesthetic agents, unfamiliarity with drugs, respiratory obstruction and misinterpretation of depth of anaesthesia. In cats, complications following endotracheal intubation and mask induction of anaesthesia were identified as risk factors.

The death rate for dogs and cats with pathological but not immediately life-threatening conditions was estimated to be 1 in 31. Most of these animals died while undergoing diagnostic radiography. This highlights the need for careful physical examination prior to investigation and the need to anticipate potential anaesthetic problems.

Although it is unlikely in veterinary anaesthesia that a similar death rate to that in man will be achieved, the rate of 1 in 679 leaves considerable room for improvement.

A new Confidential Enquiry into Perioperative Small Animal Fatalities (CE-PSAF) is being launched in the United Kingdom in summer 2002, and it will be interesting to see whether continuing advances in anaesthetic technique, equipment, drugs and education have reduced the incidence of perioperative fatalities in small animals.

REFERENCES

Clarke, K.W. & Hall, L.W. (1990) A survey of anaesthesia in small animal practice: AVA/BSAVA report. *Journal of the Association of Veterinary Anaesthetists* **17**, 4–10.

Lunn, J.N. & Mushin, W.W. (1982) Mortality associated with anaesthesia. *Anaesthesia* **37**, 856.

RCVS (2002) *List of Veterinary Nurses 2002*. Veterinary Nurses and the Veterinary Surgeons Act 1966, pp 81–83.

Physiology Relevant to Anaesthesia

Mary Fraser

A good understanding of normal physiological processes is essential for veterinary nurses because all anaesthetic agents affect the organ function of anaesthetised animals to a greater or lesser extent, whether healthy or otherwise. Conversely, organ dysfunction (for example, hepatopathy, renal disease) can also affect the functioning of anaesthetic agents.

RESPIRATORY SYSTEM

The main function of the respiratory system is to carry oxygen into the body and remove carbon dioxide. The respiratory tract is also used to deliver volatile and gaseous anaesthetic agents. Therefore in order to carry out successful anaesthesia the normal functioning of the respiratory system must be understood. Any disease of the respiratory system will need to be considered when deciding upon an anaesthetic regime for an individual animal.

Respiratory cycle

At rest, the lungs are held expanded in the thoracic cavity due to negative pressure in the intrapleural space. In healthy animals this is equal to −4 mmHg. Inspiration begins with movement of the diaphragm caudally. This increases the volume of the thorax, and air is pulled into the lungs. During quiet breathing, movement of the diaphragm and ribs are the main factors causing inspiration. However, during physical activity contraction of the abdominal muscles results in an increase in negative pressure within the thorax as well, and therefore an increase in the volume of air inspired.

During expiration, diaphragmatic, intercostal and possibly abdominal muscles relax. This decreases the volume of the thorax and air is forced out of the lungs. Again, when the animal is breathing more forcefully, active contraction of the intercostal muscles forces more air out of the lungs. In addition to the movement of muscles, elastic recoil of the lungs themselves also forces some air out of the airways.

MUSCLES OF RESPIRATION
- Diaphragm
- External intercostal muscles
- Internal intercostal muscles
- Abdominal muscles

The coordinated movements of diaphragmatic and intercostal muscles to produce inspiration and expiration are controlled by two main factors: first, the chemical constituents of the bloodstream such as oxygen and carbon dioxide, and second, stretch receptors located in the lungs themselves to prevent overinflation.

Chemoreceptors are located in three main sites in the body: the carotid body on each side of the carotid bifurcation; the aortic body near the arch of the aorta; and in the medulla. All of these areas have a high blood flow, so that they can easily detect any changes in the concentrations of carbon dioxide, oxygen and hydrogen ions (pH) in the bloodstream. Information from the carotid body is transferred to the medulla *via* the glossopharyngeal nerve and that from the aortic body *via* the vagus nerve.

The concentrations of gases in the body fluids are described by their partial pressure. This is the pressure exerted by an individual gas where there is a mixture of gases. The symbol P is used to denote the partial pressure of specific gases, for example, PO_2 (oxygen) and PCO_2 (carbon dioxide). If the amount of oxygen present increases then the PO_2 will increase; the same applies for carbon dioxide.

Any increase in the partial pressure of carbon dioxide (PCO_2) or in the hydrogen ion (H^+) concentration or a decrease in the partial pressure of oxygen (PO_2) will be detected by the chemoreceptors mentioned above, and will cause an increase in the activity of the respiratory centre in the medulla. Stimulation of the respiratory centre results in contraction of the muscular portion of the diaphragm and the intercostal muscles so that respiratory rate and depth are increased (hyperpnoea). Although carbon dioxide, oxygen and hydrogen ion concentration are monitored, carbon dioxide is the main controlling factor because the respiratory centre in mammals works to keep PCO_2 levels constant. This is illustrated in the following example.

If the air that an animal inhales has a low level of oxygen then the respiratory centre will be stimulated so that respiration increases. However, this increase in respiration will result in a decrease in blood carbon dioxide level due to increased expiration of carbon dioxide from the lungs. This decrease in PCO_2 will be detected by the chemoreceptors and respiration will be decreased so that blood carbon dioxide level can increase back to normal (see Fig. 2.1).

In the same way, if an animal inhales 100% oxygen, then the increased blood oxygen level will be detected by chemoreceptors and respiration will be depressed. An animal will only be given 100% oxygen if there is a potential problem with its respiration; obviously an unwanted outcome is to depress respiration to the extent that the animal stops breathing. It is important to give 100% oxygen for only relatively short periods of time so that inhibition of respiration is minimised (see Fig. 2.2).

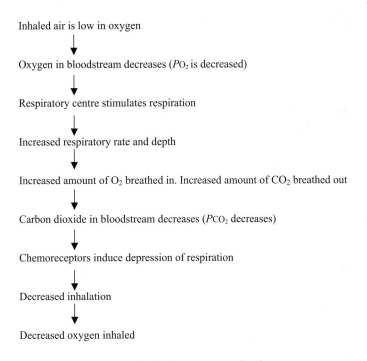

Inhaled air is low in oxygen

↓

Oxygen in bloodstream decreases (PO_2 is decreased)

↓

Respiratory centre stimulates respiration

↓

Increased respiratory rate and depth

↓

Increased amount of O_2 breathed in. Increased amount of CO_2 breathed out

↓

Carbon dioxide in bloodstream decreases (PCO_2 decreases)

↓

Chemoreceptors induce depression of respiration

↓

Decreased inhalation

↓

Decreased oxygen inhaled

Fig. 2.1 Changes in respiratory cycle due to low oxygen levels.

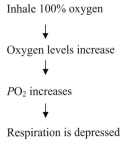

Inhale 100% oxygen

↓

Oxygen levels increase

↓

PO_2 increases

↓

Respiration is depressed

Fig. 2.2 Effect of 100% oxygen on respiration.

In conditions where animals become hypoxic, respiration will eventually increase, but only once the factors controlling carbon dioxide concentrations and hydrogen ion concentrations are overridden.

Pulmonary stretch receptors are present within the smooth muscle of the airways. When the lungs inflate the stretch receptors are activated and send impulses to the respiratory centre *via* the vagus nerve. This causes inhibition of the medullary inspiratory neurons and inspiration is stopped, thus preventing the lungs from being overinflated. Similarly, when the lungs deflate, the stretch receptors are no longer activated; inhibition of inspiratory neurons stops and inspiration can take place. This mechanism is known as the Hering–Bruer reflex.

The Hering–Bruer reflex plays an important role during intermittent positive pressure ventilation (IPPV) in anaesthetised or unconscious patients. Manual or mechanical IPPV inflates the lungs, activating airway smooth muscle stretch receptors and inhibiting spontaneous respiration.

AVERAGE NORMAL RESPIRATORY RATES
Dog: 10–30 breaths per minute (faster in small breeds)
Cat: 20–30 breaths per minute

The respiratory rate can be affected by a variety of different factors, some of which are listed in the next box.

FACTORS AFFECTING RESPIRATORY RATE
- Age
- Temperature
- Stress
- Drugs
- Exercise
- Body size
- Disease

Many of the drugs used during anaesthesia of small animals will affect the control of respiration. For example, ketamine induces characteristic changes in respiration known as an apneustic response. Here the cat or dog will inspire slowly, pause and then expire rapidly. Thiopentone and propofol can cause post-induction apnoea.

Lung volumes
Air that is present in the airways can be classified in different ways. Individuals

who administer or monitor anaesthesia need to understand these classifications as they are of practical importance (Fig. 2.3).

The simplest way of describing air in the lungs is by **tidal volume**. This is classically defined as the volume of air that is breathed in or out in one breath; note that it is *not* the sum total of the volume of air breathed in and out. In the dog the normal tidal volume is 15–20 ml/kg.

When an animal breathes out, the airway does not collapse and some air is always left in the airways. The volume of air that is left in the lungs following normal expiration is known as the **functional residual capacity**. This means that throughout the entire respiratory cycle, air is in contact with the alveoli. Hence during anaesthesia volatile or gaseous anaesthetic agents will be present in the alveoli and can continue to diffuse into the bloodstream even during expiration. Functional residual capacity allows the concentration of oxygen and volatile and/or gaseous anaesthetic agent present in the alveoli to remain constant over a short period of time instead of fluctuating between inspiration and expiration.

Although the functional residual capacity is left in the lungs at the end of normal expiration, it is still possible to force more air out of the lungs by using thoracic muscles. This volume is known as the **expiratory reserve volume**. It is possible, but not desirable, to reduce the expiratory reserve volume by pressing on the patient's chest when checking the position of an endotracheal tube following intubation. In addition to being able to force more air out of the lungs at

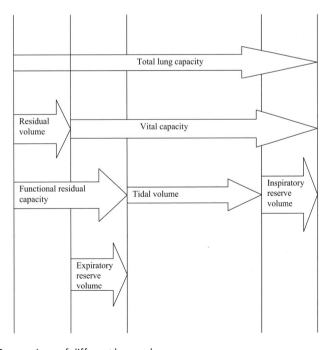

Fig. 2.3 Comparison of different lung volumes.

the end of expiration, it is possible to take more air into the lungs at the end of normal inspiration. This is known as the **inspiratory reserve volume**.

Following the most forceful expiration, some air still remains in the lungs. This is known as the **residual volume**. It is not possible to force all air out of the lungs due to the elasticity of the lungs holding the airways open and holding air within them. If all air were to be forced out of the lungs, then they would collapse!

Following the most forceful expiration, the lungs can take in more air than during normal respiration. If a patient were to breathe in as much air as possible at this point, then this volume would be the most that it could take in, in one breath. This is known as the **vital capacity**. The total volume of air present in the lungs at this time is calculated by adding the vital capacity to the residual volume and is known as the **total lung capacity** (Fig. 2.3).

The purpose of breathing is to supply the alveoli with oxygen and to remove carbon dioxide from them. However, gaseous exchange takes place at the surface of the alveoli. Therefore, although we can measure different volumes of air that pass into or out of the lungs, only a very small proportion of this air is involved in gaseous exchange.

The area within the respiratory tree, where gaseous exchange does not take place, is known as **dead space**. This can be described in different ways. The simplest is **anatomical dead space**. This is the area of the airways from the trachea down to the level of the terminal bronchioles. Anatomical dead space is relatively fixed, however it can change slightly due to lengthening or shortening of the bronchiole during respiration. In addition, atropine and other parasympatholytic agents relax airway smooth muscle, increasing anatomical dead space.

When dogs pant dead space air from the upper airways moves in and out of the body, cooling the animal by evaporative heat loss. It is important that this movement of air does not interfere with gaseous exchange because the animal would then hyperventilate and oxygen and carbon dioxide levels would be affected.

Anaesthetic apparatus (for example, an endotracheal tube extending beyond the tip of the nose) can increase the effect of dead space; the additional space is referred to as **mechanical or apparatus dead space**.

The other way of describing dead space is **physiological dead space**. This depends on the dimensions of the airways and the volume of air that enters the alveoli but does not diffuse. For example, air in the alveoli may not diffuse due to inadequate capillary perfusion of the alveoli. Therefore physiological dead space also takes into account the cardiovascular system and gives us a more accurate description of the proportion of air that is not being used by the body.

The **ventilation perfusion ratio** is used to indicate the concentrations of oxygen and carbon dioxide in the bloodstream related to the alveolar ventilation and the amount of blood perfusing the alveoli. From the point of anaesthesia, alveolar ventilation is very important because this will control the amount of volatile or gaseous anaesthetic agent that can diffuse into the bloodstream. Any increase in alveolar ventilation will increase the uptake of anaesthetic agent into the pulmonary blood.

When describing gaseous anaesthetic flow rates the term **minute ventilation** (or **minute respiratory volume**) is often used. This is defined as the total amount of air that moves in or out of the airways and alveoli in one minute, and is calculated by multiplying the respiratory rate by the tidal volume. If we assume a respiratory rate of 20 breaths per minute and an average tidal volume of 15 ml/kg, this will give a minute volume of 300 ml/kg. It should be remembered that this is an average figure. The respiratory rate will be different for different animals and hence the minute volume will be different too.

Oxygen transport

Oxygen is transported round the body in the haemoglobin of red blood cells (erythrocytes). Haemoglobin is a large molecule made up of four haem molecules and one globin molecule. Each haem molecule is associated with an atom of iron, which has the ability to combine with oxygen. Therefore, each haemoglobin molecule can transport four molecules of oxygen.

Oxygen in the alveoli diffuses across the cell membrane into interstitial water, then into vascular water (plasma) and finally into the erythrocyte (see Fig. 2.4). Within erythrocytes, oxygen is present both in the intracellular water and combined with haemoglobin. The erythrocytes then travel round the body. In areas of reduced oxygen concentration oxygen leaves the erythrocytes, enters the plasma and then passes across the cell endothelium lining the capillary into interstitial water. Finally it enters the target cell where it will be used.

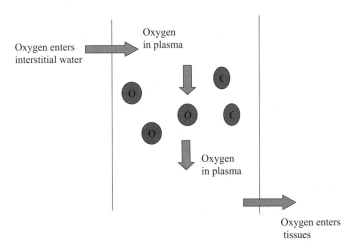

Fig. 2.4 Oxygen transport.

Oxygen is a relatively soluble gas and the amount of oxygen that is in solution is directly related to the PO_2 and the solubility coefficient for oxygen (Henry's law). The oxygen requirement of a dog or cat is 4–5 ml/kg/min and will influence the fresh gas flow rate during anaesthesia.

Carbon dioxide is much more soluble than oxygen. Carbon dioxide produced by aerobic cell metabolism diffuses from an area of high concentration in the cell to an area of low concentration in the interstitial water. The carbon dioxide then crosses into plasma and finally enters the intracellular water of the erythrocyte.

Carbon dioxide can be carried on haemoglobin, dissolved in cellular fluid or hydrated to carbonic acid (H_2CO_3). This unstable molecule breaks down to produce hydrogen ions (H^+) and bicarbonate (HCO_3^-), as shown below.

$$CO_2 + H_2O \leftrightarrow H_2CO_3 \leftrightarrow H^+ + HCO_3^-$$

This equation illustrates why carbon dioxide is important in the acid–base balance of the body. Some of the hydrogen ions can diffuse into plasma, but haemoglobin also plays a role by buffering the hydrogen ions to keep the pH constant within the cell. Once the erythrocytes reach the lungs, carbon dioxide diffuses out of the erythrocyte into plasma and into the alveoli where it is breathed out.

Where concentrations of carbon dioxide increase, some of this is converted to carbonic acid with the release of hydrogen ions. This means that increases in carbon dioxide levels will lead to a decrease in body pH and the development of respiratory acidosis.

Influence of disease or anaesthesia on respiration

Many aspects of disease can affect how well the respiratory system functions. Clearly, animals with pneumonia or bronchitis will have impaired respiration, due to secretions building up in the airways and reducing the volume of air that comes in contact with the surface of the alveoli, or the alveoli themselves becoming damaged or thickened. Healthy alveoli are one cell thick and gases can diffuse easily across them. Thickening of the alveoli will reduce the degree of gaseous diffusion that can take place causing decreased alveolar ventilation and an increased physiological shunt, that is, blood passes through the lungs but is not adequately oxygenated.

It has been noted that it is important that alveoli have an adequate blood supply. Normally, at rest, the dorsal aspects of the lungs have greater ventilation than perfusion, whereas the ventral aspects have greater perfusion than ventilation. However, in recumbent animals the position changes and there is an uneven distribution of blood flow and ventilation. This will affect the ventilation perfusion ratio and the animal may develop respiratory problems. Recumbent posture can occur for any number of reasons, such as geriatric animals or spinal disease, but is probably most important in the anaesthetised animal.

While the flow rate of oxygen and gaseous anaesthetic agents and the concentration of volatile anaesthetic agents administered to an animal may be adjusted, it is important to take account of potential inequalities of ventilation and perfusion as this will affect the uptake of gases and the depth of anaesthesia achieved. Where the recovery period is prolonged, it is important to turn the animal, so that gaseous and volatile anaesthetic agents can be removed from the lungs efficiently.

Changes in acid–base balance also affect respiration. The medulla monitors the concentration of carbon dioxide, oxygen and hydrogen ions in the bloodstream. Where an animal suffers from acidaemia or alkalaemia, the hydrogen ion concentration will have changed. One way that the body can rectify this is by altering the amount of carbon dioxide in the body. For example, in the case of metabolic acidosis (e.g. due to diabetes mellitus) the hydrogen ion concentration will have increased. Carbon dioxide can be combined with water to produce carbonic acid and hydrogen ions. This reaction can be reversed to remove hydrogen ions and produce carbon dioxide. If the animal is acidaemic hydrogen ions are removed from the circulation with the result that more carbon dioxide is produced. Therefore the respiratory rate needs to increase so that the carbon dioxide can be removed from the circulation *via* the lungs. Similarly, if an animal is affected by metabolic alkalosis, ventilation will be depressed and carbon dioxide builds up in the body. Some carbon dioxide in the bloodstream will convert to carbonic acid with a concomitant increase in hydrogen ion concentration that will neutralise the acidosis.

Changes in respiratory rate (either voluntary or during anaesthesia) will affect the body's hydrogen ion concentration. Hyperventilation results in the loss of carbon dioxide and a drop in hydrogen ions. This is known as **respiratory alkalosis**. Conversely, during hypoventilation, **respiratory acidosis** will result.

If an anaesthetised animal breathes in carbon dioxide (for example, if there is a problem in carbon dioxide removal in a closed breathing system) the animal will hyperventilate to try to remove the carbon dioxide. If carbon dioxide levels continue to increase so that the level of carbon dioxide in the alveoli reaches that of the bloodstream, it becomes difficult for the animal to excrete carbon dioxide. This will result in a state of **hypercapnia**. Hypercapnia can cause depression of the central nervous system, and will result in coma if not corrected.

CARDIOVASCULAR SYSTEM

The heart is responsible for pumping blood around the body and consists of four chambers: two atria and two ventricles. Vessels carrying blood from the heart are called arteries, while those carrying blood to the heart are called veins. Lymphatics assist in returning fluid from the interstitial spaces to the blood.

The cardiovascular system works in conjunction with the respiratory system to ensure delivery of oxygen and nutrients to the body tissues and removal of carbon dioxide and other waste products from the tissues.

Muscle contraction is dependent on a flow of electrical charge across muscle cell membranes. Heart or cardiac muscle is no exception. At rest the interior of cardiac muscle cells are negative relative to the exterior so that the resting membrane potential is −90 mV.

The electrolytes sodium, chloride, potassium and calcium are all important for normal cardiac function. Initial depolarisation of the cell takes place when sodium channels in the cell membrane open, increasing sodium permeability. The resting membrane potential becomes less negative due to an influx of positive sodium ions. The cell begins repolarising when the sodium gates close and negatively charged chloride ions begin to move into the cell. Calcium channels open, allowing influx of these ions. During final repolarisation calcium channels close and potassium permeability increases. At this time the interior of cardiac muscle cells are negative relative to the exterior once again. Thus any deviation from normal plasma concentrations of these electrolytes can affect cardiac muscle function.

All cardiac muscles have the potential to contract, but the normal heart beats automatically and rhythmically. For the heart to function effectively in this manner, depolarisation and thus contraction must occur in an ordered and controlled fashion. This is achieved by the **conduction system** of the heart (Fig. 2.5).

The sino-atrial node (SAN, a small area of specialised cardiac muscle located in the wall of the right atrium) initiates the heartbeat. Impulses from the SAN spread to the atrioventricular node (AVN, located in the intraventricular septum). Impulses to the rest of the heart are transmitted *via* the bundle of His, the bundle branches and the Purkinje fibres. If any part of the cardiac muscle becomes damaged then these impulses will not be transmitted in a synchronised fashion. This can lead to irregular heart contractions and a reduction in cardiac output. Damaged areas of the heart can continue to contract, but will follow their own inbuilt pacemaker rather than the SAN.

- Sino-atrial node
- Atrioventricular node
- Bundle of His
- Bundle branches
- Purkinje fibres

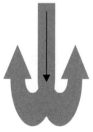

Fig. 2.5 Conduction system of the heart.

The sino-atrial node acts as an intrinsic cardiac pacemaker and controls the rate of heart contractions. Both the parasympathetic and sympathetic nervous systems innervate the SAN. Nervous system mediators – acetylcholine and nor-adrenaline – affect sodium, calcium and potassium channels and can increase or decrease depolarisation. Conditions such as stress (for example, during handling or anaesthesia) may cause the production of adrenaline, increasing the heart rate. Various drugs used as pre-anaesthetic medications or sedatives can affect heart rate. For example alpha-2 agonists such as xylazine or medetomidine decrease the heart rate; anticholinergics such as atropine directly increase the heart rate. In these situations heart rates need to be monitored.

The sequence of events that occur during one complete heartbeat is referred to as the **cardiac cycle:**

- Blood flows into the atria from the venae cavae and pulmonary veins.
- The atrioventricular (mitral and tricuspid) valves open when atrial pressure exceeds ventricular pressure.
- Blood flows into the relaxed ventricles (ventricular diastole).
- Atria contract to complete filling of the ventricles.
- Atria relax and begin refilling.
- Ventricles contract (ventricular systole) and atrioventricular valves close as ventricular pressure exceeds atrial pressure.
- Ventricular contraction generates sufficient pressure to overcome arterial pressure and blood flows out of the ventricles through the semilunar (aortic and pulmonic) valves.
- Ventricles begin to relax and arterial pressures exceed ventricular pressures, closing the semilunar valves.

During systole (ventricular contraction) blood pressure will be at its highest. During diastole blood pressure will be at its lowest. Normal blood pressure in the dog is 120/70 mmHg and 140/90 mmHg in the cat. It is important that blood pressure is maintained within this normal range.

Systemic arterial pressure (arterial blood pressure) is determined by cardiac output (predominantly controlled by the heart) and resistance to flow (predominantly controlled by the blood vessels). **Baroreceptors** are present in numerous sites throughout the cardiovascular system including the carotid sinus, aortic arch, walls of the left and right atria, left ventricle, and pulmonary circulation.

Any alteration in blood pressure within the cardiovascular system is detected by the baroreceptors and the circulatory system is stimulated to respond *via* the medulla. If the blood pressure increases, the baroreceptors will be stimulated and there will be a decrease in the sympathetic outflow to the heart, arterioles and veins. Conversely, the parasympathetic outflow to these organs will increase. This will result in vagal inhibition of the heart, causing bradycardia and vasodilation so that the blood pressure will fall, ideally to within a normal range. Drugs such as halothane can also cause bradycardia because they decrease vagal tone.

Cardiac output depends on the rate and the force of heart contractions. The sino-atrial node controls the heart rate and is innervated by both the sympathetic and parasympathetic nervous system. The force of heart contractions depends on a number of factors. Starling's law explains that the degree of stretch that the heart muscle undergoes will affect the force of contraction – the greater the degree of stretch, the greater the force of contraction. Thus, if a large blood volume fills the heart during diastole then the force of contraction will be increased, as will the cardiac output. Blood volume will also affect blood pressure. This will influence the volume of venous blood that returns to the heart, diastolic volume, stroke volume and therefore cardiac output.

In addition to neural mechanisms controlling blood pressure, a number of chemical mediators influence blood vessel diameter and hence the resistance to flow. For example, vasoactive substances such as kinins present in the bloodstream can cause venodilation, lowering blood pressure. Drugs such as the phenothiazines (for example, acepromazine) also cause vasodilation. Alternatively, substances such as antidiuretic hormone and adrenaline can cause vasoconstriction and increase blood pressure.

Whether an animal is lying down or standing up will have an effect on the baroreceptors and on blood pressure. If humans stand up suddenly, the blood supply to the head is decreased. This is detected by baroreceptors and the heart rate increases to compensate. A similar mechanism operates in animals.

Pathological causes of increased blood pressure include:

- decreased arterial oxygen concentration
- increased arterial carbon dioxide concentration
- decreased blood flow to the brain
- increased intracranial pressure.

In contrast visceral pain causes a decrease in blood pressure. Many anaesthetic agents can affect blood pressure (see chapter 6).

The blood supply to body tissues is affected by a number of factors: those that affect the cardiovascular system in general and local regulatory mechanisms. General controlling factors (which have been discussed already) are those that alter the output of the heart, change the diameter of blood vessels and alter blood pooling in the venous system.

Local controlling factors will cause vasodilation or vasoconstriction of specific areas of blood vessels. For example vasodilation can be caused by:

- a decreased oxygen tension due to: reduced oxygen in inspired gases, reduced alveolar ventilation, ventilation perfusion inequalities, anaemia or pyrexia, causing increased oxygen demands;

- decreased pH (acidaemia), for example, due to respiratory or metabolic acidosis;
- increased carbon dioxide concentrations due to: increased carbon dioxide in inspired gases, increased production of carbon dioxide or hypoventilation;
- increased temperature.

Local vasoconstriction can be caused by chemicals released by injured arteries and arterioles to reduce blood loss.

Anaesthesia often causes hypotension, reducing the blood supply to organs such as the kidney, damaging the kidneys and impairing excretion of anaesthetic agents. Blood supply to the lungs will also be affected during anaesthesia because the animal will be recumbent. This affects the ventilation : perfusion ratio and hence the uptake of gaseous agents, so it is important to monitor blood pressure during anaesthesia and ensure that it remains within normal range.

Blood–brain barrier

The blood–brain barrier restricts the movement of molecules into the brain. Only water, carbon dioxide and oxygen can enter or leave the brain easily by crossing this barrier. Other molecules cross into the brain more slowly. The rate is dependent on molecular size and lipid solubility; smaller molecules and those with high lipid solubility cross the barrier most rapidly. Anaesthetic agents must cross the barrier in order to exert their effect on the brain. Most of the inhalational anaesthetic agents used in veterinary practice are lipophilic. The more easily they can enter the brain the more potent they are; for example, methoxyflurane is the most lipophilic inhalational agent and is also the most potent.

Shock

Shock is defined as a circulatory state where the cardiac output is insufficient to maintain adequate blood flow to tissues. Causes of shock include haemorrhage, dehydration, heart failure and anaphylaxis.

In the initial stages of shock the animal will attempt to compensate for the loss in blood volume physiologically. Systemic vasoconstriction and increased heart rate attempt to maintain cardiac output and blood supply to major organs. Antidiuretic hormone is released from the pituitary gland to stimulate resorption of water and electrolytes, which will also maintain blood pressure.

As shock progresses, these changes cannot maintain blood volume. The heart rate continues to increase and vasoconstriction of the vascular beds of the skin and muscle takes place. Fluid from the interstitial space moves into plasma, resulting in clinical dehydration. Blood supply to heart, kidney and central nervous system is also impaired.

If the loss in blood volume continues then the animal will develop irreversible shock. The animal will have a low cardiac output and low blood pressure.

Hypovolaemia will result in a prolonged circulation time and reduced peripheral circulation. This means that the brain will receive an increased proportion of the blood, and relative to the rest of the body the brain will actually receive more anaesthetic agent. Decreased splanchnic flow means that redistribution, metabolism and excretion of drugs will be decreased.

KIDNEYS AND CONTROL OF FLUID

The kidneys have a number of important functions with regard to anaesthesia. They are involved in the excretion of many anaesthetic agents and control blood volume, blood pressure and electrolyte balance. During anaesthesia blood supply to the kidneys is often reduced and it is therefore important that kidney function is checked before anaesthesia to ensure that it can withstand any additional demands that are put upon it (see chapter 3).

The kidneys control the excretion and retention of electrolytes such as sodium, chloride, potassium, hydrogen and bicarbonate, in addition to controlling the excretion of water. The commonest electrolyte imbalance is probably metabolic acidosis, due to, for example, chronic vomiting, diarrhoea or diabetes mellitus. Here the plasma concentration of hydrogen ions is increased. The kidney increases the excretion of hydrogen ions into the urine in exchange for sodium that is reabsorbed from the urinary filtrate. The kidney also increases bicarbonate resorption from the filtrate so that body fluids become more alkaline.

In respiratory acidosis, carbon dioxide is retained and converted to carbonic acid with an increase in hydrogen ion concentration. In this situation, the kidney also increases hydrogen ion excretion so that acidosis is reduced.

Plasma pH will affect the actions of anaesthetic drugs such as thiopentone. If the animal is acidotic, the amount of active thiopentone in the circulation will be increased and therefore lower doses are often required.

Renal disease can cause both metabolic acidosis and electrolyte imbalances, especially affecting potassium concentration. Renal disease can also cause hypoalbuminaemia due to protein loss through the kidney. As many of the anaesthetic drugs are present in the circulation bound to albumin, there will be reduced protein binding and therefore more active drug in the circulation. Hence animals will require lower doses of anaesthetic agents such as thiopentone. In kidney disease, renal excretion of many anaesthetic agents will be decreased, meaning that the drug half-life will be increased.

The kidney is involved with the endocrine system. Alterations in blood pressure result in the release of renin from the kidney, which then results in the production of aldosterone from the adrenal gland. Aldosterone will act on the kidney, causing retention of sodium and water.

The kidney also produces erythropoietin in response to a fall in packed cell volume. Erythropoietin will induce the production of red blood cells by the bone marrow. Animals suffering from kidney disease can therefore be anaemic because of a lack of erythropoietin.

The kidney produces prostaglandins such as PGE which can decrease systemic blood pressure, increase blood flow in the renal medulla and increase urinary sodium excretion. Non-steroidal anti-inflammatory drugs (NSAIDs) are often administered to animals undergoing surgery. It is important to be aware that as NSAIDs block prostaglandin production (see chapter 7), this will reduce renal blood flow and can cause varying degrees of renal damage. The extent to which renal prostaglandin production is decreased varies with different NSAIDs but it is an important consideration when NSAIDs are administered to an animal undergoing anaesthesia.

LIVER

The liver is important in anaesthesia for a number of reasons.

Drug transport

Many anaesthetic agents such as thiopentone are transported in the bloodstream bound to albumin, a protein produced by the liver. Liver disease may cause decreased levels of albumin in the bloodstream (hypoalbuminaemia) and consequently a greater proportion of thiopentone will be free and active in the circulation. Thus animals with low albumin levels may require reduced doses of anaesthetic agents.

Drug metabolism

Anaesthetic agents can directly affect the blood supply to the liver. For example, halothane reduces liver blood supply by 30%.

The liver is involved in the metabolism of many anaesthetic agents including thiopentone or propofol. Liver disease, including endocrine disease, decreases the liver's ability to metabolise and excrete many anaesthetic drugs, and dosage may need to be reduced to avoid overdose. Liver function in diseases such as diabetes mellitus, Cushing's syndrome, and hypothyroidism is impaired, mainly due to the accumulation of fat within the liver. Even when suitable precautions are taken, animals suffering from liver disease (acquired or congenital) may take longer to recover from an anaesthetic than healthy patients.

Breeds such as sighthounds are particularly sensitive to thiopentone. It is possible that this is because these dogs are usually very thin and recovery from thiopentone anaesthesia initially is by redistribution of the drug into fat. However, it is also possible that these dogs lack particular liver enzymes involved in the metabolism of thiopentone.

Colloid oncotic pressure

Proteins (especially albumin) produced by the liver help to retain fluid in the circulation. If the liver is diseased then albumin levels fall and fluid is lost from the circulation as the colloid oncotic pressure is no longer adequate to counteract the effects of hydrostatic pressure. This can present clinically as oedema and ascites.

NERVOUS SYSTEM

The nervous system can be divided up into the somatic nervous system (involving voluntary actions such as that of skeletal muscle) and autonomic nervous system (involving involuntary actions such as that of the viscera).

The main transmitter substance in the somatic nervous system, transmitting impulses between nerves and skeletal muscle, is acetylcholine (ACh). Acetylcholine is released by the motor axon at the neuromuscular junction, travels across the synapse, binds to the muscle cell surface and causes depolarisation of the muscle (Fig. 2.6). Acetylcholine has a very short-acting effect because it is rapidly degraded by the enzyme acetylcholinesterase. The speed of transmission of this impulse can be affected by anoxia, anaesthetics and some drugs.

Many muscle relaxants act on cholinoreceptors. For example, competitive neuromuscular blocking drugs such as atracurium compete with acetylcholine to reversibly combine with cholinoreceptors, resulting in flaccid paralysis. However, the skeletal muscles can be flaccid or contracted due to suxamethonium.

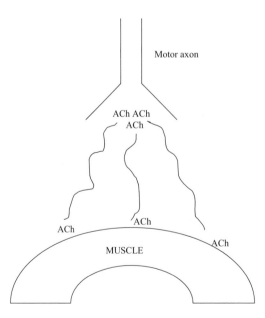

Fig. 2.6 Action of acetylcholine. ACh released by motor axon crosses synapse and binds to surface of muscle cell, causing depolarisation.

In order for acetylcholine to be released from the nerve cell, sufficient levels of calcium are required. Therefore, if the animal is hypocalcaemic (for example, in cases of lactational hypocalcaemia), less acetylcholine is released so muscle contraction may not occur and the animal will demonstrate varying degrees of weakness.

The autonomic nervous system transmits impulses between nerves and effector organs in a method similar to that described above. Postganglionic nerve fibres release either acetylcholine or noradrenaline. The transmitter that causes an effect distinguishes receptors. Those receptors that respond to acetylcholine are known as cholinergic and those that respond to noradrenaline are known as adrenergic.

Cholinergic receptors are present in both the parasympathetic and sympathetic branches of the autonomic nervous system. Some acetylcholine receptors will bind the substance muscarine. The effects of muscarine will mimic those of acetylcholine and these receptors are therefore known as muscarinic receptors. Atropine will compete with acetylcholine to bind to muscarinic receptors so that acetylcholine cannot bind to them. Thus atropine is often given as a preanaesthetic medication to inhibit the effects of the parasympathetic nervous system, and is variably referred to as a parasympatholytic or anticholinergic or antimuscarinic agent.

Adrenergic receptors can be further divided into alpha or beta receptors, dependent on the type of effect that these receptors have. For example alpha-adrenergic receptors are present where noradrenaline has an excitatory activity, except in the alimentary tract where noradrenaline has an inhibitory effect. Beta receptors are present at junctions where noradrenaline relaxes smooth muscle or excites cardiac muscle.

Alpha receptors can be further divided into α_1 and α_2 groups. Alpha-2 agonists such as medetomidine are discussed later (see chapter 6).

OVERVIEW OF AVIAN RESPIRATORY PHYSIOLOGY

The avian respiratory system is different to that of mammals in a number of ways and is extremely complicated. The description that follows is a simplified version of that to be found in Fedde (1983).

The most notable difference between birds and mammals is that the lungs of birds are rigid structures, attached to the underside of the thoracic vertebrae. To allow air to move back and forth, the bird has a series of thin-walled elastic air sacs that act as bellows. On average there are nine air sacs – a cervical air sac in the lower neck, paired clavicular air sacs (at the neck inlet), cranial thoracic air sacs, caudal thoracic air sacs and abdominal air sacs. These expand by contraction of the external intercostal muscles which pull the ribs laterally and cranially, and the movement of the sternum ventrally and cranially. These actions increase the volume of the body cavity (known as the coelomic cavity;

there is no division into a thorax and abdomen) and allow the air sacs to inflate. Reversal of the process by dorsal and caudal movement of the sternum, and contraction of the internal intercostal muscles moving the ribcage medially and caudally, decreases body cavity size. In association with the natural elastic recoil of the air sacs, air is thus expelled, allowing expiration to occur.

On inspiration fresh air is inhaled. The inspired air and the air already in the dead spaces may largely bypass the lung structure and go straight to the most caudal air sacs in the abdomen. Air already in the airways is displaced cranially through the gaseous exchange portion of the lung structure and on into the cranial air sacs in the thorax and cervical areas. During the following expiration, air in the caudal air sacs (abdominal and caudal thoracic) is passed again through the portions of the lung responsible for gaseous exchange. This allows the bird to extract oxygen from air on both inspiration and expiration, but if the chest or abdomen are in any way constricted, the ribs cannot move and the air sacs cannot work and so the bird will rapidly asphyxiate.

The air sacs are important in that they can be cannulated directly to supply air to the bird if there is a physical obstruction to the trachea. It does not matter whether the air sac cannulated is a cranial air sac or an abdominal air sac, as air flow through the airways does not alter the bird's ability to extract oxygen from it. The air sacs will also accumulate anaesthetic gases, so recovery may be more prolonged with certain gaseous anaesthetics in comparison with mammals.

Many anaesthetic agents suppress respiration in birds. One such drug is halothane, which will depress the intrapulmonary chemoreceptors' ability to detect a rising PCO_2 level during anaesthesia, which can lead to respiratory suppression and anoxia.

REPTILE PHYSIOLOGY RELEVANT TO ANAESTHESIA

Reptiles are ectothermic, that is, they rely on external heat to maintain their body temperature at a physiologically optimum level. Each reptile has a preferred body temperature (PBT) at which it functions most effectively. To enable it to maintain its PBT the reptile must be kept in a temperature zone covering this PBT so that it may regulate its body temperature by movement within the temperature gradient provided. This temperature is known as the preferred optimum temperature zone (POTZ). As all metabolic processes are enhanced by increasing the temperature at which they work, it can be seen that to ensure safe recovery from an anaesthetic, particularly from an anaesthetic which has to be metabolised by the body in order for the reptile to recover, the reptile must be kept at or near its PBT during the recovery period.

Other factors to be considered in reptile anaesthesia include the ability of many species to hold their breath. This is particularly true for members of the Chelonia family. They may breathe so slowly, and utilise anaerobic respiration so effectively, that some species can survive for many hours without breathing oxygen at all. This makes induction of anaesthesia using volatile anaesthetic agents futile in these species. In addition, the stimulus for reptiles to breathe is based on a decrease in the PO_2 and not an increase in the PCO_2. Thus placing a reptile in an oxygen-enriched atmosphere will inhibit breathing rather than enhance it.

Finally, many reptiles possess a unique blood flow pattern in the caudal half of their bodies, which has a bearing on where drugs such as injectable anaesthetics should be administered. The renal portal system is a blood drainage system whereby the blood from the caudal limbs and tail may be passed through the renal parenchyma before returning to the heart. This pattern of blood flow may not occur at all times, but the fact that it occurs at all should make the operator wary of administering any nephrotoxic drug into the caudal half of a reptile's body. In addition, anaesthetic agents excreted by the renal route may be discharged from the body before they have had a chance to work. Injectable medications should therefore be administered, if possible, into the cranial half of reptiles.

REFERENCES AND FURTHER READING

Detweiler, D.K. (1993) Control mechanisms of the circulatory system. In: *Dukes' Physiology of Domestic Animals* 11th edition (eds M.J. Swenson & W.O. Reece). Cornell University Press, Ithaca, New York and Comstock, London.

Fedde, M.R. (1993) Respiration in birds. In: *Dukes' Physiology of Domestic Animals* 11th edition (eds M.J. Swenson & W.O. Reece). Cornell University Press, Ithaca, New York and Comstock, London.

Ganong, W. F. (1989) Cardiovascular regulatory mechanisms. In: *Review of Medical Physiology* 14th edition. Prentice Hall, USA.

Preoperative Assessment and Preparation of the Patient

Joan Duncan

The perfect anaesthetic drug would induce reversible unconsciousness, analgesia and muscle relaxation without depression of the heart and lungs. It would not require metabolism and would be non-toxic to the patient. Although the anaesthetic agents used for veterinary patients have improved greatly in recent years, they still fall short of this ideal. Consequently, careful pre-anaesthetic assessment of patients before sedation and anaesthesia is essential to identify physiological, pathological or drug-related factors which may complicate the anaesthetic management or the surgical procedure, the expected outcome of surgery, or the management of the patient. This chapter reviews the components of the pre-anaesthetic assessment and the actions that may be required to investigate or stabilise any abnormalities.

It is essential to collect a detailed medical history and perform a thorough physical examination before any procedure. On the basis of these examinations, further diagnostic tests may be recommended, or the perioperative management tailored to the individual's needs (Fig. 3.1). Initial assessment of the patient is often performed by the veterinary surgeon when surgical options are being outlined to the client. Examination at this time means that any further tests which may be required can be discussed with the pet owner. Assessment of the patient should be repeated on admission of the animal, to ensure that nothing has been overlooked.

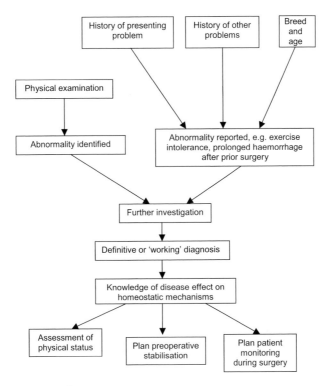

Fig. 3.1 Components of assessment.

ASA (AMERICAN SOCIETY OF ANESTHESIOLOGISTS) CLASSIFICATION SCHEME

I   Healthy patient
II Mild systemic disease; no functional limitation
III Severe systemic disease; definite functional limitation
IV Severe systemic disease that is a constant threat to life
V   Moribund patient unlikely to survive 24 hours with or without surgery
E   Added to the above classification if the patient is presented on an emergency basis; denotes additional risk inherent in rushing into a procedure

HISTORY

A standard approach to recording a medical history is essential to ensure that important factors are not missed. The most important topics are outlined below, but it can be difficult to gain accurate information from some pet owners.

General considerations

(1) Confirm identity of patient. This may include practice details, e.g. case number, in addition to general information such as species.

(2) Confirm age of patient. Both very young and geriatric ($\geq$ 75–80% of life span) patients are more susceptible to the effects of anaesthetics.

(3) Breed: Many owners of purebred animals are concerned about breed sensitivities to selected anaesthetic drugs. Currently, there is little scientific information to support these fears although many breed websites perpetuate the concerns. However, it is important to consider disease susceptibility in specific breeds, for example, von Willebrand's disease in the Dobermann pinscher. The increased susceptibility of brachycephalic and large breed dogs to acepromazine is well recognised, and the increased susceptibility of sighthounds to thiopentone. Other, more general, breed-related concerns might have to be considered during the anaesthetic period such as the possibility of upper airway obstruction in brachycephalic breeds.

(4) Entire or neutered? If the patient is an entire female, then when was her last season? In entire females consider the possibility of pregnancy and the effects the gravid uterus may have on cardiovascular and respiratory function. Additionally, it is important to consider the effect of the chosen anaesthetic agents on the foetus, e.g. teratogenicity, abortion.

(5) Prior adverse reactions to drugs or anaesthetic agents: Review any previous anaesthetic records available for the patient.

(6) Prior medical history.

(7) Recent and current drug therapy: Diuretic therapy may have significant effects on body water content and electrolyte concentrations, while long-term glucocorticoid treatment can impair the ability of the patient to mount an appropriate stress response. The administration of some antibiotics can affect the action of anaesthetic agents, for example, aminoglycoside antibiotics can affect the action of non-depolarising muscle relaxants. Other drugs that may affect the course or outcome of the anaesthetic include digoxin, phenobarbitone, cimetidine and other H_2 blockers, beta blockers, insecticides, calcium channel blockers, ACE inhibitors, bronchodilators, glucocorticoids and non-steroidal anti-inflammatory drugs. In general, drug therapy should be continued as normal, ensuring administration before premedication.

(8) Main complaint and history.

Cardiovascular history

- Exercise tolerance: one of the most useful indicators of cardiac 'fitness'. It is advisable to investigate reported exercise intolerance before surgery, and stabilise any identifiable cardiopulmonary disease.
- Coughing?
- Difficulty breathing?

Gastrointestinal history

- Persistent, recurrent or recent vomiting?
- Persistent, recurrent or recent diarrhoea?
- Altered water intake? Investigation of polydipsia and polyuria (PUPD) should be considered before surgery since many of the causes of PUPD would also be associated with increased anaesthetic risk, for example, renal disease, feline hyperthyroidism.
- Altered appetite?

Neurological history

- Prior seizures or collapsing episodes. Acepromazine may decrease the seizure threshold in epileptic patients and induce seizures.
- Muscle twitching.

Dermatological history

- Masses or swellings present? Recently noticed? Rapidly enlarging? Record any erythema or pain on handling the lesion. Mast cell tumours can release histamine when handled that can cause hypotension.
- Confirm with owner, and record, the location of lesions for investigation or removal.

General history

- Behavioural changes?
- Signs of pain?
- Sleeping position: may indicate respiratory compromise, e.g. animals with bilateral pleural effusions often sleep upright.

'Red alert' answers or evasions

In many patients with systemic disease the owner has identified significant changes (for example, in appetite or exercise tolerance) but may have failed to recognise the significance of these changes, or perhaps attributed them to the ageing process. Careful physical examination is particularly important in geriatric patients and where the owner has reported exercise intolerance, coughing and polydipsia.

PHYSICAL EXAMINATION

The physical examination of a patient may be performed in many ways but it is important to establish a routine, which ensures that all body systems are examined.

Cardiovascular assessment
- Heart rate and rhythm.
- Pulse rate and quality: Ensure that there is no pulse deficit present, that is, each heart beat should generate a palpable pulse.
- Murmurs: Gallop rhythms and murmurs in cats must be taken seriously since these patients may be poor anaesthetic candidates.
- Mucous membrane colour.
- Capillary refill time: Not a sensitive indicator but reflects poor circulation or hypovolaemia if the refill time is > 2 sec.
- Temperature of extremities.
- Jugular vein examination: Check for distension or presence of a jugular pulse.

Respiratory assessment
- Respiratory rate (normal dog: 10–30 breaths per minute; normal cat: 20–30 breaths per minute).
- Respiration character: Rapid, shallow breathing can be noted in pulmonary disease or the presence of pleural effusion (air or fluid), while a slow respiration rate with increased effort can be noted with airway obstruction, for example, tracheal collapse.
- Pulmonary auscultation.
- Percussion to assess thoracic resonance, for example, dullness on percussion could reflect the presence of free pleural fluid.

Oral examination
- Examination for masses, ulceration (possibly associated with uraemia) and petechiation (most commonly associated with thrombocytopenia).

Lymph nodes
- Generalised or localised lymphadenopathy? Cytological examination of a fine needle aspirate or histological examination of a biopsy would be required for further investigation.

Abdominal palpation
- Renal size.
- Abdominal mass present?
- Abdominal pain present?

Dermatological examination
Examination for:

- masses or swellings;
- discoloration, including petechiation and bruising;
- other skin lesions, for example, pustules, erythema, scale.

Reproductive system
- Examination of the vulva in an entire bitch.
- Check mammary glands or testicles for swellings or masses.

General assessment
- Body condition: Obesity compromises cardiovascular system and demands an increased respiratory effort. Obese patients should receive drug dosages calculated on ideal body weight. Cachexic patients are physiologically stressed and have little metabolic or homeostatic reserve. They may have a reduced ability to metabolise injectable anaesthetic agents because of impaired hepatic function. Care should be taken during the anaesthetic procedure to minimise heat loss and to pad pressure points in these patients.
- Demeanour: The veterinary surgeon may choose different pre-anaesthetic or general anaesthetic drugs for patients that are very excitable, nervous or aggressive compared to those for a quiet, relaxed patient.

Hydration status
The results of the following observations are important in the identification of dehydration and/or hypovolaemia:

- skin elasticity;
- pulse rate and quality;
- mucous membrane colour: mucosal pallor may reflect hypovolaemia, poor circulation or anaemia (however, in chronic anaemia the mucosal colour may appear relatively normal);
- capillary refill time;
- respiratory rate;
- temperature of extremities;
- mental alertness.

THE SIGNIFICANCE OF ABNORMALITIES

The common causes of some of the most important abnormalities detected during patient assessment are listed in Table 3.1.

Further assessment or investigation, before surgery, is warranted for many of these clinical presentations, but this is especially true for exercise intolerance, coughing, polydipsia, suspected hepatic encephalopathy and bleeding disorders. Many of the causes of these presenting signs could have a significant impact on both anaesthetic and surgical procedures. A brief guide to the procedures, which may be required for further investigation, is given in Table 3.1, but in some cases it is not possible to fully investigate the signs, or establish a diagnosis, before anaesthesia or surgery. However, even without a definitive diagnosis, steps can still be taken to stabilise the patient, or provide a more suitable anaesthetic protocol, for example, preoperative oxygenation and shortened surgical procedures for animals with possible cardiopulmonary disease.

Table 3.1 Pre-anaesthetic abnormalities, possible causes, and the tests often used to investigate these clinical presentations. Anorexia may be associated with many systemic diseases and is not listed here.

Clinical abnormalities noted or reported	Possible causes	Further tests often required to reach a diagnosis
Exercise intolerance	Cardiac disease	Thoracic radiography
	Respiratory disease	ECG
	Systemic disease	Ultrasound examination
	including anaemia	Haematology and biochemistry screen
Respiratory embarrassment	Pleural effusion	Thoracocentesis
	Diaphragmatic rupture	Radiography
	Pulmonary disease	
Coughing	Cardiac disease	Thoracic radiography
	Respiratory disease	Bronchoscopy
		Tracheal wash
		Therapeutic trials, e.g. diuretic therapy
Episodic collapse	Cardiac disease	Radiography
	Pulmonary disease	ECG
	Neurological disease	Ultrasound examination
	Hypoglycaemia	Biochemistry profile
Vomiting	Gastric disease	Radiography
	Intestinal disease	Biochemistry screen (including electrolytes)
	Pancreatic disease	For pancreatitis: amylase, lipase and canine
	Pyometra	pancreatic lipase immunoreactivity (dogs)
	Renal disease	Feline TLI (cats)
	Liver disease	Endoscopic examination
	Feline hyperthyroidism	Biopsy
	Diabetes mellitus	
	Hypoadrenocorticism	
Diarrhoea	Intestinal disease	Faecal examination
	Feline hyperthyroidism	Biochemistry screen (including electrolytes)
	Liver disease	TLI, folate, cobalamin
	Hypoadrenocorticism	Breath hydrogen test
		Intestinal permeability tests, e.g. sugar probes
		Biopsy (intestinal or hepatic)

Table 3.1 (Continued)

Clinical abnormalities noted or reported	Possible causes	Further tests often required to reach a diagnosis
Polydipsia	Renal disease Liver disease Pyometra Feline hyperthyroidism Diabetes mellitus Hyperadrenocorticism Hypercalcaemia Hypoadrenocorticism Diabetes insipidus Psychogenic polydipsia	Urinalysis, haematology and biochemistry screen (including calcium and electrolytes) Feline thyroxine (T4) Bile acid stimulation test (hepatic function) Low dose dexamethasone suppression test or ACTH stimulation test (for hyperadrenocorticism)
Petechiation/ bruising	Thrombocytopenia Coagulation defects Trauma Vasculitis	Haematology profile with film examination Coagulation profile, e.g. ACT, PT, APTT
Lymphadenopathy	Reactive lymphoid hyperplasia Metastatic neoplasia Lymphadenitis	Examination of drainage region of enlarged nodes Cytological examination of fine needle aspirate Histological examination of biopsy
Neurological signs or behavioural changes	Primary neurological disease Hepatic encepholopathy, e.g. congenital portosystemic shunt Hypoglycaemia Hypocalcaemia	Biochemistry screen Diagnostic imaging Cerebrospinal fluid analysis Serology

PREOPERATIVE MANAGEMENT OF SYSTEMIC DISEASE

For most of the diseases listed in Table 3.1 it is important to establish a diagnosis or narrow the differential diagnosis list before anaesthesia. Where anaesthesia is required in an emergency then consideration should be given to all the possible causes of physical abnormalities or reported signs. For many diseases, anaesthesia may be required to perform the procedures necessary to make a diagnosis, for example, radiography, bronchoscopy and liver biopsy. The following sections briefly describe the effects of specific conditions on homeostatic mechanisms relating to anaesthesia, and highlight some of the methods for stabilising patients before anaesthesia or surgery.

Dehydration

Dehydration or hypovolaemia should be suspected if the following are reported in the history: vomiting, diarrhoea, sepsis, trauma and diuretic treatment. In addition to absolute volume depletion, there may be other abnormalities:

- reduced tissue perfusion (this is particular important as many drugs are metabolised by the liver and excreted by the kidneys);
- electrolyte disturbances;
- acid–base disturbances;
- reduced oxygen-carrying capacity where there has been haemorrhage.

When possible, hypovolaemia should be corrected before surgery. It may be necessary to replace fluid losses and correct electrolyte disturbances during and after surgery but it is recommended that hypoglycaemia and hypo- and hyperkalaemia be corrected before anaesthesia. Calculation of fluid requirements should take into consideration the degree of dehydration, gastrointestinal losses, e.g. vomiting, blood loss, and insensible losses (Welsh 1999).

Trauma and anaemia

In addition to assessment of obvious injuries, consider:

- Severity: Suspect internal haemorrhage if there are multiple fractures.
- Onset and duration: Some internal consequences such as pulmonary contusions may not be evident for 24–48 hours. If possible anaesthesia should be delayed until the contusions have resolved.
- Blood loss: The packed cell volume (PCV) and total protein concentration are initially within the reference range. After 12–24 hours, redistribution of body water into the vascular space (to maintain blood volume) produces a decline in total protein concentration, and then PCV. Initially, therefore, the PCV is not a reliable indicator of the amount of blood lost. Decreased PCV will affect the total oxygen-carrying capacity of the blood and demands more critical interpretation of SaO_2 results obtained by pulse oximetry. Small changes in SaO_2 are of greater significance in anaemic patients than in non-anaemic individuals. For chronic and acute anaemia, blood transfusion (Knottenbelt & Mackin 1998) or administration of bovine haemoglobin (Rentko 2000) may be required to maintain the oxygen-carrying capacity of the blood.

- Possibility of ruptured diaphragm.
- Possibility of ruptured bladder.

Cardiac disease

Where possible, make an accurate diagnosis so that specific effects can be predicted and the perioperative management tailored to the individual patient. Anaesthesia should be avoided in uncontrolled cardiac disease. When anaesthesia is undertaken the following should be considered:

- Lower dosage and slower infusion rates of injectable agents may be required.
- Possibility of reduced renal clearance and hepatic removal of drugs.
- Pulmonary oedema should be treated before surgery since it decreases oxygenation.
- Noxious stimuli (including anaesthesia) initiate the stress response, which in most circumstances is a lifesaving mechanism. However, sodium retention and water conservation are features of the stress response that could complicate anaesthesia in patients with cardiac disease.
- Take care with administration of fluids to patients with cardiac disease. Frequent monitoring is essential to detect pulmonary oedema.
- Frequent physiological monitoring is essential during the perioperative period.

Pulmonary and thoracic disease

Anaesthesia is frequently required in patients with chronic pulmonary disease to facilitate radiography, bronchoscopy, collection of material for cytological examination and collection of material for culture. Many patients have suffered chronic hypoxia and have blood gas abnormalities with altered uptake of gaseous anaesthetics. In these individuals, and in animals with severe disease, therapy may be required to stabilise the patient before investigative procedures. Stabilisation may require antibiotic therapy, diuretics and bronchodilators, which may, unfortunately, have some effect on the cytological features of the disease and the culture results. Procedures should be as short as possible and some (for example, transtracheal wash), may be performed without chemical restraint or with light sedation alone. Increasing the oxygen content of inspired air before induction can be helpful for patients with pulmonary disease.

In cases of trauma, especially where there are multiple fractures, there should be an increased suspicion of pulmonary contusions. The full extent of pulmonary lesions associated with both trauma and smoke inhalation is likely to develop over 24–48 hours and may be missed on initial presentation. Where pleural fluid is suspected, this should be drained by thoracocentesis before anaesthesia.

Hepatic disease

The following are potential consequences of hepatic disease, which may impact upon anaesthetic or surgical procedures:

- prolonged action of anaesthetic agents which require hepatic metabolism, e.g. thiopentone;
- hypoalbuminaemia results in a relative overdosage of albumin-bound drugs, e.g. thiopentone;
- hypoalbuminaemia may increase risk of pulmonary oedema;
- ascites may impair respiration;
- hypoglycaemia;
- hepatic encephalopathy;
- electrolyte disturbance;
- clotting defects;
- platelet dysfunction.

Diagnosis of liver disease

For patients undergoing anaesthesia for biopsy of the liver, it is likely that a large amount of information is available. The tests and investigations commonly performed are listed in Table 3.2.

A wide range of extrahepatic diseases and drugs can affect the liver enzymes (see box) and care should be taken in the interpretation of pre-anaesthetic blood profiles which include liver enzymes.

Table 3.2 Laboratory tests and other procedures commonly used in the investigation of liver disease in the dog and cat.

Liver enzymes	Liver function tests	Other tests
Alanine aminotransferase (ALT)	Bilirubin	Total protein
Aspartate aminotransferase (AST)	Albumin	Glucose
Alkaline phosphatase (ALP)	Urea	Haematology
Gamma-glutamyl transferase (GGT)	Cholesterol	Radiography
	Bile acids	Ultrasound examination
	Ammonia	Fine needle aspirate

Confirmation of primary hepatic disease is likely to require:

- measurement of liver function indicators;
- exclusion of extrahepatic disease on basis of clinical signs and history;
- exclusion of extrahepatic disease on basis of further tests;
- diagnostic imaging;
- liver biopsy.

INFLUENCES ON LIVER ENZYMES

Extrahepatic conditions

Intestinal disease
Pancreatic disease
Cardiac disease
Shock
Hypothyroidism
Hyperthyroidism
Diabetes mellitus
Hyperadrenocorticism
Severe dental disease
Pyometra
Abscess
Trauma

Drugs

Glucocorticoids
Anticonvulsants

Preoperative management of liver disease

It is advisable to stabilise patients with hepatic encephalopathy by medical means before any surgical intervention, for example, for ligation of a shunt vessel. Ascites should also be treated medically before surgery since large amounts of abdominal fluid can cause respiratory embarrassment. Medical management is preferred, but slow manual drainage may be required if there is significant respiratory distress.

Liver dysfunction, and obstruction of the bile duct can produce coagulation defects secondary to impaired synthesis of coagulation factors and failure of vitamin K absorption, respectively. It is therefore essential to check the clotting times before biopsy of the liver. Parenteral treatment with vitamin K for 12–24 hours before surgery corrects the vitamin K deficiency associated with biliary obstruction, but infusion of fresh or fresh frozen plasma or fresh whole blood (administered within 6 hours of collection) would be required to replace the coagulation factor deficiency of liver dysfunction. Any whole blood for transfusion must be fresh, since ammonia accumulates in stored blood, and may precipitate hepatic encephalopathy.

Significant platelet dysfunction can be associated with liver disease and is identified using the buccal mucosal bleeding time, a test of primary haemostatic function (see box and Fig. 3.2). Abnormal results are a consequence of thrombocytopenia, platelet dysfunction or von Willebrand's disease.

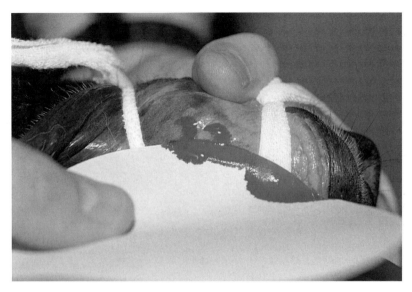

Fig. 3.2 Performance of a buccal mucosal bleeding time (BMBT).

PERFORMANCE OF BUCCAL MUCOSAL BLEEDING TIME (BMBT)

Equipment

- Simplate-II (a spring-loaded device which delivers two incisions of standard length and depth to a mucosal surface)
- Length of bandage to tie around the everted upper lip and maxilla
- Filter paper, blotting paper or tissue

Method

- Evert the upper lip and tie it so that the mucosal surface is exposed.
- Place the Simplate-II against the mucosal surface and trigger the device, delivering two incisions to the lip. Ensure the device is not close to large blood vessels.
- Blood oozing from the incisions is blotted. Blot the area next to the incision and do not disturb the wound.
- Record the time taken for bleeding to stop. A marked difference in bleeding times for the two incisions usually reflects laceration of a blood vessel by one blade.

Results

In normal, sedated or anaesthetised dogs and cats the BMBT is less than 4 minutes.

Renal disease

The following factors should be considered in patients with renal disease:

- Uraemia increases the sensitivity of the patient to anaesthetic drugs.
- Decreased renal perfusion during anaesthesia may precipitate clinical disease in individuals with pre-existing subclinical disease.
- Anaemia (associated with chronic renal failure) reduces tolerance to decreased tissue perfusion.
- Hypertension may be noted with chronic renal failure.
- Hypoproteinaemia (secondary to proteinuria) increases the risk of pulmonary oedema during fluid therapy.
- Postrenal obstruction, for example, feline lower urinary tract obstruction, may cause dehydration, hyperkalaemia, uraemia and acidosis.

Diagnosis of renal disease

Renal failure is defined as an inability of the kidneys to maintain normal homeostatic functions and is noted when approximately 75% of normal function is lost. Diagnosis usually relies upon identification of azotaemia (raised urea and creatinine concentrations) and a failure to maximally concentrate urine (Fig. 3.3). Care must be taken when interpreting the urea and creatinine concentrations, since increases can be associated with pathological processes other than primary renal failure (Table 3.3). Raised urea and creatinine commonly reflect pre-renal disease (hypovolaemia) and need not indicate primary renal disease. In addition, the creatinine concentration in any individual is related to the muscle mass and glomerular filtration rate (GFR). Therefore, in patients with reduced muscle mass (common in geriatric cats), the creatinine concentration may be within the reference range, even in patients with renal disease. The urine specific gravity is used to assess tubular function and provides additional supportive evidence of renal disease where other causes of tubular dysfunction (e.g. hypercalcaemia, pyometra, hyperadrenocorticism) have been excluded (Fig. 3.3).

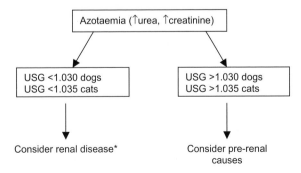

Fig. 3.3 Interpretation of urea and creatinine concentrations and the urine specific gravity (USG). Ideally, urine should be collected at the time of blood sampling. *Other diseases, which impair tubular function, will also produce urine that is not maximally concentrated, e.g. hypercalcaemia, hypoadrenocorticism.

Table 3.3 Causes of raised urea in the dog and cat.

Cause	Additional useful tests
Dehydration	Physical examination and history
	PCV
	Total protein concentration
	Urine SG
	Electrolytes
Cardiac disease	Physical examination and history
	Diagnostic imaging
Recent high-protein meal	History
Intestinal haemorrhage	History
	Haematology profile (to identify an iron deficiency anaemia secondary to chronic blood loss)
	Faecal occult blood test (patient must be on a meat-free diet)
Postrenal obstruction	History and physical examination

Preoperative management

The aim of management is to avoid reduced renal perfusion that can precipitate clinical disease in patients with subclinical disease and cause deterioration in patients with recognised disease:

- Maintain fluid balance.
- Avoid non-steroidal anti-inflammatory agents.
- Avoid water deprivation.
- Maintain normotension.

Treatment of hyperkalaemia in postrenal obstruction should be undertaken before anaesthesia, and may require fluid therapy, administration of sodium bicarbonate and peritoneal lavage with potassium-free fluid (Waterman-Pearson 1999).

Endocrine disease

The body responds to noxious stimuli, including anaesthesia and surgery, by initiating the stress response. The stress response ensures sufficient energy for tissues, facilitates water conservation and allows for healing (by increased protein synthesis) in the time following the noxious stimulus. Many patients with endocrine disease cannot mount an appropriate stress response. Most endocrine diseases, therefore, can have major implications for the perioperative management of patients (Table 3.4).

Table 3.4 Management considerations for patients with endocrine disease.

Disease	Anaesthetic considerations
Diabetes mellitus	Correct ketoacidosis and fluid deficits prior to surgery
	Place IV cannula for easy access
	Follow patient's normal insulin-feeding regime as closely as possible
	Give half dose insulin at premedication
	Detect hypoglycaemia by frequent blood glucose measurements during and after surgery. Collect blood sample for glucose estimation at a different site from fluid administration
	Expect upset glycaemic control for a few days after surgery
Insulinoma	Risk of massive insulin release after tumour has been handled
	Place IV cannula for easy access
	Monitor blood glucose frequently. Collect blood sample for estimation at a different site from fluid administration
	Avoid large boluses of glucose to correct hypoglycaemia – these may stimulate further insulin secretion. Use of intravenous dextrose (2.5%) solutions prevents significant hypoglycaemia
	Increased risk of postoperative pancreatitis and hyperglycaemia
Hyperadrenocorticism (Cushing's disease)	Increased risk of pulmonary thromboembolism
	Increased skin fragility
Hypoadrenocorticism (Addison's disease)	Inability to mount a stress response
	Replacement glucocorticoids required (in addition to maintenance mineralocorticoids)
Hyperthyroidism	Hypertrophic cardiomyopathy, hypertension, impaired renal function, poor body condition and aggression
	Medical management for 3–4 weeks prior to surgery, in order to achieve euthyroidism. Check T4 and renal function prior to surgery since establishment of euthyroidism can lead to deterioration in renal function
	Check for postoperative hypocalcaemia after thyroidectomy. Signs include increased vocalisation, restlessness, muscle twitching and seizures
Hypothyroidism	Obesity, bradycardia, laryngeal paralysis. May also have other endocrine disease, especially diabetes mellitus or hypoadrenocorticism
	Delayed recovery and risk of hypothermia

Ocular disease
The following are considerations when planning ocular surgery:

- Avoid drugs that induce vomiting and therefore an increased intraocular pressure.
- Patients for cataract surgery may have diabetes mellitus and require specific planning for the timing of surgery, perioperative management of insulin therapy and intraoperative blood glucose measurements (Table 3.4).
- Mannitol may be given before surgery, to decrease intraocular pressure.

GERIATRIC PATIENTS

Individuals are considered to be geriatric when they are older than 75–80% of their expected life span. They have an increased risk of age-related disease and particular care must be taken when obtaining the patient's history and performing the physical examination. Reports of exercise intolerance and increased thirst are of concern since these could reflect cardiac disease and early renal disease, respectively. The physiological factors, which may be important in any geriatric patient, include:

- Decreased drug elimination secondary to reduced hepatic mass and blood flow.
- Decreased dose of injectable anaesthetics required.
- Decreased renal perfusion. Consideration should be given to administration of fluid therapy routinely in older patients. However, care must be taken in patients with cardiac disease.
- Potential for decreased oxygenation.
- Increased physiological monitoring including blood pressure, if possible.
- Long procedures (e.g. dental surgery) present an increased risk of hypothermia.

PREOPERATIVE BLOOD TESTS

The aim of preoperative blood testing in apparently healthy patients is to identify disease processes which may progress as a consequence of the patient's management (e.g. subclinical renal disease), diseases which would benefit from preoperative stabilisation, and those which may have an impact on the anaesthetic regime (e.g. hypoalbuminaemia). There is some controversy over how many tests and which tests should be included in a pre-anaesthetic profile, but most clinicians are in agreement over the baseline tests listed in Table 3.5. Other tests are included on the basis of abnormalities identified on physical examination or history. In the older cat, hyperthyroidism is a major concern

Table 3.5 Tests included in a baseline pre-anaesthetic blood profile.

Test	Reason for inclusion

PCV or haemoglobin (Hb)	Indicator of:
	
	  oxygen-carrying capacity of blood
	  hydration status
	  chronic hypoxia
	
	Chronic anaemia is often difficult to detect on the basis of mucosal colour alone, and measurement of the PCV is required

Visual appraisal of serum or plasma	Check for changes which could reflect systemic disease:
	
	  lipaemia
	  haemolysis
	  icterus

Total protein	Indicator of:
	
	  hydration status
	  inflammatory disease
	  hypoproteinaemia (haemorrhage, hepatic, renal or gastrointestinal disease)

Albumin	Indicator of:
	
	  hydration status
	  hypoalbuminaemia (hepatic, renal or gastrointestinal disease)

Urea and creatinine	Used as indicators of glomerular function, but can be affected by other processes (see Table 3.3)
Glucose	Hypo- and hyperglycaemia create metabolic disturbances which interfere with anaesthetic management and risk neurological damage

regarding anaesthetic risk and thyroxine is commonly included, especially where signs could be compatible.

In addition to disease, a number of physiological, error-related and statistical factors may cause results to be outside the reference interval in healthy patients (Table 3.6).

GENERAL PREPARATION GUIDELINES AND ADMISSION

On admission, it is advisable to confirm the patient's identity, weigh the patient accurately and perform a physical examination. Check that the patient has been fasted and that the owner and the practice are in agreement over the details of the surgical procedures to be performed (especially if the presenting problem is unilateral, for example, investigation of lameness). Obtaining the owner's

Table 3.6 Potential causes of abnormal blood results, other than disease.

Factors	Comment
Lipaemia	Interferes with assay methodologies
Glucocorticoid therapy	Increased liver enzyme activity (ALP, ALT, AST)
Anticonvulsant therapy	Increased liver enzymes (ALP, ALT, AST)
Fluid therapy	Decreased proteins and PCV
Haemolysis	Interferes with assay methodologies
Icterus	Interferes with assay methodologies
Breed	Reference intervals are usually not breed-specific. Some breeds have characteristics variation, e.g. raised PCV in greyhounds
Age	Reference intervals are usually not age-specific. This is of particular importance for puppies and kittens
Sample error	Sample incorrectly labelled
Preparation error	Sample preparation, e.g. failure to completely separate serum may affect phosphorus result
Operator error	Staff must have sufficient training for operation of equipment. Always take care to analyse the correct sample and follow the SOP
Equipment error	Probability of equipment error is reduced by adequate maintenance and implementation of a quality control scheme
Reagent failure	Follow SOP for preparing, diluting and storing reagents. Check and record freezer and refrigerator temperatures at regular intervals
Clerical error	Transcription of results into wrong patient record
Reference ranges	For many assays, 5% of healthy patients have one test result outside the reference interval

consent for procedures to be performed is important, but does not provide legal protection if the veterinary staff are found to be negligent (see chapter 1).

Pre-anaesthetic fasting is recommended to reduce regurgitation and aspiration of gastric contents and minimise the development of tympany (bloat). For most patients, it is sufficient to withhold food for 6 hours before surgery. Unfortunately, this is not always possible, for example, for caesarean section or following trauma. Fasting is not recommended for young animals, small mammals and birds because this can cause hypoglycaemia. Fresh water should be provided until pre-anaesthetic medication is administered. This is particularly important in geriatric patients that may have subclinical renal disease.

It is essential to reduce the stress of admission and hospitalisation to minimise the release of catecholamines (e.g. adrenaline) into the circulation, and special housing requirements should be considered for cats, small mammals and birds.

Tranquillisers, sedatives and other pre-anaesthetic medications may be administered intramuscularly, subcutaneously or intravenously. Following administration of these drugs patients should be disturbed as little as possible to allow the full effects of the medication to develop. However, they must be observed frequently (preferably every 5 minutes) in case any unexpected events occur such as idiosyncratic drug reactions or vomiting. The veterinary nurse should ensure that the correct equipment is available and has been checked before the patient receives a general anaesthetic (box). Intravenous catheters may be placed following sedation or pre-anaesthetic medication.

EQUIPMENT CHECKLIST

- Anaesthetic trolley available: Clean. Safety checks performed (oxygen flush, alarm systems). Rotameters functional. Cylinders attached and labelled ('Full', 'Empty', 'In-use'). Piped gases attached.
- Gases (oxygen, nitrous oxide) switched on. Back-up supply available.
- Vaporiser checked. Filled with appropriate agent.
- Scavenging system available. Switch on; assemble; weigh charcoal absorbers to ensure activity.
- Endotracheal tubes selected. Cleaned; cuff checked for leaks; no luminal obstructions.
- Cuff inflator available.
- Method of securing endotracheal tube available. White open-weave bandage generally used.
- Lubricant for endotracheal tube. Water, sterile water-soluble gel or sterile silicone spray.
- Laryngoscope. Assembled. Light functional. Stylet available if required.
- Local anaesthetic spray. Available for cats.
- Mouth gag.
- Assistant. To restrain patient during placement of intravenous catheter, induction of general anaesthesia.
- Appropriate breathing system selected and assembled correctly. Check for leaks. Soda lime checked if appropriate. Attached to anaesthetic trolley.
- General anaesthetic agent. Chosen by veterinary surgeon, drawn up and labelled.
- Equipment for placement of intravenous catheter. See chapter 8.
- Scissor or clippers. Clip hair from injection site.
- Surgical scrub and alcohol. Swab or cotton wool to prepare the intravenous injection site.
- Location of emergency drugs identified and readily accessible.
- Monitoring equipment laid out.
- Non-medicated ocular lubricant. To prevent corneal drying during general anaesthesia.

SUMMARY

The preoperative assessment of a patient is an essential part of all procedures. The history and physical examination are the fundamental requirements. Based on the results of these examinations, other diagnostic tests may be performed, anaesthetic risk assessed, and specific management regimes selected.

REFERENCES AND FURTHER READING

Knottenbelt, C. & Mackin, A. (1998a) Blood transfusions in the dog and cat. Part 1. Blood collection techniques. *In Practice* **20**, 110–114.

Knottenbelt, C. & Mackin, A. (1998b) Blood transfusions in the dog and cat. Part 2. Indications and safe administration. *In Practice* **20**, 191–199.

Lumsden, J.H. (1998) Laboratory data interpretation. In: *Manual of Small Animal Clinical Pathology* (eds M.G. Davidson, R.W. Else & J.H. Lumsden), pp 27–32. British Small Animal Veterinary Association, Cheltenham.

Rentko, V. (2000) Practical use of a blood substitute. In: *Kirk's Current Veterinary Therapy XIII Small Animal Practice* (ed. J.D. Bonagura), pp 424–427. WB Saunders Company, Philadelphia.

Waterman-Pearson, A.E. (1999) Urogenital disease. In: *Manual of Small Animal Anaesthesia and Analgesia* (eds C. Seymour & R. Gleed), pp 211–216. British Small Animal Veterinary Association, Cheltenham.

Welsh, E. (1999) Fluid therapy and shock. In: *Veterinary Nursing* 2nd edition (eds D.R. Lane & B.C. Cooper), pp 568–585. Butterworth Heinemann, Oxford.

Anaesthetic Machines and Ventilators

4

Craig Johnson

The anaesthetic machine is a vital tool for inhalation anaesthesia. At first inspection its size and complexity can be intimidating, but it is essential that personnel using it understand how it provides gases to the breathing system and how to use it in such a way as to not break it. Such knowledge is imperative to ensure the safety of both the patient and the operator.

Although the anaesthetic machine is central to the practice of anaesthesia, it remains a machine and the principles that govern it are found in the realm of physics. Students of veterinary anaesthesia from different backgrounds can have very different levels of exposure to the study of physics. This chapter is therefore divided into two sections. The first section covers the anaesthetic machine without explaining the physical principles involved. In the second section, readers without a firm grounding in physics will find all the relevant processes described. It is suggested that the reader becomes familiar with the first section before embarking on the second section. Once the second section has been read, it should be possible to reread the first section with a deeper understanding of the processes involved.

THE ANAESTHETIC MACHINE

Inhalation anaesthetics are delivered by means of anaesthetic machines that may be free-standing or form part of a larger anaesthesia delivery system. They can be broken down into a number of parts (Fig. 4.1) that perform specific functions.

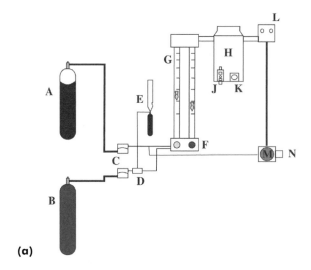

(a)

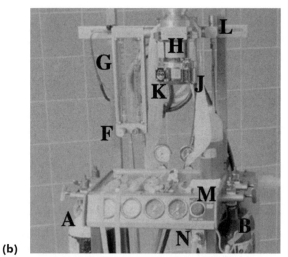

(b)

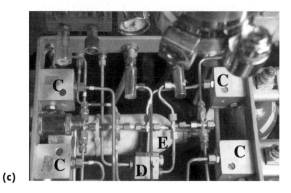

(c)

Fig 4.1 Anaesthetic machine. (a) Diagrammatic; (b) MIE Salisbury machine; (c) Salisbury with instrument tray removed. A oxygen cylinder, B nitrous oxide cylinder, C reducing valves, D nitrous oxide cut-off, E oxygen alarm, F needle valves, G rotameters, H vaporiser, J key filler, K agent level window, L pressure relief valve, M oxygen flush, N common gas outlet.

FUNCTIONS OF ANAESTHETIC DELIVERY SYSTEMS

Storage and transport of anaesthetic gases

Cylinders
Gas pipeline

Processing of anaesthetic gases and volatile agents

Pressure reduction valves
Vaporisers

Mixing of agents

Needle valves
Rotameters
Vaporisers

Delivery of gas mixture to patient

Breathing system (circuit)

Removal of gas mixture from patient and disposal

Scavenging systems

Cylinders and pipelines
(Physical principles 1 and 2; see pages 79–80)
Anaesthetised patients breathe gas mixtures that have a different composition
to room air. This means that the anaesthetic delivery system must have a store
of gases to deliver to the patient. Unfortunately, gas is inconvenient to store and
move round due to its high volume (a 20 kg dog will breathe 240 litres of gas an
hour, that is about one-and-a-half dustbins full). Anaesthetic systems usually
overcome the problem of high volume by storing gas at high pressure in metal
(molybdenum steel) cylinders. Pressurised gas has the added advantage of providing energy to push the gas through the anaesthetic machine. Gas cylinders
are available in a range of sizes (AA [smallest] to J [largest]). A full 'E' cylinder
of oxygen stores gas at approximately 13 300 kPa (133 atmospheres). This is
the equivalent of 680 litres of gas at atmospheric pressure, enough to keep a
20 kg dog supplied for almost 3 hours.

   At this pressure, accidental damage caused by, for example, knocking over
a cylinder left leaning against a wall can have dramatic effects. Cylinders have
been recorded propelling themselves along corridors and through brick walls
before coming to a halt. They can cause severe damage to buildings and are
potentially lethal. Anaesthetic cylinders should always be stored properly and
handled with care. This means that they should be stored in a secure fashion
away from busy parts of the clinic. Most cylinder stores secure the cylinders to

the wall using chains or purpose-made hoops; other systems such as racks may be acceptable. It is wise to keep the cylinder store locked so that unauthorised personnel cannot gain access and inadvertently injure themselves.

Cylinders can be removed from the gas store manually and transported to the anaesthetic machine (usually smaller cylinders), or the cylinders in the store can be connected to a pipeline that carries the gas to outlets in the clinic (usually larger cylinders). Where a pipeline system is used, two banks of cylinders of each gas used are optimal – one 'in use' and one 'in reserve'. The anaesthetic machine is plugged in to a pipeline outlet before use *via* wall- or ceiling-mounted Schraeder-type sockets. Anaesthetic machines should be able to hold two oxygen cylinders *via* specialised hanger yokes in addition to two nitrous oxide cylinders, though nitrous oxide is optional. These two systems can be compared to electrical appliances that can be operated using mains electricity or batteries. Small cylinders (batteries) cost less to set up (no installed wiring), but pipelines (mains) are cheaper to run as each litre of gas costs less. Even when a pipeline is used, it is good practice to have cylinders available as back-up in case there is an interruption in the gas supply while a patient is being anaesthetised.

Cylinders (and pipelines) are colour coded to allow gas to be rapidly identified. The United Kingdom coding for six different cylinders is shown in Table 4.1. It should be noted that colour codes in the US are different to the UK. Gases in cylinders can be stored as compressed gases (e.g. oxygen) or as liquids (e.g. nitrous oxide). When a gas is stored as a liquid it simply means that it has been compressed to such a pressure that it condenses in the cylinder. This distinction is important when determining how much gas is left in a partly used cylinder. If the contents are gaseous then the pressure in the cylinder will be proportional to the volume of gas left in the cylinder. If the contents are liquid then the pressure will remain constant until all the liquid has evaporated. At this point the cylinder will be almost empty and the pressure in the cylinder will fall rapidly from 'full' to 'empty'.

'Check' valves
These valves prevent retrograde flow of gases from cylinders 'in use' to vacant hanger yokes, allowing empty cylinders to be removed while the anaesthetic

Table 4.1 United Kingdom colour codes for medical gas cylinders.

Cylinder containing	Body of cylinder	Head of cylinder
Oxygen	Black	White
Medical air	Grey	Black and white
Carbon dioxide	Grey	Grey
Nitrous oxide	Blue	Blue
Entonox	Blue	Blue and white
Cyclopropane	Orange	Orange

machine is being used. In addition they prevent retrograde flow between 'in use' cylinders of high and low pressure.

Pressure gauge

When gas cylinders are attached to an anaesthetic machine, a pressure gauge indicates the pressure of the gas remaining within the cylinder, measured in kilopascals (kPa). For oxygen the pressure in the cylinder will be proportional to the volume of gas left in the cylinder. The length of time the remaining anaesthetic gas will last can then be calculated:

$$\text{Length of time remaining} = \frac{\text{Volume remaining in gas cylinder (litres)}}{\text{Fresh gas flow (litres/min)}}$$

OXYGEN

$$\frac{\text{Volume of gas remaining in oxygen cylinder}}{\text{Original volume of gas in cylinder}} = \frac{\text{Pressure of gas left in cylinder}}{\text{Original gas pressure}}$$

Example, for a type E cylinder:

$$\frac{\text{Volume of gas remaining in oxygen cylinder}}{680 \text{ litres}} = \frac{\text{Pressure of gas left in cylinder}}{13\,300 \text{ kPa}}$$

i.e.

Litres remaining = [current pressure/133 × 100 kPa] × 680

NITROUS OXIDE

The calculations for oxygen are not suitable for nitrous oxide. However, the weight of the cylinder can give an indication of the amount of nitrous oxide remaining in the cylinder.

Volume of gas remaining in nitrous oxide cylinder
= [weight of cylinder (kg) − empty weight of cylinder (kg)] × 534

The weight of the empty cylinder is generally stamped on the neck of the cylinder.

Pressure reduction valves

(Physical principle 3; see page 80)

As already discussed, gas at very high pressure is dangerous and difficult to work with. The first step in preparing gas for a patient to breathe is to reduce the pressure to an intermediate level. The aim is to make the flow rate of the gas easier to regulate while keeping enough pressure to drive the gas through the remainder of the anaesthetic machine. Most anaesthetic machines operate at a standard machine pressure of approximately 410 kPa (4 atmospheres), which is referred to as pipeline pressure. Gas from the cylinder is passed into a reducing valve that produces a reduced and constant supply pressure for the anaesthetic machine, i.e. a constant flow of gas is provided downstream from the valve, removing the requirement for constant small adjustments to the flowmeter as the amount of oxygen remaining in the cylinder (and thus the pressure within the cylinder) falls. The reducing valve can be part of the anaesthetic machine and difficult to identify, for use with attached cylinders, or part of the pipeline installation.

A typical pressure reduction valve is illustrated in Fig. 4.2. The pressure is reduced by passing the gas through a valve that opens against the force of a

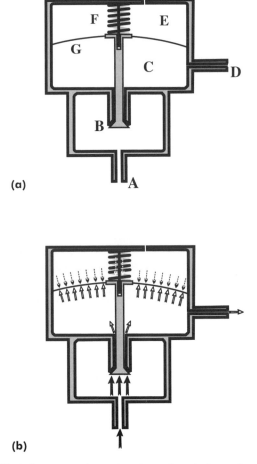

Fig 4.2 (a) Simplified diagrammatic section through reducing valve. (A) high pressure inlet, (B) high pressure chamber, (C) regulated pressure chamber, (D) regulated pressure outlet, (E) atmospheric pressure chamber, (F) spring. (b) Arrows represent forces: black arrows – forces due to high pressure gas, white arrows – forces due to regulated pressure gas, dashed arrows – forces due to atmospheric gas, dotted arrows – force due to spring.

spring. The pressure of the regulated side of the valve is compared to atmospheric pressure in order to maintain a constant pressure output.

Needle valves

(Physical principles 4 and 5; see pages 80–81)
Needle valves (Fig. 4.3) are used to regulate the flow of gas into the low-pressure part of the anaesthetic machine (vaporiser and common gas outlet) where the gases mix and are at a pressure just greater than atmospheric. Needle valves are an example of a variable orifice device. They utilise the relationship between resistance, pressure and flow to adjust the flow of gas to the patient. Adjusting the area of the valve orifice alters the resistance, the pressure is held constant by the reducing valve and so the flow is controlled.

Most needle valves are designed so that the spindle seats into the valve before the thread reaches its end. This means that the control knob should only be turned until there is no flow. If it is forced round until the end of the thread is reached, the spindle will be forced into the valve and can bend or break off. This will prevent the valve from working correctly. At best the flow of gas will no longer be altered smoothly as the valve is opened and at worst the valve will need replacing before the machine can be used again.

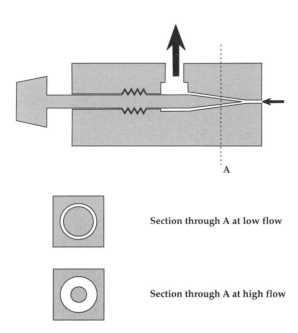

Section through A at low flow

Section through A at high flow

Fig 4.3 Diagrammatic section through needle valve. Turning the knob moves the needle into or out of its seat and alters the area through which gas may flow, thereby altering the resistance and so the flow of gas.

Rotameters

(Physical principles 4 and 5; see pages 80–81)

Rotameters are the most commonly encountered example of a number of devices which measure the gas flow. They allow precise adjustment of the total fresh gas flow and the proportions of different gases in the mixture. The rotameter (Fig. 4.4) functions according to similar principles to the needle valve. Downward force is constant (due to gravity acting on the bobbin) and the bobbin moves up or down in a graduated tube with a variable orifice. At equilibrium the upward force due to the resistance of the gas passing through the orifice is equal to the force of gravity.

Rotameters have either a float which spins in the airflow and is read from the top or a ball which tumbles in the airflow and is read from its centre (Fig. 4.5). The reading is only accurate if the float or ball is free to spin or tumble. Common causes of the rotameter not reading properly are that the tube is tilted to one side so that the float sits against the wall of the tube or that there is dirt inside the tube which is impeding the movement of the float. Floats have a dot painted on the side so that it is easy to verify that they are spinning; balls are half painted so that they can be seen to be tumbling.

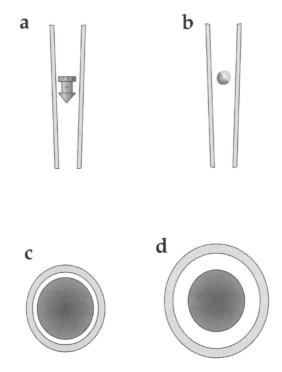

Fig 4.4 Diagrammatic representation of rotameter. (a) Vane type; (b) ball type; (c) at low flows the area of the space between the vane and the cylinder is small; (d) at high flows the area is larger.

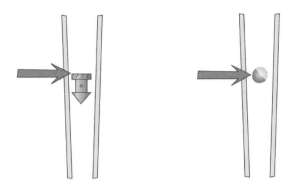

Fig 4.5 Vane rotameters should be read from the top; ball rotameters should be read from the centre of the ball. The correct level at which to read these two rotameters is indicated by the arrow.

Vaporisers

(Physical principles 6, 7 and 8; see pages 81–82)
A vaporiser adds a volatile anaesthetic agent to the gas mixture. Volatile anaesthetics are liquids that are added to the gas mixture as a vapour. There are two kinds of vaporiser: plenum and draw-over. Gas is driven through plenum vaporisers by positive pressure from the anaesthetic machine and through draw-over vaporisers by the patient's respiratory efforts. Draw-over vaporisers are uncommon in current veterinary anaesthesia.

Draw-over vaporiser (in-circuit vaporiser)

When using a circle breathing system, it is possible to mount the vaporiser either before the gas enters the breathing system (out-of-circuit) or within the breathing system itself (in-circuit). In-circuit vaporisers are draw-over vaporisers placed (usually) in the inspiratory limb of the breathing system. They must have low resistance to breathing and therefore are of relatively simple design. Their output cannot be accurately controlled as can a plenum vaporiser, but because of the manner in which they are used this is not an important consideration. The most common examples of such vaporisers in current use are found on Stephens and Komesaroff anaesthetic machines.

Each time anaesthetic gases pass around a circle system, they will be driven through the in-circuit vaporiser and pick up more volatile anaesthetic agent. This means that the greater the patient's minute volume, the more gas will pass through the vaporiser, leading to increased delivery of anaesthetic agent. Volatile anaesthetics cause respiratory depression, leading to feedback between the respiratory system and the depth of anaesthesia. If a patient comes 'light' due to insufficient anaesthetic or increased surgical stimulation, its minute volume will increase and more anaesthetic will be delivered, tending to deepen anaesthesia. Conversely if a patient becomes too deeply anaesthetised, its minute volume will decrease and less anaesthetic will be delivered, tending to lighten anaesthesia.

Whilst this automatic feedback can be useful, it should be remembered that there are a number of circumstances where this mechanism does not work:

- Any form of controlled ventilation such as IPPV removes the patient's control of respiratory function. This means that the amount of anaesthetic delivered will depend on the ventilator settings rather than changes in depth of anaesthesia.
- If the soda lime becomes exhausted during an anaesthetic, this will lead to the build-up of carbon dioxide that is a potent stimulant to ventilation. The patient's minute volume will continue to increase despite the increased delivery of anaesthetic agent.
- If the patient becomes hypoxaemic for any reason, the hypoxic drive will increase ventilation and the patient will take on more anaesthetic agent even if already deeply anaesthetised.

It is important to ensure that these circumstances do not arise when using draw-over vaporisers, as they can quickly lead to the development of a dangerous overdose of inspired anaesthetic agent.

Plenum vaporisers (out-of-circuit vaporiser)

Modern, calibrated plenum vaporisers add a very controlled amount of volatile anaesthetic to the gas mixture and have a number of compensating devices to ensure that this remains constant over a range of working conditions. In order to understand how a modern vaporiser works it is best to start by considering the factors that influence the output of a much simpler vaporiser (Fig. 4.6).

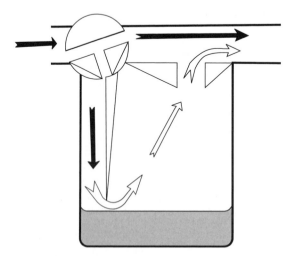

Fig 4.6 Diagrammatic representation of a simple plenum vaporiser. Anaesthetic gas passes through the vaporiser (black arrows). That which passes through the vaporisation chamber becomes saturated with volatile anaesthetic vapour (white arrows). The output of the vaporiser is altered by turning the control knob to alter the relative flow through and past the vaporisation chamber.

The gas passing into the vaporiser is divided into two channels. One passes over the anaesthetic liquid in the vaporisation chamber and the other does not come into contact with the liquid. The amount of vapour in the output of the vaporiser will depend upon the following factors.

- *Proportion of gas which goes through vaporisation chamber:* The greater the proportion of gas which passes over the liquid, the greater the partial pressure of gas in the output of the vaporiser.
- *Total flow of gas through vaporiser:* The lower the total flow, the longer the gas will remain in the vaporisation chamber and the more vapour it will pick up until it becomes saturated. The output of the vaporiser will fall with high gas flow rates (gas no longer has time to become saturated).
- *Level of liquid in vaporisation chamber:* With more liquid in the chamber, the gas will pass closer to the surface and more anaesthetic will be vaporised.
- *Temperature of liquid in vaporiser:* At higher temperatures the output of the vaporiser will rise. As anaesthesia progresses, the latent heat of vaporisation is taken from the liquid and the surrounding vaporiser. The vaporiser gets colder and its output falls.

Modern vaporisers are temperature, level and flow compensated, leaving the output of the vaporiser to be decided by the proportion of gas that passes through the vaporisation chamber. The compensating devices in a typical vaporiser (an early Bowring Medical Engineering model) are illustrated in Fig. 4.7.

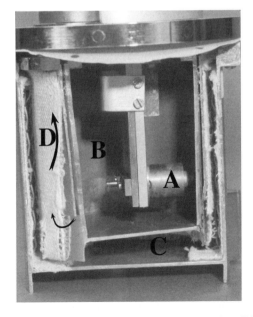

Fig 4.7 Cut-away of early Bowring Medical Engingeering vaporiser. (A) thermostatic valve, (B) bypass chamber, (C) vaporisation chamber, (D) fibrous wicks.

- *Temperature compensation:* There are two temperature compensating mechanisms. The vaporiser is constructed using a large amount of metal (brass in this instance), which acts as a reservoir and conductor for heat energy. This reduces the cooling effect of the vaporisation process. A thermostatic valve (A), which is mounted in the bypass chamber (B), gradually closes as the vaporiser cools. This reduces the proportion of gas which passes through the bypass chamber and so increases the output of the vaporiser to compensate for any fall in temperature.
- *Level compensation:* The vaporisation chamber (C) contains fibrous wicks (D) which allow the anaesthetic agent to climb by capillary action. This increases the surface area for vaporisation and means that a change in the level of liquid will have no effect on the output of the vaporiser as long as the liquid still reaches the bottom of the wicks.
- *Flow compensation:* The gas, which passes through the vaporisation chamber, is forced to take a tortuous route (arrows) which means that it remains in close proximity to the wicks for a longer period of time. This increases the maximum flow rate at which the gas can become saturated with anaesthetic agent and so reduces the effect of high gas flows through the vaporiser.

Modern vaporisers may be removed from the anaesthetic machine. Furthermore some back bars can accommodate more than one vaporiser, for example, halothane and isoflurane.

Common gas outlet
This outlet is the site of attachment of anaesthetic breathing systems.

Safety devices
In addition to parts that carry out the primary functions involved in anaesthetic delivery, anaesthetic machines are fitted with a number of safety devices.

SAFETY DEVICES ON ANAESTHETIC MACHINES
- Pin index cylinders
- Pipeline connectors
- Oxygen whistle
- Nitrous oxide cut-off
- Hypoxic gas mixture preventer
- Vaporiser key filler
- Pressure relief valve
- Emergency oxygen flush

Each device is aimed at making the use of the anaesthetic machine as safe as possible for the patient by alerting the anaesthetist to potential problems or preventing common mistakes.

Pin index cylinders

Cylinders which connect directly to the anaesthetic machine incorporate a system of holes bored into the face of the valve block. These interlock with pins on the face of the valve seat on the anaesthetic machine. The pins are placed in different positions for different gases, preventing a cylinder from being connected to the inlet for the wrong gas. A selection of pin positions for different gases is illustrated in Fig. 4.8.

Pipeline connectors

Anaesthetic machines that are supplied from a pipeline are connected by removable connectors fitted onto gas hoses. These are manufactured in such a way that it is not possible to connect the hose for one gas into a connector for any other gas. There are several such systems in use, each from different manufacturers.

Oxygen whistle

This is a device that sounds a loud whistle if the pressure in the oxygen pipeline falls during anaesthesia. It warns the anaesthetist in time to change over cylin-

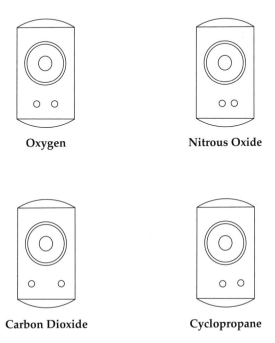

Oxygen **Nitrous Oxide**

Carbon Dioxide **Cyclopropane**

Fig 4.8 Pin index valve block system for small medical gas cylinders.

ders or connect to the pipeline before the oxygen supply to the patient runs out. There are various designs of oxygen whistle that work in different ways. Some are only functional if the nitrous oxide is connected. It is most important to be familiar with the type of oxygen alarm fitted to the machine prior to using it for the first time. The alarm should be tested once every day before the machine is used that day. An anaesthetic machine that has no oxygen alarm can be extremely dangerous and should be avoided. Such a machine should never be used with nitrous oxide.

Nitrous oxide cut-off
In addition to an oxygen alarm, many machines have an automatic nitrous oxide cut-off that prevents nitrous oxide from being delivered to the patient when the oxygen alarm is sounding.

Oxygen–nitrous oxide proportioning devices
Anaesthetic machines may be fitted with a variety of devices that proportion the flow of oxygen and nitrous oxide in such a way as to prevent hypoxic gas mixtures from being delivered to the patient. Typically, they will allow a minimum of 25% oxygen to be included in the gas mixture. If the nitrous oxide flow is increased beyond this, the flow of oxygen will be automatically increased to maintain the minimum concentration of oxygen in the gas mix.

Vaporiser key filler
Key fillers (Fig. 4.9 shows an example of a halothane filler) fit onto the caps of volatile anaesthetic bottles and provide a sealed means of filling the vaporiser. This reduces the risk of breathing in anaesthetic agent fumes during filling, however, it is still good practice to fill vaporisers at the end of the day. In addition, the filler provides two keys, one between the bottle and filler and the second between the filler and vaporiser, that prevent the vaporiser from being filled with any but the correct anaesthetic agent.

Pressure relief valve
This is a valve placed in the common gas pathway immediately prior to the common gas outlet that vents gas to the outside. It is designed to open if the pressure in this part of the system exceeds 35–70 kPa. This valve is designed to prevent gas build-up within the anaesthetic machine from reaching a pressure which could damage the machine. It is not intended to protect the patient, as an inspiratory pressure of 35 kPa is enough to prevent venous return and cause barotrauma.

Emergency oxygen flush
This is usually a well-marked button in a prominent place on the anaesthetic machine. It will deliver a rapid flow of 100% oxygen to the patient, bypassing the rotameters and vaporiser. It is very useful in an emergency to flush gas that

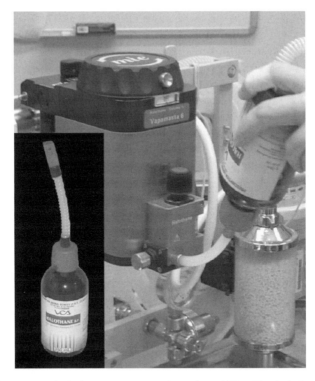

Fig 4.9 Filling an MIE halothane vaporiser using a keyed filler. The halothane bottle with the filler attached is shown in the inset.

contains anaesthetic agents from the breathing system. It should never be used in a closed breathing system without first ensuring that the expiratory valve is open.

Waste anaesthetic gas scavenging

Effective scavenging of waste anaesthetic gases, especially the volatile anaesthetic agents and nitrous oxide, is extremely important (see chapter 1). There are three methods of controlling the level of exposure of staff to waste anaesthetic gases:

- adequate ventilation in the workplace;
- good working practices;
- gas scavenging systems.

Gas scavenging systems may be classified as active, semi-passive or passive.

Active systems

Active systems are the preferred method of waste gas scavenging and basically comprise four components [1–4]. The receiving unit and transfer hose [1] system receives waste anaesthetic gases from the patient breathing system and provides a safe interface between the patient and the extraction unit. Modern transfer hoses are fitted with a pressure relief valve (10 cmH$_2$O) to provide the patient with an expiratory path in the event of the hose becoming occluded. The receiving system connects to interconnecting pipework [2]. The main plant [3] (usually a fan or a pump) finally removes the waste gases to the exterior of the building *via* a terminal outlet [4].

Passive systems

Passive systems are 'driven' by the anaesthetised patient's respiratory efforts. To minimise resistance a large-bore tube (22 mm) is used to vent waste gases from the expiratory valve, either to the outside of the building or to active charcoal absorbers. There is increased resistance when active charcoal absorbers are used and they do not absorb nitrous oxide. It is recommended that the length of the scavenge tube does not exceed 2.6 metres.

Semi-passive (active-passive) systems

Semi-passive systems use the same system of tubing as passive systems but the tube is vented into a forced ventilation system. It is important when this system is used that air removed from the anaesthetic room is not recirculated to another part of the building but vented from the building.

Although it is important to have a waste anaesthetic scavenging system in place, there are a number of simple working practices that can be adopted to minimise the exposure of staff to waste gases.

- Check both the anaesthetic machine and patient breathing systems for leaks.
- Turn on active scavenge systems and ensure charcoal absorbers are still active (by weighing). Connect scavenge tube to patient breathing system.
- Use key fillers to minimise spillage of volatile agent when filling vaporisers.
- If possible remove vaporisers from anaesthetic machine to a well-ventilated area before filling. Alternatively fill vaporiser at the end of the day or at the end of the procedure, to minimise the number of staff present.
- Wear gloves when filling vaporiser.
- Contain volatile agent spills appropriately (see chapter 1).
- Minimise the use of mask anaesthesia.
- Use endotracheal intubation and use cuffed tubes where appropriate.
- Do not turn on anaesthetic gases (other than oxygen) until the patient is attached to the breathing system.
- Turn off anaesthetic gases when the patient is disconnected from the breathing system.
- At the end of the anaesthetic period allow the patient to breathe oxygen through the breathing system before disconnecting it completely. Alternatively, purge the breathing system with oxygen before disconnecting the pa-

tient, or by occluding the patient connection and emptying the gas remaining in the reservoir bag into scavenging system.

- Allow patients to recover in well-ventilated areas.
- Service all equipment annually.
- Monitor theatre pollution periodically.

Care and maintenance of anaesthetic machines

It is advisable to have maintenance contracts for the anaesthetic machines and vaporisers used within the practice, ensuring that they are serviced once a year. However, qualified practice staff should also make daily safety checks.

- Wipe anaesthetic machine with a disinfectant solution.
- Attach anaesthetic machine to gas pipeline or ensure cylinders are attached to the machine at the appropriate yokes. Remove and replace any cylinders marked as 'empty' by cylinder neck labels.
- Open the flowmeters. No gas should flow when gases from cylinders attached to the anaesthetic machine are used. Gas flow indicates a leak in the system.
- Turn the oxygen cylinder on and check the pressure gauge. Calculate the volume of gas remaining if necessary. Turn the oxygen flowmeter to ensure flow. There should be no flow through the other flowmeters. Occlude the common gas outlet briefly. The flowmeter bobbin should dip, indicating there are no leaks downstream from the flowmeter. Turn the oxygen flowmeter off. The bobbin should return to zero, indicating the needle valve is functioning normally.
- Repeat the procedure above for nitrous oxide, but remember that the pressure gauge does not reflect the volume of gas remaining.
- Check the oxygen failure device. Turn the oxygen flowmeter on and then turn the oxygen cylinder off. The flowmeter bobbin should fall and the device should sound. This may be repeated when both oxygen and nitrous oxide are flowing through the machine. However, the health and safety aspect of releasing nitrous oxide into the system without anaesthetic waste gas scavenging should be considered.
- Turn on the oxygen flowmeter and occlude the common gas outlet. Initially the pressure relief valve should open and vent.
- With all flowmeters turned off, check oxygen flows when the emergency oxygen flush button or lever is operated.
- With all flowmeters turned off, check that the vaporiser dial moves freely and returns to the off position. This is particularly important to avoid inadvertent administration of volatile agent and when more than one vaporiser is attached to the back bar.
- Check level of volatile agent in vaporiser and fill if necessary.

At the end of the day or following completion of the daily anaesthetic list, the following points should be remembered.

- Turn off all gases at the cylinder. This prevents damage to the pressure reduction valves. Remove and replace empty cylinders. Alternatively disconnect gas pipelines and store hoses appropriately.
- Vent all gases remaining in the anaesthetic machine by either using the emergency oxygen flush button or opening the flowmeters. This prevents damage to the pressure gauge and ensures that no one uses the anaesthetic machine in the mistaken belief that the gas cylinders are turned on because of the readings on the pressure gauges.
- Turn all flowmeters off. This prevents the bobbin being forced up the flowmeter tube where it may become lodged when the gas cylinders are turned on.
- Remove vaporisers for filling and replace. Ensure dial is turned to 'off'.
- Remove all organic debris from the anaesthetic machine using a mild soapy solution. Wipe anaesthetic machine with a disinfectant solution.

VENTILATORS

Conscious, healthy patients breathe spontaneously. Under general anaesthesia most patients continue to breathe spontaneously once connected to the chosen breathing system. However, it is advisable to 'sigh' or 'bag' these patients at 5- to 10-minute intervals. This is performed either by closing the expiratory valve of the patient breathing system or by briefly increasing the fresh gas flow and compressing the reservoir bag (or by pinching the end of the open-ended reservoir bag in the modified Ayre T-piece). In-circuit vaporisers should be switched off. The degree of lung inflation desired should inflate the chest wall slightly beyond that observed in the spontaneously breathing anaesthetised patient and mimic the level of chest expansion of the conscious patient (maximum of 20 cmH$_2$O). 'Sighing' allows assessment of pulmonary and thoracic compliance, facilitates detection of breathing system disconnection or occlusion and limits pulmonary atelectasis (collapse), hypercapnia and hypoxia. Following sighing, the expiratory valve should be reopened or the fresh gas flow returned to normal and the in-circuit vaporisers switched back on. All anaesthetic breathing systems may be used in this fashion.

Manual ventilation also can be used either to assist ventilation (i.e. to increase frequency of 'sighing'), or to control ventilation where the anaesthetist controls both respiratory rate and tidal volume. The Lack and Magill breathing systems are not suitable to be used with manual ventilation because expired gases would be rebreathed at standard calculated fresh gas flow rates.

Ventilators provide a mechanical means of inflating the patient's lungs during anaesthesia. There are many types and models of ventilator available and their internal workings and operation can be complicated. In addition, the act of artificially ventilating a patient can have profound and complex effects upon respiratory and cardiovascular physiology, which can dramatically alter the course of an anaesthetic.

What follows is a brief description of the ways in which ventilators are categorised, which it is hoped will enable the reader to make further study of specific ventilators and the physiology of ventilation.

Positive and negative pressure ventilation

There are two possible ways to artificially inflate the lungs. A negative pressure can be applied to the outside of the thoracic cavity. This will cause the chest wall to move outwards and the lungs to expand, drawing in air. The pressure changes using this system are very similar to those found in natural breathing and so this is a physiologically sensible way to ventilate a patient. Unfortunately, in order to perform negative pressure ventilation, the patient's chest must be fully enclosed in a rigid, sealed container, which can make surgical access difficult. Hence negative pressure ventilation is rarely used in anaesthesia.

Positive pressure ventilation requires the lungs to be inflated by applying a positive pressure to the airway. Providing the airway is sealed by an endotracheal tube or similar, this is very easy to achieve. The equipment can be as simple as a Mapleson F breathing system (with an assistant to squeeze the bag). For this reason, positive pressure ventilation of the lungs is the most common technique used in anaesthesia.

There are a variety of alternative techniques for providing ventilation or gas exchange by artificial means. These include high-frequency jet ventilation, high-frequency oscillation, differential lung ventilation, liquid ventilation and extracorporeal gas exchange. Discussion of these techniques is beyond the scope of this text.

Intermittent positive pressure ventilation

The act of ventilating an anaesthetised patient by intermittently increasing the pressure in the breathing system appears deceptively simple. Unfortunately it has many physiological effects that can be complex and can influence the patient's body function in profound ways that may or may not be beneficial.

Effects on lung ventilation

The way in which the lungs fill when pressure is applied at the airway depends on two factors: the static compliance and the time constant of the lungs. Static compliance is a measure of the elasticity of the lungs, an increase in compliance meaning that the lungs will be more full at a given airway pressure. The time constant is a measure of the resistance of the airways; increased resistance will give a longer time constant. In general, compliance is more important when the lungs are filled slowly and the time constant is more important when the lungs are filled quickly.

Both compliance and time constant vary throughout individual lungs and so the speed at which the lungs are inflated will alter the distribution of respiratory gases to different lung regions. In patients with localised areas of collapsed lung or other focal disease process, small alterations in the rate at which the lungs are inflated or the peak inspiratory pressure can dramatically alter the degree of oxygenation of the blood leaving the lungs. If most of the ventilation is directed into a region where there is little perfusion or there is disruption of gas exchange, then the patient may become hypoxaemic.

Many respiratory diseases can alter the compliance of the lungs and/or the respiratory time constant. In patients with bronchoconstriction, for example, a cat with feline asthma, the time constant is increased. In such cases it is important to ensure that the lungs are inflated slowly and that sufficient expiratory pause is allowed for the lungs to empty after each breath. In patients with diseases involving altered compliance, such as bullous emphysema, it is important that the peak inspiratory pressure is limited: the bullae are very compliant and can easily overexpand and even rupture if too much pressure is applied.

Effects on cardiovascular function
The stroke volume of the heart varies with several factors, one of which is the amount of filling that takes place during asystole (Starling's law). During normal respiration the pressure in the thoracic cavity changes little and the mean pressure is usually zero or a little negative. IPPV can raise the thoracic pressure considerably and this can reduce the venous return of blood to the heart. When thoracic pressure is greater than venous return pressure, there will be little return of blood to the heart and so cardiac output is much reduced. These effects will be pronounced in hypovolaemic patients, who tend to have a low central venous pressure.

Over a complete respiratory cycle, the effects on cardiac output will be proportional to mean thoracic pressure. The effects can be minimised by limiting peak inspiratory pressure or by increasing the expiratory pause so that there is a longer period where thoracic pressure is low. Both these techniques will reduce mean intrathoracic pressure and so preserve cardiac output; however, both can have adverse effects in their own right. When peak inspiratory pressure is reduced, the degree of filling of the lungs is reduced which leads to a decrease in minute volume. Over a period of time this may lead to the patient retaining carbon dioxide. When the expiratory pause is extended there is more potential for collapse of the smaller bronchi and this can result in areas of shunt, leading to hypoxaemia.

Effects on oxygenation
Intermittent positive pressure ventilation will often improve oxygenation in patients that are hypoxaemic, but not always. In most anaesthetised patients breathing gas containing an adequate oxygen tension, the haemoglobin in arterial blood is almost 100% saturated with oxygen. When this is the case, IPPV

will not improve the amount of oxygen in the blood. It should be remembered that the amount of oxygen delivered to the tissues is more important than the blood oxygen concentration *per se*. It is possible that the reduction in cardiac output caused by IPPV can reduce tissue oxygen delivery despite an increase in the oxygen content of the arterial blood. For this reason, PaO_2 or SaO_2 aq should not be considered in isolation when assessing the effects of IPPV in a particular patient.

Effects on carbon dioxide tension

Arterial carbon dioxide tension is the main determinant of respiratory minute volume in animals that are breathing spontaneously. An increase in $PaCO_2$ will stimulate an increased minute volume that will reduce $PaCO_2$ back to normal. Conversely a decrease in $PaCO_2$ will depress minute volume and so allow $PaCO_2$ to increase back to normal. During IPPV this homeostatic mechanism is removed and so great care should be taken that $PaCO_2$ remains within normal limits.

If the patient is not sufficiently ventilated to remove enough carbon dioxide, there will be a gradual build-up leading to a respiratory acidosis. This can have many effects that will be detrimental to the patient. Effects include an increase in sympathetic stimulation with increased arterial blood pressure and tissue perfusion; this will increase cardiac workload and oxygen consumption and may lead to the development of ventricular dysrhythmias. Intracranial pressure and intraocular pressure will be increased. There will be increased tissue perfusion which may be seen as increased bleeding at the surgical site and, in severe cases, the effects of the anaesthetic agents may be potentiated by alterations in their degree of dissociation and plasma protein binding.

If the patient is overventilated, too much carbon dioxide will be removed and a respiratory alkalosis will develop. Effects on the patient include a reduction in arterial blood pressure and a decrease in perfusion of the tissues, particularly the brain. In extreme cases it is possible for cerebral perfusion to reduce to such an extent that oxygen delivery is compromised and the patient suffers cerebral hypoxaemia with subsequent brain damage.

When $PaCO_2$ is reduced, the main stimulus for respiration is removed and it may be difficult to wean the patient from the ventilator at the end of anaesthesia. This scenario can become confusing as IPPV is often used during complicated anaesthetic procedures and it may be difficult to tell whether the absence of respiratory drive is due to hypocapnia, relative overdose of drugs such as potent opioids which cause respiratory depression, or residual neuromuscular blockade. In these situations, it is essential to take time to ascertain and treat the cause of respiratory depression before the patient is allowed to recover from anaesthesia.

Effects on anaesthesia

Intermittent positive pressure ventilation will often increase the rate at which inhalation agents are absorbed from the respiratory gases. This means that when a patient is ventilated they will often require less anaesthetic than when breathing spontaneously. The use of IPPV will also allow drugs that normally cause severe respiratory depression such as potent opioids and neuromuscular blocking agents to be used as part of a balanced anaesthetic protocol. This will reduce the amount of inhalation agent or other anaesthetic required and so will reduce the side effects of these agents.

Weaning from the ventilator

The regular rhythm of IPPV is in itself soporific and can contribute to respiratory depression. For this reason, it is often useful to vary the pattern of respiration when weaning the patient from the ventilator. Patients can be transferred from the ventilator to a normal circuit suitable for IPPV for weaning. This will allow the anaesthetist to give two or three rapid breaths followed by a respiratory pause. The pause allows a small degree of hypercapnia to develop that acts as a stimulant to respiration; the rapid breaths break the rhythm of the ventilator and so make the patient more likely to take over breathing spontaneously. When the patient is breathing normally, the anaesthetist must be absolutely sure that respiratory function has returned to normal before the patient is allowed to recover from anaesthesia. The best way to ensure this is to monitor end-tidal carbon dioxide for a few minutes to ensure that the patient does not become hypercapnic. Alternatively, a pulse oximeter can be used to monitor SaO_2 aq but in this case monitoring should be continued when the patient is breathing room air to ensure that they do not become hypoxaemic as the inspired oxygen tension falls.

Beneficial or detrimental?

As outlined above, IPPV is a complicated technique and should be carried out with care. It is undoubtedly of great benefit to many patients (see box), but can have significant complications (see Table 4.2), which can be avoided with careful monitoring, attention to detail and a good understanding of the underlying physiological processes.

INDICATIONS FOR IPPV

To facilitate balanced anaesthesia

Apnoea

Hypoventilation causing hypercarbia and/or hypoxia

Decrease patient's work of breathing, e.g. disease, elderly patients

Respiratory arrest

Cardio-respiratory arrest

Thoracotomy

Laparotomy for diaphragmatic hernia repair

Delicate surgical procedures where a regular respiratory pattern is preferred, e.g. portosystemic shunt dissection

Table 4.2 Complications of intermittent positive pressure ventilation.

Complications	Aetiology	Comment
Reduce venous return and cardiac output	Increased intrathoracic pressure	These effects can be minimised by having a shorter inspiratory time : expiratory time ratio. A ratio of 1 : 2 is generally used with an inspiratory time of 1.5–2 sec
Respiratory alkalosis	Overventilation reduces CO_2	A respiratory rate of 8–12 breaths per minute is usually used
Pneumothorax, pneumomediastinum, air embolism, emphysema	Excessive lung inflation causes alveolar septal rupture	Inflation pressure and tidal volume should be the minimum required to maintain oxygenation and normocapnia. Inflation pressure should not exceed 18–20 cmH_2O. Pre-existing pulmonary disease, e.g. bullous emphysema and recent pulmonary trauma, can predispose to this problem
Re-expansion pulmonary oedema	Excessive lung inflation following a period of atelectasis	Inflation pressure should not exceed 18–20 cmH_2O. This is particularly a problem following prolonged periods of lung collapse, e.g. in chronic diaphragmatic rupture
Monitoring more difficult	If neuromuscular blocking agent (NBA) used	NMB drugs will abolish many of the cranial nerve reflexes used to assess anaesthetic depth
Additional equipment required	Mechanical ventilators	
Additional person required	Manual ventilation	
Increased intracranial pressure (ICP)		This occurs due to increased venous resistance. However, IPPV can also decrease $PaCO_2$ that conversely will decrease ICP

Minute volume dividers and bag-in-bottle ventilators

Ventilators used in anaesthesia are divided into two main classes. Although they both provide IPPV, they function in ways that have very different consequences for the control of respiratory function.

Minute volume dividers take the fresh gas flow from the anaesthetic machine and divide it into breaths that they deliver to the patient in a regular pattern. The ventilator controls can adjust each individual breath in a variety of ways, but the respiratory rate is controlled indirectly by the rotameters on the anaesthetic machine. When the ventilator has stored enough gas for a breath, it delivers that breath to the patient and then begins to store the next breath. At the end of inspiration the breath is channelled from the patient with no possibility of rebreathing. Minute volume dividers comprise the entire connection between the anaesthetic machine and the patient; they do not work with a separate breathing system. Examples of this kind of ventilator include the Manley and the Flomasta.

As the name suggests, bag-in-bottle ventilators (also known as bag squeezers) work in a similar manner to manually compressing the reservoir bag of a breathing system. They do not form the entire connection between patient and anaesthetic machine, but are attached to a conventional breathing system. Care should always be taken that these ventilators are used with a system which is suitable for IPPV such as a Mapleson DEF or a circle, they should never be used in conjunction with a Mapleson A breathing system. When a bag-in-bottle system is used, it takes on the functional appearance of the system to which it is connected. This may or may not allow rebreathing and may or may not allow carbon dioxide tensions to be altered by changing the ventilator settings or the fresh gas flow through the system. For example, if such a ventilator is used as part of a circle system, carbon dioxide removal will be by soda lime absorption. Altering the fresh gas flow at the rotameters will have no effect, but altering the respiratory rate or tidal volume may have a dramatic effect. Conversely, if the ventilator is used with a Mapleson D system, carbon dioxide removal will be by dilution with fresh gas. Here altering the respiratory rate and tidal volume may have little or no effect on carbon dioxide, but altering the fresh gas flow may have a dramatic effect. The behaviour of the various anaesthetic systems during IPPV is discussed in chapter 5. Examples of bag-in-bottle ventilators include the Carden Ventmasta and the Vetronics Small Animal Ventilator.

Respiratory cycling of ventilators

Respiration is divided into inspiratory and expiratory phases. One of the most important distinctions in ventilator function is what triggers the ventilator to start and finish the inspiratory phase. Ventilators may be cycled by volume (inspiration continues until a set tidal volume is delivered), pressure (inspiration continues until a set airway pressure is reached) or time (inspiration continues for a set time).

Ventilators that are cycled in different ways can give very different responses to alterations in respiratory variables. The following examples are two situations where differently cycled ventilators respond in different ways.

A volume-limited ventilator will deliver the same tidal volume under all circumstances whereas a pressure-limited ventilator will deliver the same peak inspiratory pressure under all circumstances. This means that a volume-limited ventilator must be adjusted for every new patient (tidal volume depends on weight), but a pressure-limited ventilator can be connected to patients of varying weight without adjustment (peak inspiratory pressure is similar regardless of weight).

Once set up a volume-limited ventilator will deliver the same tidal volume whatever the circumstances and will give little warning of disconnection or bronchospasm. A pressure-limited ventilator will not end inspiration if the patient becomes disconnected, as the airway pressure will not increase to the preset limit. In the case of bronchospasm, the limit will be reached almost immediately and the inspiratory period will be noticeably short. These alterations may alert the anaesthetist to changes in respiratory function.

VENTILATOR CYCLE TYPE
Pressure cycled: Gas supplied to pre-set pressure, e.g. 18–20 cmH$_2$O
Volume cycled: Tidal volume selected (15–20 ml/kg)
Time cycled: Duration of inspiration selected, e.g. 1.5–2 sec

---

PHYSICAL PRINCIPLES

1 The three perfect gas laws

The perfect gas laws describe how gases behave under conditions of changing temperature, pressure and volume. They can be combined into the following equation:

$$\frac{P_1 V_1}{T_1} = \frac{P_2 V_2}{T_2}$$

where P_1, V_1 and T_1 are the pressure, volume and temperature of the gas before a change and P_2, V_2 and T_2 are its temperature, volume and pressure after the change.

This equation can best be understood if one of the three variables is kept constant; thus if the temperature of a gas is kept constant and its volume changes (by compressing it into a cylinder, for example), then the pressure will rise. In practice, it is unusual for one of the variables to remain constant. If a gas is compressed, then both its volume will reduce and its temperature increase (a bicycle pump will get hot when it is used to inflate a tyre).

2 Critical temperature in a gas

Elements can exist in three states: solid, liquid and gaseous. The phase in which an element exists will depend upon the prevailing conditions of temperature and pressure. The critical temperature is the temperature above which a given element can only exist in the gaseous phase no matter how high the pressure. For example, the critical temperature of nitrous oxide is 37°C. This means that it can (and does) become a liquid at room temperature if it is compressed to a high enough pressure. In contrast, the critical temperature of oxygen is –128°C.

This means that it can never become a liquid at room temperature no matter how much it is compressed.

3 Pressure, force and area

The relationship between pressure (P), area (A) and force (F) is:

$$P = \frac{F}{A}$$

A reducing valve makes use of this relationship by allowing a valve to be opened in the high-pressure chamber by atmospheric pressure plus the force exerted by a spring. This is achieved by making the valve opening into the high-pressure chamber very small (Fig. 4.3). The force exerted on the valve by the high-pressure gases is small (a high pressure multiplied by a very small area) in comparison to the forces exerted by the regulated pressure gas (a moderate pressure multiplied by a large area), atmospheric air (a lower pressure multiplied by the same large area) and the spring. At equilibrium, the force due to the regulated pressure will equal and oppose the force due to atmospheric pressure and the spring. The pressure in the high-pressure chamber will have almost no effect on this equilibrium. In practice, the valve is always more or less at equilibrium and the pressure of the gas that comes out of the low-pressure side is constant over a range of flows and cylinder pressures.

4 Flow of fluids

Fluid flow (liquids and gases are both fluid) can be laminar or turbulent. In laminar flow, all the molecules move in the direction of bulk flow in an orderly fashion. In turbulent flow, the molecules swirl in all directions in addition to the direction of bulk flow. Most flow in an anaesthetic machine is laminar for most of the time.

During laminar flow (in a circular tube to keep the equation simple!), the Hagen-Poiseuille equation applies:

$$\dot{Q} = \frac{\pi P d^4}{128 \eta l}$$

where $\dot{Q}$ is flow, P is pressure drop along the tube, d is the diameter of the tube, l is the length of the tube and η is the viscosity of the fluid.

5 Variable orifice devices

The force exerted on an object in the path of a given flow can be estimated by substituting 'force divided by area' for pressure (area is the area of the object presented to the flow) into the Hagen-Poiseuille equation and rearranging it.

In the real world, other things such as the density of the fluid, the shape of the object and the coefficient of friction get in the way, but the substitution will do to demonstrate that the force increases as the area decreases. A variable orifice device makes use of this by either adjusting the flow of fluid by altering the area (needle valve) or measuring the flow by altering the area through which it passes against a constant force (the force due to gravity on the float or ball in a rotameter).

The force exerted on the bobbin at a particular height up the column will depend on both the density and viscosity of the gas. For this reason, rotameters should only be used to measure the flow of the gas for which they were designed. In general rotameters are usually only accurate over the upper 90% of their range. A 10 l min^{-1} rotameter, for example, should not be considered accurate at flows of less than 1 l min^{-1}.

6   Vaporisation

A vapour is a substance that is a gas despite being below its boiling point. For example, on a humid day the air is full of water vapour, but water as a gas (steam) comes out of a kettle. A liquid will tend to become a vapour (evaporate) into a gas until it reaches its saturated vapour pressure. Saturated vapour pressure of a given liquid increases with temperature and is usually expressed as a partial pressure at a specified temperature. For example, the saturated vapour pressure of halothane is 32% at 20°C. A specific amount of energy is required for a substance to evaporate. This is known as the latent heat of vaporisation. This heat energy is usually removed from the surroundings of the molecules that evaporate. This means that a liquid and its container tend to get cooler as some of the liquid evaporates.

7   Specific heat capacity

The specific heat capacity of a substance is the amount of energy required to raise the temperature of 1 gram of the substance by 1°C. Substances with high specific heat capacities are good conductors of heat. In general, their temperature will be less influenced by changes around them compared to poor conductors (with low specific heat capacities). If a fluid evaporates from an expanded polystyrene cup, the temperature of the liquid in the cup will cool and little heat will be brought in from the cup. If the cup is made of metal, heat will be conducted into the evaporating liquid and it will not cool as much. Vaporisers tend to be made from substances with high specific heat capacities so that the temperature of the anaesthetic agent in the vaporiser remains stable as the agent evaporates.

8   Capillary action

The molecules of liquids are attracted to each other and to some other molecules. This means that water, for example, will tend to stick to or wet some surfaces (e.g. paper), but not others (e.g. grease). When a liquid comes into contact with a vertical surface of a wettable material it will climb up the surface until the attractive force between the surface and the liquid equals the force of gravity on the liquid that is lifted. This forms a meniscus. If the surface forms a narrow tube or series of channels such as a capillary tube or the spaces between fibres of a fabric, the liquid can climb for a considerable distance. This climbing is said to be by capillary action.

SUMMARY

The anaesthetic machine is one of the workhorses in small animal practice; used daily and essential to the practice of inhalational anaesthesia. Understanding how the individual components of the machine contribute to the overall function of the machine allows the veterinary nurse to care for and use the machine not only efficiently but also safely.

FURTHER READING

Ward, C.S. (1997) *Ward's Anaesthetic Equipment* 4th edition. WB Saunders, London.
Seymour, C. & Gleed, R. (eds) (1999) *Manual of Small Animal Anaesthesia and Analgesia*. British Small Animal Veterinary Association, Cheltenham.
Parbrook, G.D., Davis, P.D. & Parbrook, E.O. (eds) (1990) *Basic Physics and Measurement in Anaesthesia* 3rd edition. Butterworth Heinemann, Oxford.

Breathing Circuits and Airway Management

5

Craig Johnson

Anaesthetised animals are usually provided gas to breathe from an anaesthetic machine (see chapter 4). This machine allows control over the inspired concentration of gasses in the fresh gas mixture, but supplies this gas at a constant flow rate, which must be delivered to the patient in individual breaths. The anaesthetic breathing circuit is placed between the patient and the anaesthetic machine in order to achieve this.

BREATHING SYSTEMS

Breathing systems (circuits) come in various shapes and sizes, but they must all perform the same three functions: supply of oxygen to the patient; removal of carbon dioxide from the patient; and supply of inhalation and/or volatile anaesthetic agents to the patient.

Supply of oxygen to the patient

During anaesthesia it is usual to supply at least 30% inspired oxygen to the patient. Above the point at which the haemoglobin becomes fully saturated (usually less than 30% oxygen in the inspired gas), oxygen supply to the body depends on the blood flow through the lungs rather than oxygen supply to them. This means that except during rebreathing the performance of a circuit is not critical to the supply of sufficient oxygen to oxygenate the blood.

Normally the reservoir bag on patient breathing systems should be capable of holding 3–6 times the patient's tidal volume.

Removal of carbon dioxide from the patient

It is not normal for an animal to breathe carbon dioxide in fresh gas. The physiological regulation of breathing depends on the tension of dissolved carbon dioxide in arterial blood (see chapter 2). This means that the way in which a breathing system deals with the carbon dioxide that a patient breathes out is critical to its performance. Breathing systems are designed with the removal of carbon dioxide and the elimination of rebreathing of carbon dioxide in mind. The way to understand breathing systems is to understand the flow of carbon dioxide through them.

Supply of inhalation and/or volatile agent to the patient

The supply of inhalation and/or volatile agent to the patient is important as the required clinical anaesthetic concentration of these agents is usually within a narrow concentration band. When a non-rebreathing system is used at an appropriate fresh gas flow rate then the concentration of anaesthetic breathed by the patient will be the same as that delivered by the vaporiser. When a rebreathing system is used then the concentration breathed by the patient can be markedly different from the vaporiser setting (see below).

Classes of circuit

There are several different ways of classifying breathing systems. Some are anatomical and are based on how the system has been built. Some are functional and are based on how the system is being used. The anatomical classifications are useful for deciding how a system will work and in which situations it is likely to be useful. The functional classifications are useful for describing how a system is being used in a given situation. A system that falls into a single anatomical classification may be placed into different functional classes depending on how it is being used.

Anatomical classifications of systems include the overall classification in general use in the UK (open, semi-open, semi-closed, closed) and the Mapleson classification (A to F). Functional classifications include the overall classification in use in the USA (open, semi-open, semi-closed, closed) and the descriptive terms (rebreathing and non-rebreathing). When attempting to classify systems, it should be remembered that it may be confusing to rely too heavily on the classification systems, especially as some use the same terms with alternative meanings. It is more important to be able to describe a given breathing system and to understand how it works and what its limitations are. A selection from some of the more widely used classifications now follows.

UK GENERAL CLASSIFICATION (HALL AND CLARKE)

Open: The anaesthetic agent is vaporised from a swab held close to the airway. An example of this is a jamjar ether system.

Semi-open: The anaesthetic agent is vaporised from a swab held over the airway. An example of this is a Cox's mask.

Semi-closed: The patient inhales gas from an anaesthetic machine. Expiratory gas is voided to the atmosphere. An example of this is a Magill system.

Closed: The system incorporates chemical absorption of carbon dioxide. An example of this is a circle system.

US GENERAL CLASSIFICATION (DRIPPS, ECHENHOFF AND VANDAM)

Open: The patient inhales gases directly from the anaesthetic machine and exhales to the atmosphere with no rebreathing. An example of this is the E valve assembly.

Semi-open: Exhaled gases flow out of the system and also to the inspiratory limb. There is no chemical absorption of carbon dioxide. Rebreathing depends upon the fresh gas flow. An example of this is a Magill system.

Semi-closed: Part of the exhaled gas passes to the atmosphere and part mixes with the fresh gas and is rebreathed. Chemical absorption of carbon dioxide takes place. An example of this is a circle system used with higher fresh gas flows.

Closed: Here there is complete rebreathing of expired gas with carbon dioxide absorption by chemical means. An example of this is a circle system used at low fresh gas flows.

MAPLESON CLASSIFICATION (MAPLESON)

Mapleson classified the non-rebreathing systems into five categories, A to E. Mapleson F was added later to include the Jackson–Rees modification of the Ayre T-piece (Mapleson E). The most commonly used Mapleson systems in veterinary anaesthesia are the Mapleson A (Magill and Lack), the Mapleson D (modified as the Bain) and the Mapleson F (Jackson–Rees modification of the Ayre T-piece). These systems are illustrated in Figs 5.1–5.7 and will be discussed in detail below.

Non-rebreathing versus rebreathing

Table 5.1(a) and (b) compares non-rebreathing systems with rebreathing systems.

Non-rebreathing systems eliminate carbon dioxide by flushing it to a waste or exhaust system. The Mapleson systems are usually considered to be non-

Table 5.1(a) Advantages and disadvantages of non-rebreathing systems.

Advantages	Disadvantages
• Economical purchase price	• High fresh gas flows required
• Simple construction	(–cost)
• Rapid changes in concentration of inspired volatile agents possible	• Increased use of volatile agents (–cost)
• The concentration of anaesthetic breathed by the patient will be the same as that delivered by the vaporiser	• Increased potential for contamination of atmosphere by waste anaesthetic gases
• Soda lime not required	• Dry, cold gases delivered to patient
• Suitable for a large range of patients	
• Nitrous oxide may be used safely	
• Denitrogenation not necessary	
• Low resistance to breathing	

Table 5.1(b) Advantages and disadvantages of rebreathing systems.

Advantages	Disadvantages
• Economy of fresh anaesthetic gases	• Initial purchase price high
• Economy of volatile agents	• Denitrogenation required
• Warms and humidifies inspired gases	• Slow changes in concentration of inspired volatile agents in closed and low-flow systems
• Reduced contamination of atmosphere by waste anaesthetic gases	• The concentration of anaesthetic breathed by the patient will not be the same as that delivered by the vaporiser
	• Valves increase resistance to breathing
	• Soda lime is irritant to tissues
	• Soda lime canister increases resistance
	• Soda lime canister contributes to mechanical dead space
	• Nitrous oxide may only be used when FIO_2 can be monitored

rebreathing systems. It should, however, be remembered that rebreathing can occur using a Mapleson system at low fresh gas flows (refer to the use of a Bain system with IPPV, page 94). Rebreathing systems eliminate carbon dioxide by chemical absorption, allowing the same gas to be breathed by the patient on more than one occasion. To-and-fro systems and circle systems are usually considered to be rebreathing systems.

CARBON DIOXIDE REMOVAL BY SODA LIME

The rebreathing systems remove carbon dioxide from the expired gas by chemical absorption. The gas is passed through a canister containing granules of soda lime. Soda lime is made up of 90% calcium hydroxide, 5% sodium hydroxide, 1% potassium hydroxide and 4% silicate. Silicate acts as a stabiliser and stops the granules turning to powder. Barium hydroxide lime will also absorb carbon dioxide but is rarely used in the UK.

Soda lime canisters contain approximately 50% air around and within the granules. Thus the total volume of the canister should be at least double the tidal volume of the patient anaesthetised to ensure efficient absorption of carbon dioxide from expired gases. Some circle systems incorporate a switch that allows the gases within the system to bypass the soda lime canister. If this switch is in the 'off' position in fully closed or low-flow systems, carbon dioxide can accumulate to life-threatening levels.

Fresh soda lime contains 35% water by weight and opened containers of soda lime may dehydrate and lose absorptive capacity, as water is essential for the chemical reaction involved in scavenging carbon dioxide.

The soda lime reacts with the carbon dioxide in the gas as follows:

$$CO_2 + Ca(OH)_2 \Rightarrow CaCO_3 + H_2O$$
$$CO_2 + 2NaOH \Rightarrow Na_2CO_3 + H_2O$$

This reaction traps the carbon dioxide in the solid phase of the soda lime and releases not only water vapour but also heat, as the chemical reaction is exothermic. Following this reaction the granules of soda lime become hard and cannot be crushed easily. The rise in temperature may be as great as 40°C. Cold dry gases passing through soda lime canisters are thus warmed and humidified.

Soda lime is highly alkaline and caustic and irritant to tissues, especially when wet. The eyes, skin and respiratory tract are at particular risk. When refilling a soda lime canister, gloves and a mask should be worn, and the canister should be refilled over a waste bin to prevent loss of dust to the floor.

Most soda lime contains a pH indicator (e.g. ethyl violet), which shows if it is still active. Different manufacturers use different indicators. The most common are:

- White soda lime that becomes purple when spent (inactive).
- Pink soda lime that becomes white when spent.
- White soda lime that becomes blue when spent.

Unfortunately, the indicators can return to their unspent state even in spent soda lime if this is allowed to stand. For this reason, a note should be kept of when the soda lime was last changed and it should be changed prior to an anaesthetic if there is any doubt as to its freshness. In general, the soda lime within a canister should be changed when 50% of the soda lime has undergone a change in indicator colour. If double canisters placed in series are used (i.e. the gas passes first through one and then the other), the soda lime should be changed in both when the soda lime in the first (usually the top one) is exhausted.

System details
Mapleson A (Magill and Lack)

Mapleson A systems are designed to be efficient when the patient is breathing spontaneously. They become very inefficient if used with IPPV. The Magill is illustrated in Fig. 5.1 and its advantages and disadvantages are listed in Table 5.2. The Lack (Fig. 5.2 and Table 5.3) is functionally similar to the Magill and only differs in that the expiratory valve is on an extended expiratory limb, allowing it to be sited close to the anaesthetic machine rather than close to the patient. This helps to minimise drag on the endotracheal tube and facilitates head and neck surgery. Lack systems may be coaxial (tube inside tube) or parallel (Fig. 5.2). The reservoir bag is sited on the inspiratory limb of the coaxial Lack.

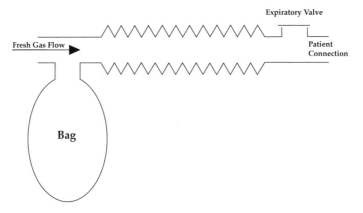

Fig 5.1 Magill breathing system.

Table 5.2 Advantages and disadvantages of Magill breathing system.

Advantages	Disadvantages
• General advantages of non-rebreathing system	• General disadvantages of non-rebreathing system
• Efficiency unaffected by breathing pattern	• Not suitable for long-term IPPV
• FGF = ≥ 1 × MV	• Valve close to patient, increasing drag and limiting access

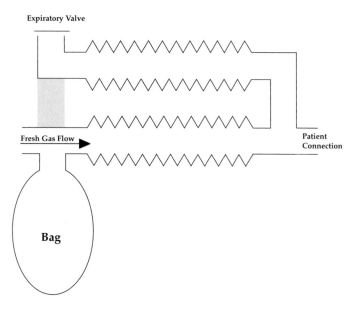

Fig 5.2 Parallel Lack breathing system.

Table 5.3 Advantages and disadvantages of Lack breathing system.

Advantages	Disadvantages
• General advantages of non-rebreathing system	• General disadvantages of non-rebreathing system
• Efficiency unaffected by breathing pattern	• Not suitable for long-term IPPV
• FGF = ≥ 1 × MV	• Disconnection of inner tube possible in coaxial system and difficult to identify
• Valve close to gas outlet, increasing access and reducing drag	• Increased bulk with parallel system

The inner tube of the coaxial Lack may become disconnected and can lead to rebreathing of expired anaesthetic gases and vapours. Unfortunately there is no easy method of checking the integrity of the inner tube connections. The parallel Lack does not have this problem but is more unwieldy because of the greater amount of tubing.

The function of Mapleson A systems under spontaneous ventilation is illustrated in Fig. 5.3 using the example of the Magill. The fresh gas flow passes from the anaesthetic machine into the inspiratory limb of the circuit and fills the breathing bag. During the inspiratory period, the patient takes gas from the inspiratory limb (Fig. 5.3A) and the bag empties. During the early part of expiration (Fig. 5.3B) gas passes back into the inspiratory limb until the bag is full. The pressure in the system then rises, causing the expiratory valve to open and gas to pass into the expiratory limb and out to the scavenge system (Fig. 5.3C). During the expiratory pause, more gas is flushed out of the system

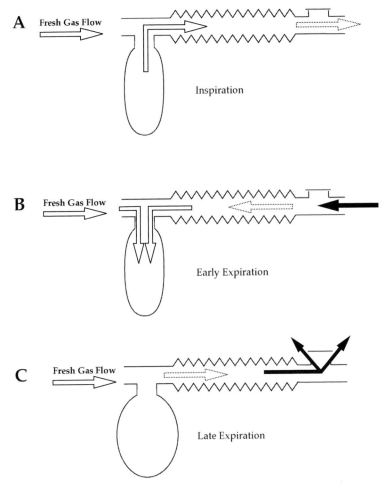

Fig 5.3 Mapleson A system during spontaneous ventilation. Gas flows through the system are illustrated in (A) inspiration; (B) early expiration; (C) late expiration. White arrows – fresh gas; black arrows – rebreathed gas containing carbon dioxide; dotted arrows – gas which has entered the anatomical dead space but has not undergone gas exchange and so does not contain carbon dioxide. See text for a full explanation.

by the constant fresh gas flow. It should be noted that the first gas to be exhaled is the gas from the upper respiratory tract that has not undergone gas exchange and contains no carbon dioxide. This gas is the last to be flushed from the system in the expiratory pause. By the beginning of the next breath all expired gas (containing carbon dioxide) will have been removed from the system and the patient will only breathe fresh gas. For this to occur the fresh gas flow used has to be equal to or greater than the patient's alveolar minute volume, although the Lack will function efficiently at lower fresh gas flow rates.

When these systems are used with IPPV, the expiratory valve must be partially closed to allow sufficient inspiratory pressure to inflate the lungs. The pressure rise in the system occurs during inspiration rather than expiration. This means that expired gas passes back into the inspiratory limb during expiration to a much greater extent than during spontaneous respiration, and also that no gas can be voided from the system during the expiratory pause. The system must be cleared of rebreathed gas between breaths by opening the expiratory valve, flushing the expired gas out of the system and closing the expiratory valve before the next breath. This is inefficient in terms of fresh gas flow and the activity required by the anaesthetist to effect proper ventilation. Consequently, these breathing systems should not be used for long-term IPPV (e.g. during thoracotomy) but are suitable for assisted ventilation (e.g. during post-induction apnoea).

Modified Mapleson D (Bain) and Mapleson F (Jackson–Rees modified Ayre T-piece)

These systems all function in a similar manner. The Bain (Fig. 5.4 and Table 5.4) is designed to be used with IPPV, but requires a very high fresh gas flow if used during spontaneous respiration in larger patients. The Bain is a coaxial system with fresh gas travelling down the inner tube and the reservoir bag situated on the expiratory (outer) limb.

Unlike the Lack the integrity of the inner tube connections may be checked prior to use:

- Attach the Bain breathing system to the fresh gas outlet of the anaesthetic machine.
- Set the oxygen flowmeter to 2–6 litres.
- Occlude the inner tube of the Bain.
- If the inner tube connections are intact the oxygen flowmeter bobbin will dip briefly.
- Immediately remove occlusion from inner tube.

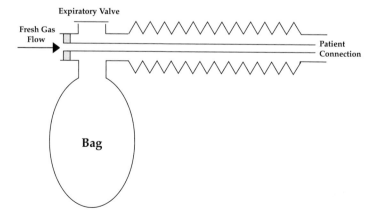

Fig 5.4 Bain breathing system.

Table 5.4 Advantages and disadvantages of Bain breathing system.

Advantages	Disadvantages
• General advantages of non-rebreathing system	• General disadvantages of non-rebreathing system
• Compact coaxial system	• Disconnection of inner tube possible in coaxial system leading to large increase in mechanical dead space
• Minimal dead space	
• Valve close to gas outlet, increasing access, reducing drag and facilitating scavenging of waste gases	• Efficiency affected by breathing pattern
• Suitable for long-term IPPV	• Highest resistance to breathing of all Mapleson systems
• Integrity of inner tube connections easy to check	• FGF = ≥ 2.5–$3 \times$ MV
• Some warming of inspired gases as they pass through the inner tube	

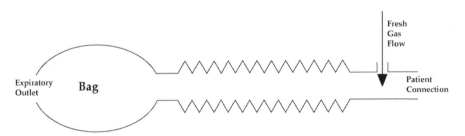

Fig 5.5 Jackson–Rees T-piece.

Table 5.5 Advantages and disadvantages of Ayre T-piece breathing system.

Advantages	Disadvantages
• General advantages of non-rebreathing system	• General disadvantages of non-rebreathing system
• Compact system	• Efficiency affected by breathing pattern
• Minimal dead space	• Difficult to scavenge waste gases efficiently
• Low resistance to breathing	
• No valves	• Reservoir bag may twist (Jackson–Rees modification)
• Suitable for long-term IPPV	• FGF = ≥ 2.5–$3 \times$ MV

The T-piece (Fig. 5.5 and Table 5.5) has no valves and so is ideal for use in very small patients. Here the high fresh gas flows in terms of multiples of minute volume are of little consequence as the total gas flow required is still small.

The function of these systems under spontaneous ventilation is illustrated in Fig. 5.6 using the T-piece as an example. During the inspiratory phase

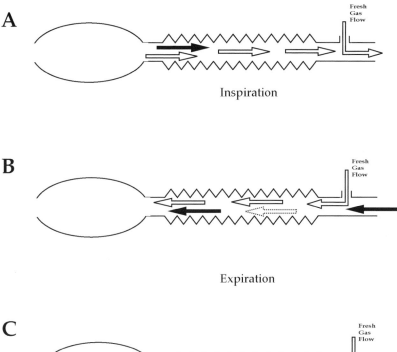

Inspiration

Expiration

Expiratory Pause

Fig 5.6 Mapleson DEF system during spontaneous ventilation. Gas flows through the system are illustrated in (A) inspiration; (B) expiration; (C) expiratory pause. White arrows – fresh gas; black arrows – rebreathed gas containing carbon dioxide; dotted arrows – gas which has entered the anatomical dead space but has not undergone gas exchange and so does not contain carbon dioxide. See text for a full explanation.

(Fig. 5.6A), fresh gas is taken from the expiratory limb of the system and directly from the fresh gas flow supplied by the anaesthetic machine. During expiration Fig. 5.6B), gas containing carbon dioxide is expired into the expiratory limb of the system and mixes with the gas from the anaesthetic machine. This means that any fresh gas provided during expiration becomes contaminated with carbon dioxide and so is wasted. During the expiratory pause (Fig. 5.6C) sufficient gas must be supplied to flush this mixed gas from the system and so ensure that the patient breathes only fresh gas at the next breath. The fresh gas flow requirement to prevent rebreathing with this system is dependent on the ratio of expiratory time to expiratory pause and inspiratory time. It is much higher than that required by the Mapleson A systems.

When used with IPPV, the Mapleson DEF systems are much more efficient. The function of these systems under IPPV is illustrated in Fig. 5.7. The expira-

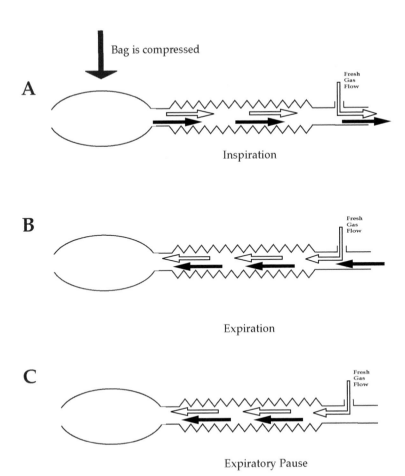

Fig 5.7 Mapleson DEF system during IPPV. Gas flows through the system are illustrated in (A) inspiration; (B) early expiration; (C) late expiration. White arrows – fresh gas; black arrows – rebreathed gas containing carbon dioxide; dotted arrows – gas which has entered the anatomical dead space but has not undergone gas exchange and so does not contain carbon dioxide. See text for a full explanation.

tory valve is set partly closed so that a suitable peak inspiratory pressure can be achieved when the bag is squeezed. Gas escapes from the system when the pressure rises during inspiration (Fig. 5.7A), but because the valve is on the expiratory limb the gas that escapes is expired gas. In effect, the act of squeezing the bag moves a column of gas from the expiratory limb of the system into the patient and back into the expiratory limb. This gas contains carbon dioxide, but it is constantly diluted by fresh gas from the anaesthetic machine that contains no carbon dioxide. Above a certain limit of alveolar ventilation, the alveolar carbon dioxide tension depends not on alveolar minute volume, but on the amount of fresh gas provided to the system. This relationship is illustrated graphically in Fig. 5.8.

The function of the Mapleson DEF systems with IPPV is useful as maintenance of normocapnia is separated from alveolar minute volume and so the

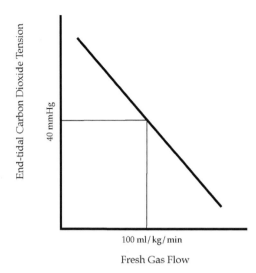

Fig 5.8 Changes in $PaCO_2$ with fresh gas flow using a Mapleson DEF system under IPPV. Graph of fresh gas flow against end-tidal carbon dioxide tension in a dog during IPPV ventilation using a Mapleson D, E or F breathing system (adapted from JFR Hird & F Carlucci (1977) The use of the coaxial circuit to control the degree of rebreathing in the anaesthetised dog. *Proc Ass Vet An G Br & Ir* **7**).

rate of ventilation and mean intrathoracic pressure can be adjusted independently of end-tidal carbon dioxide. Similarly, end-tidal carbon dioxide can be adjusted by altering fresh gas flow without affecting alveolar minute volume or ventilation rate. It is important to note that when these systems are used in this manner there is a significant amount of rebreathing. This is a good example of a system that is considered to be non-rebreathing being used with rebreathing.

To-and-fro (Water's canister)

This system (Fig. 5.9 and Table 5.6) functions in much the same way as a circle system, the details of which are described below. Compared to the circle system, it has the disadvantages of having the soda lime canister near to the patient. As well as being inconvenient this means that there is little chance for the heat created by the absorption of carbon dioxide to dissipate. In addition, soda lime dust can pass through the wire mesh and be inhaled by the patient (soda lime is extremely irritant and can damage the respiratory mucous membranes). The canister is usually horizontal and if not fully packed can allow soda lime to settle to one side, creating a low resistance pathway through which gas can travel without coming into contact with soda lime and having its carbon dioxide removed (tracking or streaming of gases) (Fig. 5.10). In normal use the soda lime nearest to the patient is used first and the absorption front moves along the canister in the direction of the rebreathing bag. This means that the dead space of the system gets progressively larger as anaesthesia proceeds; the system

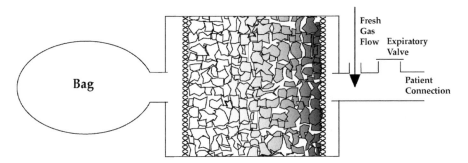

Fig 5.9 Water's canister (to and fro) breathing system.

Table 5.6 Advantages and disadvantages of to-and-fro breathing system.

Advantages	Disadvantages
• General advantages of rebreathing system	• General disadvantages of rebreathing system
	• Bulky system
	• Less efficient absorption of CO_2 by soda lime because of potential tracking of gases
	• Increasing dead space as soda lime becomes exhausted
	• Soda lime canister close to patient, increasing drag and potential for inhalation of irritant soda lime dust

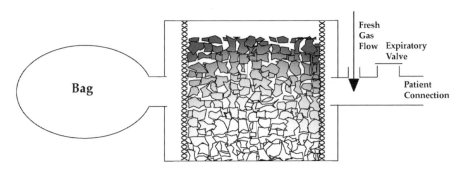

Fig 5.10 Soda lime settled to one side in poorly filled Water's canister.

should only be used with patients with a large enough tidal volume to move the majority of their alveolar gas right through the canister.

Circle

The circle system (Fig. 5.11 and Table 5.7) is the most complex in common veterinary usage. It has a soda lime canister that is away from the patient and is usually vertically orientated to prevent settling to one side. The gas is delivered to and from the patient through two tubes which can be parallel or coaxial and

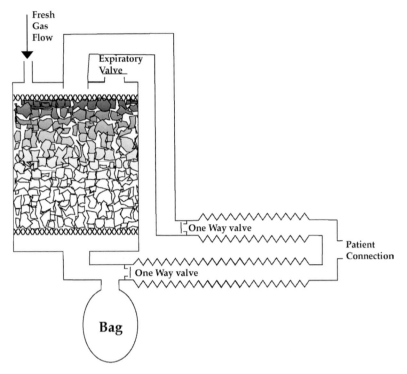

Fig 5.11 Circle breathing system.

Table 5.7 Advantages and disadvantages of circle breathing system.

Advantages	Disadvantages
• General advantages of rebreathing system	• General disadvantages of rebreathing system
• More efficient absorption of CO_2 by soda lime	
• Constant dead space	• Complex construction prone to malfunction
• Soda lime canister distant to patient reducing drag and potential for inhalation of irritant soda lime dust	• Bulky system
	• Expensive to purchase
• Suitable for IPPV	

two one-way valves are incorporated on either side of the patient which ensure that gas flows in one direction only.

The usual components of the circle system are:

- rebreathing or reservoir bag;
- soda lime canister;
- two one-way (or unidirectional) valves, e.g. Reubens valve;
- expiratory or overflow valve, e.g. Heidebrink valve;
- fresh gas inlet.

In addition, some circle systems incorporate an in-circuit vaporiser. As long as one of the one-way valves is in the inspiratory limb and the other in the expiratory limb, the components can be arranged in almost any configuration. Different arrangements will function slightly differently, but the details of this are beyond the scope of this text. The circle breathing system may be easily checked for leaks using the following procedure:

- Connect the circle breathing system to an anaesthetic machine.
- Close the expiratory valve.
- Occlude the patient port.
- Using the oxygen flush valve, fill the reservoir bag to a system pressure of 30 cmH$_2$O.
- The pressure should not fall by more than 20 cmH$_2$O in 10 sec.

The general function of a circle system is as follows. The gas passes round the system in a circle. When it is breathed in by the patient some of the oxygen is removed and replaced by carbon dioxide. If the respiratory quotient is 1 then the same amount of carbon dioxide will be added as oxygen is removed and there will be no change in the overall volume of gas in the system (this is rarely the case, but is usually assumed to be so when explaining the function of a circle system). The expiratory gas passes over the soda lime and the carbon dioxide is removed. The lost volume is replaced by gas from the fresh gas inlet. If the fresh gas flow is greater than the rate of carbon dioxide removal then gas will pass through the overflow valve and will be lost from the system. If the fresh gas flow is less than the rate of carbon dioxide removal then the rebreathing bag will empty. If the fresh gas flow is the same as the rate of carbon dioxide removal then neither of these will happen. The consequence of this is that (assuming a respiratory quotient of 1) the minimal fresh gas flow is equal to the patient's metabolic oxygen consumption, i.e. the rebreathing circle system is operating fully closed.

The **respiratory quotient** (RQ) is the ratio of the volume of carbon dioxide produced by an organism during respiration to the volume of oxygen consumed. The RQ varies with the type of organic material being metabolised. The RQ for carbohydrates is 1 and for fats 0.7.

The **metabolic oxygen requirement** of healthy conscious dogs and cats can be estimated as follows:

- Metabolic oxygen requirement = 10 ml/kg/min

Oxygen consumption will vary depending on the metabolic status of the animal, i.e. factors such as species, age, temperature, drugs administered, muscle tone and response to surgery in addition to certain diseases, e.g. hyperthyroidism can affect the metabolic oxygen requirement.

Unlike non-rebreathing systems, the concentration of inhalation agent inspired by the patient is not necessarily the same as that set on the vaporiser. This is because under almost all circumstances the patient will absorb inhalant with each breath and so will breathe out gas that contains less inhalant than that which was breathed in. This gas will mix with fresh gas from the anaesthetic machine that contains the concentration of inhalant set on the vaporiser. The inhalant concentration of the patient's next breath will depend on:

- the amount of inhalant absorbed by the patient;
- the minute volume of the patient;
- the vaporiser setting;
- the fresh gas flow.

Although the concentration of inhalation agent cannot be known (unless it is measured using an agent monitor), the use of a higher fresh gas flow will tend the inspired concentration towards that set on the vaporiser (at the expense of an increase of gas voided through the overflow valve). For this reason, a high fresh gas flow is usually used at the start of an anaesthetic and this is reduced as the rate of absorption of inhalation agent reduces later in the course of the anaesthetic, e.g. 100 ml/kg/min for 10–15 min then reduced to 10 ml/kg/min.

Room air is composed of 79% nitrogen and at the start of the anaesthetic period patients expire this gas. If the nitrogen is not removed from the circle breathing system at this time it will recirculate within the system and dilute the oxygen, anaesthetic gases and vapours. This may lead to hypoxia. High fresh gas flows used initially in circle systems, as described above, facilitate denitrogenation.

Nitrous oxide is relatively insoluble in blood compared to other inhalation agents. This means that it reaches equilibrium in the body rapidly, after which it will no longer be absorbed. Once the stage of little absorption has been reached, the partial pressure of nitrous oxide can build up in a rebreathing system. This will lead to a reduction in the inspired oxygen tension and can even lead to the patient breathing a hypoxic gas mixture despite an adequate partial pressure of oxygen being delivered by the anaesthetic machine. Thus, unless the inspired oxygen tension can be monitored using an airway gas monitor, nitrous oxide should never be used in a closed rebreathing system.

Humphrey ADE breathing system

The Humphrey ADE is a hybrid breathing system that has recently been introduced to veterinary anaesthesia. A removable soda lime canister is incorporated into the system, which allows it to be used as either a rebreathing or non-rebreathing system.

A control lever at a metal block (Humphrey block) connecting the breathing system to the fresh gas outlet controls the movement of the fresh gases entering the system. The reservoir bag is situated at the fresh gas inlet end of the circuit, and gas is conducted to and from the patient down the inspiratory and expiratory limbs of the circuit. Fresh gases pass through either the expiratory valve or the ventilator port. When the lever is 'up' the reservoir bag and the expiratory valve are used, creating a Mapleson A type circuit. When the lever is in the 'down' position the bag and valve are bypassed and the ventilator port is opened, creating a Mapleson D system for controlled ventilation. If no ventilator is attached and the port is left open the system will function like an Ayre's T-piece (Mapleson E). The reader is referred to the relevant sections of this chapter discussing the Mapleson A, D and E systems. This serves as a reminder that this hybrid circuit is a sum of its component parts rather than a circuit in its own right.

The manufacturer of the Humphrey ADE claims a number of advantages for the system, including economy and simplicity – one piece of apparatus can be used safely for patients of 100 kg or less.

In-circuit vaporisers

Some anaesthetic apparatus combines the breathing system as an integral part of the machine. These are usually based on circle systems and include the Stephens and Kommisarov anaesthetic machines. The most noticeable difference between these and conventional circle systems is the in-circuit vaporiser.

In-circuit vaporisers (see chapter 4) allow respiratory gases to come into contact with the inhalation agent each time they go round the circle system. The gas is moved through them by the patient's ventilatory efforts and so they must be of low resistance, necessitating a simple design. The idea behind in-circuit vaporisers is based on the fact that respiratory depression that is a feature of most inhalational agents. As anaesthesia lightens, the patient's minute volume increases and so more gas passes through the vaporiser. This increases the amount of anaesthetic that is introduced into the system and so will deepen anaesthesia. As anaesthesia deepens, the patient's minute volume reduces and so less gas passes through the vaporiser. This decreases the amount of anaesthetic that is introduced into the system and so will lighten anaesthesia. This variation in the amount of anaesthetic agent which is vaporised into the circuit makes these systems to some extent self-regulating, but this feature must never be relied upon and animals anaesthetised using these systems must be monitored as closely and as carefully as those anaesthetised using any other system.

Fresh gas flow requirements of anaesthetic breathing systems

Almost every textbook on anaesthesia will contain different recommendations about the minimum fresh gas flow requirements for anaesthetic breathing systems. Table 5.8 is intended as a guideline, but it is important to remember that each patient must be treated as an individual and that not all anaesthetised patients will be 'normal'. Many will have physiological and/or pathological changes that will alter their requirement for fresh gases under anaesthesia.

Table 5.8 Fresh gas flow requirements.

Mapleson classification	Common name	Rebreathing or non-rebreathing	General classification	Fresh gas flow requirement	Size of patient
A	Magill; Lack (parallel or coaxial); Mini Lack; Mini Bain	Non-rebreathing	Semi-closed	$\geq 1 \times MV$	≥ 7 kg ≤ 7 kg
D	Bain (coaxial)	Non-rebreathing	Semi-closed	$\geq 2.5{-}3 \times MV$	≥ 10 kg
E	Ayre T-piece	Non-rebreathing	Semi-closed	$\geq 2.5{-}3 \times MV$	≤ 10 kg
F	Ayre T-piece and mini Ayre T-piece (Jackson–Rees modification)	Non-rebreathing	Semi-closed	$\geq 2.5{-}3 \times MV$	≤ 10 kg
	To-and-fro	Rebreathing	Closed	100 ml/kg/min for 10–15 minutes then 10 ml/kg/min	≥ 20 kg*
	Circle	Rebreathing	Closed	100 ml/kg min^{-1} for 10–15 minutes then 10 ml/kg min^{-1}	≥ 15 kg*

*These weight recommendations are for the full-sized to-and-fro and circle systems. 'Mini' versions are available that are suitable for use in much smaller patients.

Careful monitoring of the anaesthetised patient is essential and devices such as end-tidal carbon dioxide monitors can be invaluable in establishing the correct fresh gas flow.

The patient's minute volume may be calculated as follows:

$$\text{Minute volume (MV)} = \text{Tidal volume (TV)} \times \text{Respiratory rate (RR)}$$
$$\text{Tidal volume} = 15\text{--}20 \text{ ml/kg}$$

Alternatively minute volume may be estimated as follows:

$$\text{Minute volume (MV)} = 200 \text{ ml/kg/min (range of } 150\text{--}250 \text{ ml/kg)}$$

AIRWAY MANAGEMENT

Airway management is one of the most important skills in anaesthesia. Because an anaesthetised patient is not able to protect its airway from occlusion or the aspiration of foreign material, the anaesthetist must ensure that the airway is kept clear and open at all times. General anaesthesia has the following effects that can place the airway at risk of occlusion or aspiration:

- Relaxation of the pharyngeal muscles making the tissues of the upper airway more likely to collapse inwards. This is of particular importance in animals which have loose tissue in the pharynx, e.g. bulldog.
- Relaxation of the upper and lower oesophageal sphincters, increasing the likelihood of regurgitation of gastric contents into the pharynx.
- Inability to swallow saliva. This is especially important in animals such as ruminants which produce copious saliva.
- Contamination of the upper respiratory tract with material from the surgical procedure such as blood, calculus and tooth fragments when performing a dental procedure.
- Direct occlusion of the airway with medical equipment such as an endoscope during bronchoscopy.

There are several methods of airway management that can be used in these situations. The two most commonly employed in veterinary anaesthesia are the use of a mask and the use of an endotracheal tube, both of which may be attached to any standard breathing system.

Mask anaesthesia

Because of the variability of face shapes encountered in veterinary practice, masks are not commonly used for maintenance of anaesthesia. They have their own set of disadvantages, but their advantage lies in being non-invasive with little of the potential of endotracheal tubes for iatrogenic damage.

When mask anaesthesia is employed, the anaesthetist should pay particular attention to the airway throughout the procedure. A close-fitting mask should be used and care should be taken to maintain a good seal between the mask and the face. This is important to minimise the loss of anaesthetic gases and vapours into the atmosphere and to ensure optimal delivery of the gases and vapours to the patient. The patency of the airway should be monitored by almost continual observation of the movements of the reservoir bag. Airway patency can be improved by ensuring that the tissues of the pharynx are under a degree of tension so that the pharyngeal arches are held open. Depending on the species, this can be achieved by extending the neck, protruding the mandible by gentle rostral pressure, or gently pulling the tongue out between the canine teeth (Fig. 5.12). A mask can be useful during recovery from anaesthesia following the removal of an endotracheal tube to provide supplemental oxygen.

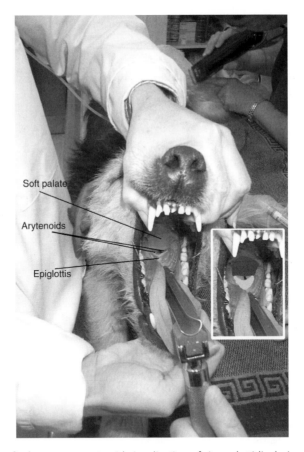

Fig 5.12 Use of a laryngoscope to aid visualisation of rima glottidis during endotracheal intubation. This picture was taken after the epiglottis was disengaged from the soft palate using the tip of the endotracheal tube. The rima glottidis (entrance to the trachea) is located caudodorsal to the epiglottis, caudoventral to the soft palate and between the two arytenoids.

Table 5.9 Advantages and disadvantages of mask anaesthesia.

Advantages	Disadvantages
• Easy to use • Useful for short procedures • Useful for small and exotic species that are not easily intubated	• Mask will tend to leak anaesthetic gases into operating room • Airway is not secure • IPPV is difficult or impossible • Mask must be held against face throughout procedure • Surgical access to mouth and face is restricted

Uses of face masks

Face masks are used (1) for pre-anaesthetic oxygenation, (2) as a method of supplementing inspired oxygen, (3) for induction and maintenance of anaesthesia. Table 5.9 lists some factors to consider.

Following induction of anaesthesia using a mask to deliver the anaesthetic gases and vapours, patients may be intubated.

There are two main types of face mask, malleable opaque black rubber and rigid transparent plastic with a rubber sealing ring. The latter are available in a wide variety of sizes. After use the mask should be cleaned and disinfected or sterilised in a similar way to endotracheal tubes (see below). Rubber masks that show signs of perishing should be discarded.

Endotracheal intubation

Endotracheal intubation involves the passage of a tube down through the mouth into the trachea (orotracheal intubation). It is routinely performed during anaesthesia. The mechanics of endotracheal intubation varies with species. In small animals it is most often performed under direct visualisation of the rima glottidis. In some animals such as the cat and rabbit there is a risk that spasm of the larynx will occur as the endotracheal tube is passed. This results in closing the vocal cords and leads to respiratory obstruction. In these animals a method of desensitising the larynx should be employed prior to placement of the tube. The most commonly used method is by the application of a spray of local anaesthetic to the vocal cords. The cords will become insensitive after about 30 sec and the endotracheal tube can then be passed safely.

There are several different models of endotracheal tube available (Fig. 5.13). The most commonly used is the Magill tube. This is a cuffed tube that is formed into the shape of an arc. It can be manufactured from rubber (reusable) or clear plastic, often with a radio-opaque strip incorporated (polyvinyl chloride – PVC) (disposable). The end is bevelled to aid placement and some tubes have an opening in the side wall a short distance from the end. This is a Murphy eye and is intended to provide an alternative passage for respiratory gases if the tube is placed such that the wall of the trachea occludes the bevel. Similar tubes are also available made of silicon rubber and are designed for repeated

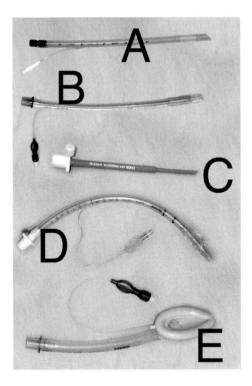

Fig 5.13 A selection of endotracheal tubes. A cuffed reusable silicon tube; B armoured tube – the wall of the tube is reinforced with a wire spiral; C Coles pattern uncuffed tube, note the narrowing of the tube at its distal end; D single-use cuffed tube; E laryngeal mask airway.

use. These are more flexible and have the advantage that they can be sterilised in an autoclave.

An alternative model is the Coles tube. This is uncuffed and has a short narrow section at the end that is placed through the rima glottidis, the remainder of the tube remaining in the mouth and pharynx. The purpose of this tube is to restrict the length of the narrowest section and so reduce the resistance to breathing. The Coles tube is uncuffed and so is rarely used in animals where regurgitation of gastric contents may be a problem.

In addition to the above, special endotracheal tubes are available for use in particular situations. These include such models as the armoured (or spiral) tube that incorporates a spiral of wire or nylon reinforcement in the wall of the tube. The spiral prevents the tube from causing respiratory obstruction by kinking when the airway is manipulated. It is especially useful for cisternal myelography where the neck must be flexed to allow placement of the spinal needle. Other endotracheal tubes that are useful in specific situations include the double-lumen tube that allows independent ventilation of the two lungs, e.g. during thoracoscopy, and moulded tubes such as the nasotracheal tube which facilitates placement *via* the wall of the pharynx to keep the mouth clear for oral surgery.

When intubating an animal it is important to select a tube of a suitable diameter. Endotracheal tubes are supplied in sizes that relate to the internal diameter. Commonly used tubes for small animals range from 3.5 mm in very small cats up to 16 mm in giant dogs. Endotracheal tubes for large animals are supplied with diameters of up to 40 mm. Tubes of 25 mm and 30 mm are commonly used in adult horses. In small exotic animals intravenous cannulae can be adapted for use as endotracheal tubes.

The selection of a suitably sized tube for an individual patient depends on experience. There is considerable variation in the diameter of the trachea in different breeds of animal. Some patients also present with conditions such as tracheal hypoplasia that results in a much narrower trachea than normal. To ensure that a suitable tube is always to hand it is good practice to place two or three tubes on the anaesthetic machine before inducing anaesthesia. There should be a tube of the estimated size together with progressively smaller sizes in case the trachea is smaller than expected. Endotracheal tubes should always be checked prior to use to ensure that the airway cuff is working properly and that the tube is clean and patent.

The most commonly used endotracheal tubes have an airway cuff. This is connected to a pilot tube and balloon that allows inflation of the cuff once the tube is placed. Cuffed tubes provide a complete seal between the airway and the breathing system and, when correctly placed, ensure that there can be no aspiration of foreign material. The complete sealing of the airway also prevents the contamination of the operating theatre with anaesthetic gases and allows IPPV to be performed efficiently. Airway cuffs are generally high-volume low-pressure cuffs designed to distribute the pressure applied to the tracheal mucosa by the cuff over a large area of the tracheal wall.

Cuffed tubes have the disadvantage that the pilot tube takes up some space in the trachea and so means that a slightly smaller diameter tube must be used. This can be problematic in very small animals such as cats, as a reduction in the diameter of a small tube will dramatically increase its resistance (resistance of a tube is inversely proportional to the fourth power of its diameter) and so increase the work of breathing. Fortunately in these very small animals the tube will leave a very narrow space between the trachea and the outside wall of the tube. This will result in a high resistance to gas leaking round the tube and means that an uncuffed tube can usually be used without problem.

Table 5.10 summarises the advantages and disadvantages of endotracheal intubation.

When endotracheal tubes are used on more than one occasion, they must be cleaned carefully after each use. Cleaning will prevent the transmission of infectious diseases between patients and also reduce the chance of occlusion due to the build-up of debris and secretions within the tube. Potentially irritant substances such as hibitane should be avoided, as residues on the tube can cause inflammation and swelling of the tracheal mucosa, which can lead to respiratory obstruction in extreme cases. Endoscope cleaning fluid containing

Table 5.10 Advantages and disadvantages of endotracheal intubation.

Advantages	Disadvantages
• Provides an airway that is secure against the inhalation of vomitus or other material that may get into the pharynx during anaesthesia	• Intubation may damage airway structures (less likely if tube is lubricated)
• Prevents respiratory obstruction by the pharyngeal tissues	• Airway cuff may damage tracheal mucosa
• Prevents the escape of anaesthetic gases into the operating room (COSHH)	• Kinking or blockage of tube will result in complete respiratory obstruction
• Allows IPPV to be performed	• Misplacement of tube (in bronchus or oesophagus) may endanger patient
• Frees personnel from holding mask in place	• Use of incorrect tube may increase resistance to breathing
• Allows easier access to face and mouth for surgeon	
• Reduces mechanical dead space	

peracetic acid or disinfectants based on sodium hypochlorite are suitable. The endotracheal tube should be cleaned and rinsed thoroughly before disinfection to remove organic debris, and rinsed and air-dried after disinfection before further use. It is especially important to inspect the inside of the tube to ensure that no residues are building up which may occlude the tube or become dislodged and inhaled during anaesthesia. Endotracheal tubes may be sterilised by cold chemical sterilisation.

EQUIPMENT LIST FOR ENDOTRACHEAL INTUBATION
Selection of endotracheal tubes:
- Rubber tubes (check for signs of cracking which may cause leakage or tracheal trauma). Oil-based lubricants should not be used with these tubes.
- Polyvinyl chloride (PVC) tubes (check flexibility: these tubes can become stiff and this can increase tracheal trauma).
- Silicone-coated PVC tubes.
- Ensure appropriate 15 mm connector is attached to reduce risk of disconnection of connector from tube.
- Check for evidence of organic debris such as dried saliva or blood.
- Check patency of lumen.
- Check pilot balloon and airway cuff integrity and volume. Ensure no distortion of the airway cuff when inflated.
- Method of occluding pilot tube and balloon. Newer PVC endotracheal tubes have spring-loaded one-way valves preventing deflation of the pilot balloon.

(Continued)

Tube tie, e.g. white open-weave bandage.

Airway cuff inflator: Syringe. Mitchell's cuff inflator.

Mouth gag.

Laryngoscope: Select appropriate blade size and shape for animal. Check that batteries are charged and light is functioning.

Lubricant: Sterile water-soluble lubricant to reduce friction between tube and mucosa. Single-use sachets are available. Water-soluble lubricant containing lignocaine can be used.

Local anaesthetic spray: This is essential for cats.

Assistant.

Laryngeal mask airway

The laryngeal mask airway (LMA) was developed in human anaesthesia as an alternative to the mask or endotracheal tube. This device consists of a tube which ends in a shaped, inflatable airway cuff. The LMA is placed into the pharynx and the cuff is inflated. The aim is to secure the airway from the risk of aspiration without entering the larynx with the attendant risk and stimulation of this manoeuvre.

There has recently been interest in the LMA for veterinary anaesthesia. The shape of the airway cuff means that it will only be useful in certain species, but it may provide a useful alternative to endotracheal intubation in animals which have sensitive larynges or are difficult to intubate, such as cats or rabbits.

Difficult intubation

It is often said that patients are never killed by failure to intubate them, but often by persistent efforts at intubation in the face of regurgitation or hypoxaemia. Some animals are difficult to intubate, but the risk of harming a patient by failure can be minimised by formulating a protocol for failed intubation in advance of the situation arising. Potentially difficult intubations can usually be spotted at pre-anaesthetic clinical examination, where any of the following may increase the index of suspicion:

- species, e.g. rabbit, guinea pig
- breed, e.g. bulldog
- previous or current facial or neck trauma
- stertor
- swellings or masses in pharyngeal area
- inability to open mouth.

In these cases careful preparation should be made prior to the induction of anaesthesia and the equipment for several alternative techniques of intubation should be at hand. The following is an example of a difficult intubation drill.

The inclusion and order of different techniques will vary according to the experience and preferences of the anaesthetist, the equipment available and the reason that difficult intubation is thought likely:

Failed intubation drill
(1) Direct intubation;
(2) Laryngoscopic assistance;
(3) Call for help;
(4) Guidewire intubation;
(5) Endoscopic intubation;
(6) Allow to regain consciousness (oxygen by mask);
(7) Reschedule with appropriate planning, e.g. elective tracheostomy.

Aborting the anaesthetic procedure and allowing the patient to regain consciousness represents a positive step in the management of the patient. It is better to abandon anaesthesia so that the information gained by the attempts to intubate (details of pharyngeal anatomy, and so on) can be used to formulate an alternative plan without the pressure of an anaesthetised patient. It is better to be able to intubate the patient quickly at the second anaesthetic than to continue protracted attempts at intubation as the patient becomes hypoxaemic.

Techniques of intubation
There are a number of different methods of tracheal intubation available: direct orotracheal intubation; laryngoscopy; guidewire intubation; endoscopic intubation; retrograde intubation; pharyngeal intubation; nasotracheal intubation; and tracheal intubation (via an elective tracheotomy using a cuffed tracheotomy tube).

Direct intubation
An orotracheal (endotracheal) tube of a suitable diameter is selected and cut to an appropriate length. If the tube is held against the animal with the circuit end level with the tip of the nose, the far end of the tube should reach about three-quarters of the way down the neck so that the airway cuff will be well past the larynx, but the end of the tube will not pass as far as the thoracic trachea. This minimises mechanical dead space. After induction of anaesthesia, the patient is placed in either sternal or lateral recumbency. The mouth is opened either by an assistant or with the aid of a gag. Some veterinary surgeons and nurses prefer to hold the mouth open themselves. The lubricated endotracheal tube is passed between the epiglottis and the soft palate. This may require the epiglottis to be disengaged from the soft palate using the tip of the tube. The tube is passed ventral to and between the arytenoid cartilages of the larynx and advanced into the trachea. Care should be taken as the tube is advanced into the trachea, as the narrowest part of the tracheal lumen is usually at the level of the cricoid cartilage a few centimetres past the rima glottidis. If the tube jams at this level

it should be removed and intubation repeated with a smaller tube. Under no circumstances should the passage of the tube be forced.

Once placed, the tube is secured in place and the airway cuff inflated. It is important to secure the tube prior to inflating the cuff as the inflated cuff may damage the tracheal mucosa if it is allowed to slide up and down. The tube should be tied at the breathing system connector by a method that does not allow it to move and so apply traction to the trachea through the inflated cuff. The tube can be tied to the upper or lower jaw, tied behind the occipital process or secured with an adhesive dressing, depending on the patient and procedure to be undertaken.

Correct placement of the endotracheal tube within the tracheal lumen may be checked by attaching the patient to the selected breathing system, closing the expiratory valve and squeezing the reservoir bag while checking for movement of the chest wall. In a similar way the endotracheal tube airway cuff can be gently inflated while the reservoir bag is squeezed (to a maximum pressure of 20 cmH$_2$O). The smallest volume of air that prevents an audible leak of gas around the endotracheal tube should be used to inflate the cuff. Overinflation of the endotracheal tube cuff can cause tracheal haemorrhage, tracheitis, tracheal mucosal ulceration and tracheal fibrosis or stricture formation. In addition, overinflation of the airway cuff in silicone rubber tubes can cause compression of the lumen of the endotracheal tube, and furthermore it has been suggested that diffusion of nitrous oxide into the cuff can compound this effect.

During prolonged periods of anaesthesia the endotracheal tube cuff can be deflated periodically (e.g. every 90–120 min), moved slightly and the cuff reinflated. This may minimise the effects of constant pressure applied to a limited area of tracheal mucosa.

Laryngoscopy

A laryngoscope combines a means of retracting the tongue and other soft tissues of the mouth and pharynx with a light that is directed at the rima glottidis. Whilst a laryngoscope is not required for the routine intubation of the majority of veterinary species (with the possible exceptions of pigs, sheep and goats) it can be very useful when intubating moderately difficult airways. A variety of blades are available, but the straight blades such as the Miller are the most useful in veterinary patients. A blade of suitable length for the patient is connected to the handle and is advanced along the ventral surface of the oral cavity until the tip lies in the vallecula ventral to the epiglottis. The structures of the floor of the mouth and pharynx can then be retracted ventrally, which will dramatically improve the view of the rima glottidis. Care must be taken to keep the laryngoscope blade parallel to the floor of the mouth rather than hinging it towards the upper incisors as that will restrict the view and place the light in the wrong place. Although a laryngoscope is not required for routine intubations, it is a good idea to use one from time to time so that its use is familiar when it is required for a difficult airway.

Guidewire intubation

In some circumstances an endotracheal tube cannot be advanced into the trachea directly. If a narrow tube or wire such as a stomach tube or catheter guide can be placed into the trachea then the tube can be threaded over this guide. This can be useful where the pharynx is narrow or obscured by a mass and there is not room for the laryngoscope blade and the endotracheal tube. A well-lubricated tube can be advanced over a guidewire with a rotating motion. This will tend to part the tissues as the tube advances, whilst ensuring that the tube can only go into the trachea as it must follow the guide. It is important to ensure that the guide is long enough to hold at the tip before the endotracheal tube enters the mouth, otherwise the guide can be carried down into the respiratory tree by the endotracheal tube and can be difficult to retrieve.

Endoscopic intubation

An endotracheal tube is threaded over an endoscope, and this is then inserted into the trachea. Once the endoscope is in place, the tube is advanced in the same manner as when using a guidewire. Either a flexible or a rigid endoscope can be suitable for this procedure, depending on the size of the patient and the structure of its upper airway.

Retrograde intubation

A sterile large gauge hypodermic needle is introduced into the proximal trachea and a guidewire is passed through the needle and directly rostrally to pass out of the trachea through the larynx and into the mouth. The endotracheal tube is threaded over the guidewire and passed through the larynx into the trachea. The needle and wire are removed. It is important that the cuff of the tube is located distal to the puncture site to limit the development of subcutaneous emphysema, pneumomediastinum and pneumothorax.

This technique may be useful in animals with pharyngeal masses.

SUMMARY

Veterinary nurses must be familiar with the more common techniques used for airway management in dogs and cats because control of the patient airway is a crucial component of anaesthetic patient management.

Breathing systems are designed to deliver both oxygen and anaesthetic gases and vapours to patients, and to remove excess carbon dioxide from the breathing system. However, the key to understanding how individual breathing systems work is to understand how the breathing system deals with carbon dioxide rather how it handles other gases and vapours. There are many different breathing systems available to the veterinary anaesthetist, and care should be taken to select an appropriate system for each individual patient rather than adopting a recipe-book approach.

REFERENCES AND FURTHER READING

Ward, C.S. (1997) *Ward's Anaesthetic Equipment*, 4th edition. WB Saunders, London.

Seymour, C. & Gleed, R. (1999) *Manual of Small Animal Anaesthesia and Analgesia*. British Small Animal Veterinary Association, Cheltenham.

Parbrook, G.D., Davis, P.D. & Parbrook, E.O. (1990) *Basic Physics and Measurement in Anaesthesia*, 3rd edition. Butterworth Heinemann, Oxford.

Hird, J.F.R. & Carlucci, F. (1977) The use of the coaxial circuit to control the degree of rebreathing in the anaesthetised dog. *Proc Ass Vet An GBr & Ir 7*.

Anaesthetic Drugs

6

Derek Flaherty

Veterinary nurses administer anaesthetic and analgesic drugs to patients, on a daily basis. Although this is under the guidance and instruction of a veterinary surgeon, it is essential for the nurse to have a thorough understanding of the actions and side effects of each of the agents being used, so that an abnormal response can be readily identified and appropriately treated. While safety of the anaesthetised patient and management of perioperative pain ultimately lie with the veterinary surgeon, veterinary nurses play an important role, as they are usually responsible for intra-operative monitoring, and for assessment of analgesic efficacy in the postoperative period.

A wide variety of drugs may be administered to patients as part of an anaesthetic protocol, but they can generally be subdivided into those used for premedication (or simply for sedation, if the patient is not to be anaesthetised), agents used for induction of general anaesthesia, those administered for maintenance of general anaesthesia, and those used to provide analgesia.

PREMEDICATION OR SEDATION

Premedication is widely used prior to general anaesthesia, with the agent(s) chosen affecting the whole course of events. The aims of premedication can be summarised:

(1) *To calm the patient:* This reduces stress, not only for the animal, but also for the anaesthetist. A patient struggling at induction will have high circulating levels of catecholamines (adrenaline, noradrenaline), and since several of the commonly used anaesthetic drugs sensitise the heart to the

effects of catecholamines, there is, generally, a lower incidence of cardiac arrhythmias at induction if the animal has received a tranquilliser or sedative.

> **Tranquillisers** relieve anxiety but do not cause the patient to become drowsy; **sedatives** calm the patient *and* make them sleepy. There is commonly a degree of overlap between the two drug types, (particularly depending on the dose used), and in veterinary anaesthesia, the terms are frequently used interchangeably.

(2) *To reduce the total dose of anaesthetic:* Drugs used for premedication will reduce not only the dose of induction agent but also the amount of maintenance agent required. With commonly used doses, acepromazine results in around a 33% reduction in maintenance requirements, while medetomidine leads to about a 50% (or greater) reduction.

(3) *To reduce autonomic side effects:* Parasympathetic effects, such as salivation and increased vagal tone leading to bradycardia, may be encountered under anaesthesia, and some of the premedicant drugs administered, particularly the antimuscarinics, are used to prevent these. Additionally, some agents used in premedication (particularly acepromazine) may reduce the incidence of catecholamine-induced cardiac arrhythmias.

(4) *To relieve pain:* In general, if a patient is in pain before anaesthesia (for example, having sustained a fracture), adequate calming will only be achieved if an analgesic is included as part of the premedication regimen. Even if the animal has no pain before surgery, there are good reasons to include an analgesic with premedication, since it has been shown that postoperative pain is much easier to control if analgesics are administered before the onset of the painful stimulus; this phenomenon is known as **pre-emptive analgesia** (see later).

(5) *To smooth the recovery period:* Many of the agents used for premedication will last into the recovery period, and calm animals as they regain consciousness. This is particularly important when drugs such as methohexitone or 'Saffan' are used for induction, since stormy recoveries are sometimes associated with these agents.

(6) *To reduce other side effects of anaesthesia:* Nausea and vomiting are common side effects associated with anaesthesia in humans, and although postoperative vomiting is not common in veterinary patients, it is difficult to be sure that nausea is not present. Acepromazine is a good anti-emetic drug, and will reduce the incidence of postoperative nausea and vomiting.

Drug groups commonly used for premedication include antimuscarinics, phenothiazines, alpha-2 adrenoceptor agonists, benzodiazepines and opioids.

Antimuscarinics (anticholinergics, parasympathetic antagonists; parasympatholytics, 'drying agents')

Although antimuscarinics were commonly administered as a standard part of premedication for many years, the tendency more recently has been to move towards reserving their use for specific defined situations. This has arisen because these drugs are not without side effects, and, therefore, routine administration is no longer considered tenable.

It has been suggested that antimuscarinic drugs should be included as part of premedication, to prevent salivation and decrease respiratory secretions. Although older general anaesthetic agents, such as ether, did induce these effects, this is not seen with any of the modern inhalational agents. Ketamine may increase salivation in some patients, but this is seldom problematic when it is combined with other drugs, such as α_2 adrenoceptor agonists. However, there is an argument that cats and other small patients have such narrow airways that any excess secretion may predispose to obstruction. It is argued that even the presence of an endotracheal tube does not guarantee airway patency in these patients, as secretions can accumulate at the distal end of the tube, leading to blockage. For this reason, many veterinary anaesthetists recommend that all small patients receive an antimuscarinic before general anaesthesia.

Similarly, some argue that antimuscarinics should be administered routinely to prevent vagally mediated bradycardia during general anaesthesia. However, in the majority of patients most modern inhalational agents have a tendency to induce a slight to moderate increase in heart rate. The exception to this is halothane, which may slow heart rate through an increase in vagal tone. However, significant bradycardia under halothane anaesthesia occurs in only a small percentage of patients, and it is difficult to justify the 'routine' use of antimuscarinics to prevent a complication that generally does not occur anyway.

Brachycephalic dog breeds (boxers, bulldogs, pugs, and so on) have pre-existing high vagal tone, and these animals may become bradycardic when anaesthetised. For this reason, antimuscarinics are commonly administered to these patients before anaesthesia. In addition, these breeds have small airways relative to their body size, and it has been suggested that the drying effect induced by antimuscarinics may also be beneficial.

In addition, some surgical procedures, especially surgery of the eye or larynx, are associated with increases in vagal tone, and this may cause severe bradycardia. The classical example is that of enucleation, when traction on the extra-ocular muscles may lead to dramatic slowing of the heart, or even cardiac arrest. This appears to be an uncommon situation, and it has recently been shown that the dose of anticholinergic agent required to obliterate this response is so high that it will cause dramatic side effects. Thus, it is preferable with surgical procedures of this type, to be aware that bradycardia may occur, and be ready to administer antimuscarinics if the need arises.

Adverse effects

- *Tachycardia:* If these drugs are administered to treat a bradycardic patient, the resulting tachycardia can actually be more problematic than the original low heart rate.
- *Cardiac arrhythmias:* It has been shown that the incidence of ventricular arrhythmias under anaesthesia is higher in patients who have been given antimuscarinics. In addition, atropine (but not glycopyrrolate) commonly causes an initial, short-lived **bradycardia**, prior to the onset of the expected tachycardic phase. There may also be a period of second-degree atrioventricular blockade with either of these agents. Both of these effects appear to be more common following intravenous administration.
- *Increased airway dead-space:* The antimuscarinics cause bronchodilation, and this increases anatomical dead space.
- *Pupillary dilation (mydriasis):* The pupils commonly become widely dilated following antimuscarinic administration, and this is often particularly marked in cats. This may cause some animals to panic, because vision can no longer accommodate. Pupillary dilation may also trigger acute glaucoma (increased intra-ocular pressure), in predisposed patients. Mydriasis is more common with atropine than glycopyrrolate.
- *Confusion:* Postoperative confusion is a well-recorded side effect of antimuscarinics in elderly human patients, and it is possible that a similar situation occurs in animals.
- *Dry mouth:* The dry mouth which follows antimuscarinic administration is reportedly extremely unpleasant in humans, and is likely to be similar for animals.

Two antimuscarinics are used in veterinary anaesthesia.

Atropine

By far the most commonly used antimuscarinic in anaesthesia, atropine can be administered by subcutaneous (SC), intramuscular (IM) or intravenous (IV) routes. The dose is approximately 0.02–0.04 mg/kg, although there is a wide variation in accepted dose rates. Marked overdosage results in central stimulation and seizures.

Glycopyrrolate or glycopyrronium

Although more expensive than atropine, this agent may offer some advantages. It has a longer duration of action, and, in humans, less commonly causes the marked tachycardia that sometimes results from administration of atropine, but at the same time appears equally effective in preventing vagally induced bradycardia. Whether glycopyrrolate is less likely to precipitate severe tachycardia in animals is disputed. There is less pupillary dilation with glycopyrrolate, and it has a more potent anti-sialogogue (blocking salivation) effect. A dose of 0.005–0.01 mg/kg IM or IV is usually used; however, this drug is not licensed for veterinary species. Glycopyrrolate is a quaternary ammonium compound that does not cross the blood–brain barrier; therefore, central side effects are not usually seen.

ANTIMUSCARINICS – SUMMARY

Indications

Absolute indications are limited!
Routinely in cats or small patients?
? Brachycephalic dogs
Treatment of vagal bradycardia or AV block

Side effects

Tachycardia
Cardiac arrhythmias
Pupillary dilation
Increased airway anatomical dead space

Contraindications

Pre-existing tachycardia
Glaucoma

Phenothiazines

The phenothiazines are a group of drugs that provide tranquillisation, with sedation appearing at higher doses. The only member of this group in use in veterinary anaesthesia in the UK is **acepromazine** (**ACP**), which forms the mainstay of premedication in most patients. The major beneficial effects of ACP are:

(1) *Tranquillisation and sedation:* In general, this agent provides reliable tranquillisation in quiet or nervous subjects, but the effects are much less predictable in vicious animals. There is a poor dose–response relationship in that, if low to moderate doses are ineffective, increasing the dose appears mainly to increase the duration of sedation and the incidence of side effects, without a concomitant increase in depth of sedation. Combining ACP with an opioid drug can produce much more effective and reliable sedation.

(2) *Cardiac anti-arrhythmic effects:* It has been consistently shown in experimental studies that ACP protects the heart against catecholamine-induced arrhythmias, resulting in a more stable cardiac rhythm under general anaesthesia. The precise mechanism through which this action is mediated is unclear, but may be due to a membrane-stabilising effect on the heart.

(3) *Anti-emetic effect:* The phenothiazines as a group are relatively potent anti-emetics, and are commonly used in humans to manage both postoperative nausea and vomiting (which is extremely common), and chemotherapy-induced vomiting. General anaesthesia rarely provokes frank emesis in animals, but it is not known whether veterinary patients develop nausea associated with anaesthesia and surgery.

(4) *Antihistamine activity:* ACP has a relatively weak antihistamine effect. Since a number of anaesthetic and analgesic drugs ('Saffan', morphine, pethidine) commonly cause histamine release, ACP may be useful in decreasing this to a minor extent. The antihistamine activity of ACP precludes its use for sedation in animals undergoing intradermal skin testing.

(5) *Smooth muscle spasmolytic:* This effect is probably not of great significance in the vast majority of patients, but ACP can reduce spasm associated with urethral obstruction, which may make it easier to dislodge calculi. A similar action is elicited in the gastrointestinal tract, so care should be taken when interpreting radiographic contrast studies, as ACP will increase gastrointestinal transit times.

Response to ACP varies from breed to breed. Giant breeds such as St Bernards and Great Danes are particularly sensitive, and require tiny doses. Even with these lower doses, sedation may last for a prolonged period (over 24 h, in some cases). Deep-chested breeds such as Irish setters and greyhounds are also fairly sensitive to the drug, and will usually be well sedated with moderate doses. Terrier breeds and cats, on the other hand, are relatively resistant, and higher doses of ACP are needed to obtain similar degrees of sedation.

Boxers are known to be unduly susceptible to ACP, and occasionally respond to the drug by collapsing with profound hypotension and bradycardia. The drug can be used safely in this breed if doses at the lower end of the spectrum are used and if the animal is additionally given an antimuscarinic.

ACP has negligible effects on the respiratory system, although in dyspnoeic patients the sedation produced by the drug may worsen the respiratory compromise.

Adverse effects

• *Hypotension:* The main side effect of ACP is a fall in arterial blood pressure, as a result of vasodilation induced by α_1 adrenergic blockade. The drug is generally well tolerated by healthy animals, but this effect is usually more marked in excited patients. Patients who are dehydrated or hypovolaemic can only maintain arterial blood pressure by vasoconstriction, and thus, when these animals are given ACP, they may respond by exhibiting dramatic hypotension and collapse. Therefore, the drug should be avoided in patients in this category.

• *Decreased ictal (seizure) threshold:* There is much controversy over the effects of ACP on seizure threshold. It has traditionally been taught that ACP will lower the ictal threshold, predisposing susceptible patients to fits. For this reason, ACP is contraindicated in epileptic animals or those undergoing myelography (since this procedure itself can induce seizures). However, there is little clinical evidence to support this belief unless excessive doses are used.

● *Hypothermia:* ACP may predispose patients to hypothermia, partly due to increased peripheral vasodilation allowing increased heat loss from the body, and partly due to direct effects on the hypothalamus.

Dosage
In general, the dose range for ACP in dogs is 0.01–0.05 mg/kg, by IM (preferable), SC or IV routes, with the lower doses being utilised for older patients, giant breeds and boxers, and where the IV route of administration is used. There is little point in exceeding 0.05 mg/kg, due to the poor dose–response relationship with this drug, and this author virtually never exceeds 1 mg no matter how large the dog.

Cats are more resistant to the sedative effects of ACP, and doses up to 0.1 mg/kg by IM or SC routes are usually used. Even with these higher doses, sedation is not as marked as in the dog, but the drug is still useful in smoothing recovery from anaesthesia.

ACEPROMAZINE – SUMMARY

Indications

Premedication and sedation

Side effects

Hypotension
Decreased seizure threshold
Hypothermia

Contraindications

Hypovolaemia or dehydration
? Epilepsy

Benzodiazepines
Although no members of this group are licensed for use in animals, they are used widely in veterinary anaesthesia and intensive care. The benzodiazepines bind to specific receptors within the CNS, resulting in:

(1) Anti-anxiety effects (anxiolysis)
(2) Minimal effects on cardiovascular and respiratory system

(3) Muscle relaxation
(4) Anticonvulsant effects
(5) Appetite stimulation.

Unfortunately, in healthy patients, the anxiolytic effects of benzodiazepines tend to produce a state of paradoxical excitement. This can be masked to some extent by administering these drugs in combination with an opioid, but even under these circumstances it is not unusual to see mild degrees of excitement in healthy animals. Even if sedation is not apparent, there will still be a reduction in the dose of anaesthetic induction agent, and maintenance requirements.

Sick patients, on the other hand, tend to become sedate following the use of these drugs, and excitement is rarely a problem. The benzodiazepines, therefore, are extremely useful in critically ill animals, because sedation can be achieved without the degree of cardiorespiratory depression associated with ACP or the α_2 adrenoceptor agonists. Like ACP, there is some evidence that the benzodiazepines may protect the heart against arrhythmias.

Benzodiazepines frequently cause some appetite stimulation in animals, and small IV doses are widely used in the management of anorexia in cats. The precise mechanism of this action is unclear.

Although a wide range of benzodiazepines are utilised in human anaesthesia, only two are used with any degree of frequency in animals.

Diazepam
Diazepam is the more commonly used of the two agents, and is available in two different formulations. The solution preparation of diazepam contains propylene glycol as a solubilising agent, and may be associated with thrombophlebitis, following intravenous administration. For this reason, it is preferable to use the emulsion preparation of diazepam – 'Diazemuls' (Dumex Ltd) – which is devoid of venous sequelae. Diazepam is painful when administered IM, and because it also has poor absorption from this site, it should probably be restricted to the intravenous route. A dose of 0.2–0.5 mg/kg IV is usually used.

Midazolam
Midazolam is a water-soluble benzodiazepine, with about twice the potency of diazepam, but a shorter duration of action. It does not cause thrombophlebitis, and can be administered intramuscularly. The usual dose is 0.2 mg/kg IM or IV. Because of its shorter action, midazolam is commonly used by infusion when there is a need to maintain sedation, particularly during the recovery period.

How are benzodiazepines used clinically?
Due to the potential for excitement, the benzodiazepines are infrequently used for premedication in healthy patients; their main indication being for epileptic animals or those scheduled for myelography, where some would consider

ACP contraindicated, due to its effects on seizure threshold. Even in these two groups of animals, benzodiazepines are best used in combination with an opioid, in one of two ways.

(1) The opioid chosen is administered IM, and following a suitable period to allow its effects to develop, diazepam is administered slowly IV, immediately followed by the intravenous induction agent. If too long a time gap is left between the diazepam and the induction agent (i.e. > 1 min), excitement may be seen. Although no effects should be seen from the diazepam if the induction agent closely follows it, it will still allow a reduction in the induction drug dose. The initial administration of opioid will provide little, if any, sedation in a healthy patient, so this technique may not be ideal for boisterous or vicious animals.

(2) A combination of midazolam and an opioid can be administered IM (mixed in the same syringe), and once the effects have been allowed to develop, induction can proceed as normal, using induction doses similar to those used following ACP premedication. In this author's experience, midazolam–opioid combinations in healthy patients have unpredictable results, with some developing only minimal sedation, while others will be profoundly affected. The combination is more predictable in sick animals, where reliable sedation usually ensues.

In addition to their use for premedication of poor-risk patients, the benzodiazepines can occasionally be used for induction of anaesthesia in this same group. However, it is virtually impossible to achieve this effect in animals unless they are severely depressed. The major advantage is that, because they have such minimal effects on cardiovascular and respiratory status, induction can be achieved without the depression of these systems normally associated with the more usual induction drugs. Even if a benzodiazepine is administered to a sick patient to induce anaesthesia, and it fails, there will still be a significant reduction in the dose of whatever induction agent is subsequently used, again sparing cardiorespiratory function.

The benzodiazepines, particularly midazolam, are also commonly used in combination with ketamine, to offset the muscle rigidity that occurs with the latter drug, and to improve the quality of central nervous system depression.

Diazepam and midazolam are useful drugs when dealing with restless patients during recovery from anaesthesia, and in the intensive care setting. Provided the animal's analgesic requirements are met, small doses of diazepam (0.1–0.2 mg/kg IV; up to 1 mg/kg/h) will usually calm distressed patients. Longer-term sedation can be achieved by infusion of midazolam, using a bolus of 0.2 mg/kg IV, followed by an infusion of approximately 0.2 mg/kg/h IV. Midazolam will be inactivated by calcium-containing solutions, so should be mixed in 0.9% NaCl or 5% dextrose for administration.

A specific antagonist to the benzodiazepines is available. This drug, fluma-zenil, has been used in combination with naloxone, to reverse opioid–benzo-diazepine sedation in dogs. Like the benzodiazepines themselves, flumazenil is not licensed for use in animals. It is very expensive, and unlikely to make a huge impact in the veterinary field.

BENZODIAZEPINES – SUMMARY

Indications

Muscle relaxation
Premedication or sedation (high risk patients; epileptics; prior to myelogra-phy)
Appetite stimulation

Side effects

Paradoxical excitement
Thrombophlebitis (some diazepam formulations)

Contraindications

No absolute contraindications

Alpha-2 adrenoceptor agonists

So-called because they bind to α_2 adrenergic receptors in the central and periph-eral nervous system, this group of drugs have developed into extremely useful agents for the veterinary anaesthetist. Despite having been in use in animals since the late 1960s, there has only recently been a flurry of research regarding their use in humans. Drugs of this class are potent sedative hypnotics, and also provide good analgesia. However, they have marked effects on the cardiovas-cular system and, for this reason, their administration is usually limited to healthy patients. Two drugs, xylazine and medetomidine ('Domitor', Pfizer), are currently licensed in the UK for small animals, and, in general, their actions are similar.

- *Central nervous system:* Alpha-2 adrenoceptor agonists produce dose-de-pendent sedation and hypnosis, which can become profound. Some dogs can be endotracheally intubated following medetomidine administration, so there is a fine line between sedation and narcosis with these drugs. Caution, however, needs to be exercised even in animals that appear deeply sedated, as sudden arousal, followed by a rapid return to non-responsiveness, may be observed.

- *Cardiovascular system:* Both xylazine and medetomidine produce marked peripheral vasoconstriction in dogs and cats, through stimulation of peripheral α_2 receptors. This is evidenced clinically by mucous membranes becoming paler, and in some cases, they may be almost white. This vasoconstriction leads to an initial period of hypertension following administration of these drugs, which is more pronounced when the IV route is used. The increase in blood pressure is detected by the arterial baroreceptors, which attempt to return blood pressure towards normal by reducing heart rate, and consequently, cardiac output. In addition, α_2 adrenergic agonists also induce a reduction in central sympathetic outflow, which also tends to decrease heart rate. As a consequence of these two effects, marked bradycardia commonly occurs, and as the heart rate decreases, arterial blood pressure also declines. Thus, α_2 agonists are generally described as having a 'biphasic' effect on arterial blood pressure, in that there is an initial period of hypertension, followed by a more prolonged period of hypotension. Despite the very low heart rates and reduced cardiac output, the hypotension is not usually severe and, in many cases, arterial pressure may be relatively normal. However, even in the presence of normotension, tissue perfusion is likely to be impaired due to the marked vasoconstriction that occurs. In addition, xylazine (but not medetomidine) will sensitise the heart to catecholamines, with the result that cardiac arrhythmias are not uncommon in xylazine-sedated patients.
- *Respiratory system:* In general, α_2 agonists have relatively mild depressant effects on ventilation in dogs and cats (see Fig. 6.1). Respiratory rate usually slows, and may become intermittent in nature with deep sedation, but arterial blood gas values are fairly well maintained. Cyanosis may be seen in some animals, but is thought to be related more to peripheral sludging of the blood, due to the effects of bradycardia slowing the circulation, rather than an actual reduction in blood oxygenation.
- *Reproductive system:* Drugs of this class may cause premature parturition, so their use is contraindicated in the last stages of pregnancy.

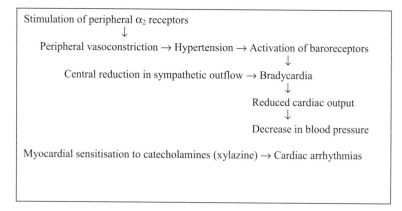

Fig. 6.1 Cardiovascular effects of α_2 agonists.

- *Urinary system:* Alpha-2 agonists exhibit a diuretic effect through two mechanisms: reduced production of antidiuretic hormone (ADH), and induction of hyperglycaemia through reduced insulin production.
- *Alimentary system:* Vomiting is not uncommon following administration of α_2 adrenergic agonists, although the incidence of emesis seems to be lower with medetomidine than with xylazine. For this reason, the drugs should be avoided in patients with mechanical obstruction of the alimentary tract. There is also a reduction in intestinal motility with these agents, making them unsuitable for use in gastrointestinal radiographic contrast studies.

Analgesic effects

It has been recognised for some time that α_2 agonist drugs provide potent visceral analgesia, and these drugs are widely used in equine practice for management of colic pain. Somatic analgesia also occurs, but appears to be less predictable.

How are the α_2 agonists used clinically?

- Sedation: Although the α_2 agonists are excellent agents for sedation in the healthy patient, their profound cardiovascular effects contraindicate their use in any sick animal. The sedation provided by these drugs is much more predictable than that of ACP. The dose range for xylazine is 1–3 mg/kg IM or IV, but this agent has largely been superseded by medetomidine in small animal practice, since the latter exhibits much greater specificity for α_2 receptors. Medetomidine can be used at 10–40 μg/kg IM, IV or SC in the dog, or up to 80 μg/kg in the cat IM, IV or SC, to produce sedation. The SC route tends to produce less predictable effects. Both xylazine and medetomidine are synergistic with opioids, so lower doses of the α_2 agonists can be used for sedation, if the two drug classes are used together.
- Premedication: The use of these drugs for premedication is more controversial. They cause a dramatic reduction in anaesthetic requirements, and because the circulation is slowed by the dramatic bradycardia, it is easy to give a second incremental dose of intravenous induction agent before the first dose has reached the brain, i.e. great care needs to be taken to avoid overdosage with other anaesthetic agents. Provided the operator is experienced in the use of α_2 agonists for premedication, and appreciates their unique effects, they are relatively safe.
- As an adjunct to ketamine: Like the benzodiazepines, the α_2 adrenoceptor agonists offset the muscle hypertonicity caused by ketamine, but supplement its central nervous system depressant effects to a greater extent.
- As a regional analgesic: In large animals (e.g. cattle, sheep and horses) the α_2 adrenoceptor agonists may be administered extradurally to provide regional analgesia.

The major advantage offered by the α_2 adrenergic agonists over other sedative drugs is the potential for complete reversal with the α_2 antagonist, atipamezole ('Antisedan', Pfizer). This solution has been formulated so that reversal of medetomidine sedation in the dog is achieved by injection of an equal volume of Antisedan to the original volume of Domitor administered while, in the cat, sedation is reversed by administration of half the volume of Antisedan to the original volume of Domitor. Despite only being licensed for reversal of medetomidine, atipamezole can also be used to antagonise xylazine.

Although α_2-mediated sedation is reversed fairly rapidly following administration of atipamezole, cardiopulmonary effects are incompletely antagonised.

ALPHA-2 ADRENERGIC AGONISTS – SUMMARY

Indications

Sedation
Premedication
? Analgesia
Concurrently with ketamine

Side effects

Profound cardiovascular effects
Milder respiratory effects
Vomiting
Diuresis
Hyperglycaemia
Premature parturition

Contraindications

Anything other than completely healthy patients

Opioids

The opioids are occasionally used in isolation for premedication (usually in 'high risk' patients), but more commonly, they are combined with ACP as part of a neuroleptanalgesic mixture. The advantage of this combination is that better sedation is achieved than with either drug alone, i.e. they are synergistic, and effects on the cardiovascular and respiratory systems are relatively mild. In addition, they offer benefits in terms of pre-emptive analgesia.

Opioid drugs may also be combined with benzodiazepines or α_2 agonists to produce sedation. A more detailed description of opioid analgesics is provided in chapter 7.

INDUCTION OF ANAESTHESIA

General anaesthesia may be induced by the use of inhalational agents, or, more commonly, by the use of injectable drugs. The latter are usually administered by the intravenous route, but some will also work when given intramuscularly ('Saffan'; ketamine). Other routes may occasionally be used (e.g. rectal, intraperitoneal, transmucosal) but, in common with all other extravenous routes, they prevent titration of the induction agent to a suitable endpoint. That is to say, with intravenous induction techniques, the drug can be given slowly to effect and administration stopped when the patient is at a suitable depth of anaesthesia for endotracheal intubation, while drugs given by other routes are administered based solely on body weight, implying that some animals will receive a relative overdose while others will be underdosed, as not all patients of a particular weight will require the same dose of anaesthetic.

Induction agents are often chosen on the basis of anticipated recovery time, effects on the cardiovascular system, and so on, but in many cases several agents may be suitable for a particular case, and personal preference and expense play a role.

Barbiturates

The barbiturates used for induction of general anaesthesia are derivatives of barbituric acid, which itself is an inert compound. However, substitution of two hydrogen atoms by organic groups produces drugs with hypnotic activity.

Thiopentone

Thiopentone is considered the 'benchmark' induction agent against which all others are measured.

Since the prepared solution is unstable, the drug is supplied as a yellow powder to be dissolved in sterile water for injection, forming a highly alkaline solution (pH > 12). It is commonly formulated to a concentration of either 2.5% or 5% for small animal use. The more dilute solution is preferable, as the drug is extremely irritant to tissues due to its high pH, and can lead to venous thrombosis when injected intravenously, and tissue sloughing if accidentally administered perivascularly. In cats and dogs < 5 kg, further dilution to 1% or 1.25% is recommended when using thiopentone, to increase the volume of solution to be injected, thereby reducing the risk of overdose. Concentrations of 10% are commonly used in large animals; these are highly irritant, and an IV catheter is mandatory.

- *Central nervous system:* Thiopentone has a rapid onset (within one arm–brain circulation time), allowing dose titration to the desired effect. Around 85% of the administered drug is carried bound to plasma albumin, and it is only the remaining 15% which exists 'free' in plasma, and is available to cross biological cell membranes and exert an effect. Similarly, thiopentone exists in both charged and uncharged forms in plasma, the ratio between the two being dictated by plasma pH. As only the uncharged form can travel across cell membranes, alterations in plasma pH can markedly influence the biological activity of thiopentone: a decrease in pH increases active drug fraction and *vice versa*. Thus, patients with acid–base abnormalities may exhibit altered sensitivity to the drug. Similarly, there will be increased active drug concentration in patients with hypoalbuminaemia, due to decreased protein binding.

- *Cardiovascular effects:* The underlying mechanisms of thiopentone's cardiovascular effects are controversial. The drug can cause hypotension (related to dose and speed of injection), probably through a reduction in myocardial contractility with a lesser contribution from peripheral vasodilation. This is partially compensated for by a baroreceptor-mediated increase in heart rate. These effects are more marked in hypovolaemic animals. In addition, thiopentone sensitises the myocardium to circulating catecholamines and commonly causes cardiac arrhythmias at induction, which are usually relatively benign in healthy patients but may take on more significance in those with cardiovascular disease. Thiopentone can cause splenic enlargement, which may be marked in some cases. While this is generally of little consequence in most patients, the drug is best avoided in animals undergoing splenectomy, or in cases of diaphragmatic rupture, where the spleen is within the thorax.
- *Respiratory effects:* Thiopentone causes dose-dependent respiratory depression, and post-induction apnoea is common. The ability to secure and protect the airway by endotracheal intubation is a prerequisite for thiopentone use.

Recovery of consciousness from thiopentone depends on redistribution from the brain to the muscles, and subsequently to adipose (fatty) tissue. As a consequence, recovery is prolonged in thin animals, with sighthounds (greyhounds, lurchers, borzois, etc.) being particularly susceptible. The drug then slowly redistributes from the fat back into the circulation over many hours, and is eventually metabolised and inactivated by the liver. Thus, the patient regains consciousness because the drug redistributes away from the brain, but there is then a prolonged hangover due to subanaesthetic doses of the drug circulating in the bloodstream, while awaiting the slow hepatic metabolism.

It has recently been suggested that sighthound breeds may also be deficient in the hepatic microsomal enzymes necessary for breakdown of thiopentone, and this may explain why these animals have much slower recoveries than other breeds which are just as deficient in body fat.

Thiopentone is licensed for induction of anaesthesia in both dogs and cats. The recommended dose is approximately 10 mg/kg IV, but this is markedly influenced by both the premedication the animal has received and its health status.

THIOPENTONE – SUMMARY

Indications

Induction of general anaesthesia

Side effects

Cardiovascular depression
Cardiac arrhythmias
Respiratory depression
Irritant to tissues
Splenic enlargement
Relatively long hangover

Contraindications

Inability to secure airway

Methohexitone
Methohexitone is approximately twice as potent as thiopentone, with a pH of approximately 11. However, it appears to be less irritant if injected perivascularly, probably because it is most often used as a less concentrated solution, usually 1%.

- *Central nervous system:* Induction of general anaesthesia with methohexitone occurs rapidly (in one arm–brain circulation time). Excitatory phenomena, such as muscle tremors and twitching, may occur at induction, particularly if the patient is underdosed.
- *Cardiovascular effects:* Methohexitone produces similar cardiovascular effects to thiopentone, although the degree of hypotension may be less, as there is generally a more marked tachycardia.
- *Respiratory effects:* Respiratory effects of methohexitone are comparable to those of thiopentone.

Methohexitone exhibits a faster recovery profile than thiopentone, due to rapid redistribution and hepatic metabolism. However, recovery may be stormy unless the patient has received adequate premedication.

Methohexitone is suitable for use in sighthounds as it is less reliant on body fat for recovery.

To a large extent, methohexitone has been superseded by propofol, and the drug has recently gone off the market in the UK.

'Saffan' (Schering Plough Animal Health)

'Saffan' is a combination of two steroids, alphaxalone and alphadolone, for-mulated in Cremophor EL (polyethoxylated castor oil), which gives it a slightly viscous texture. Its main use in veterinary practice is in cats, for intravenous induction and/or maintenance of anaesthesia, although it is also licensed for use in primates. The drug is non-irritant perivenously, and, indeed, can be given by the IM route for induction of anaesthesia. However, this entails the admin-istration of large volumes, which limits its usefulness by this route.

- *Central nervous system:* 'Saffan' provides rapid, and typically smooth, in-duction of general anaesthesia.
- *Cardiovascular effects:* 'Saffan' causes a similar degree of hypotension to thiopentone. Cardiac arrhythmias appear less common.
- *Respiratory effects:* Respiratory depression is minimal with clinical induc-tion doses of 'Saffan'.
- *Musculoskeletal effects:* 'Saffan' provides good muscle relaxation (better than the barbiturates).

Recovery from the drug occurs through redistribution as well as hepatic metab-olism. Due to rapid clearance from the body, 'Saffan' can be used by incremen-tal doses or infusion, for prolongation or maintenance of anaesthesia, without increasing recovery time. However, recovery can be stormy, even after a single induction dose, particularly if the patient is stimulated. This can be minimised by providing adequate premedication.

The drug can also be used at low infusion rates for prolonged periods of se-dation, for instance, in cats with thoracostomy tubes in place, where sedation may be required to prevent interference.

Oedema and hyperaemia of the ears and paws occur commonly in cats under 'Saffan' anaesthesia due to histamine release, but this is seldom a sig-nificant concern. However, oedema of the larynx, lungs or brain has also been reported, associated with high mortality. This appears to be an unpredictable and sporadic problem, but does negate some of the benefits of using 'Saffan' as an induction agent in cats.

'Saffan' is absolutely *contraindicated* in dogs, as Cremophor EL induces massive histamine release in this species. Nevertheless, there are numerous re-ports from Australia of the use of this drug during caesarean section in bitches, following antihistamine premedication, and anecdotal claims that the neonates are livelier than when more conventional anaesthetic techniques are utilised. However, it is difficult to justify the use of a drug with such severe side effects for general anaesthesia, particularly when safer agents are available. Indeed, even with antihistamine premedication, many dogs in the Australian studies showed evidence of bleeding from their gums – presumably an effect of hista-mine release.

'SAFFAN' – SUMMARY

Indications

Induction of general anaesthesia (cats and primates)
Prolonged sedation (cats)
? Where IV access cannot be gained

Side effects

Cardiovascular depression
(Mild) respiratory depression
Histamine release

Contraindications

Inability to secure airway
Dogs
? Cats with allergic diseases (e.g. atopy)

Propofol

Propofol belongs to a class of drugs known as the hindered phenols, and is unrelated to all other anaesthetic agents. The drug is poorly soluble in water and is supplied as an emulsion containing 10 mg propofol, 100 mg soyabean oil, 22.5 mg glycerol and 12 mg purified egg phosphatide per ml. The emulsion contains no preservative and strongly supports bacterial growth. Consequently, ampoules must be disposed of within 8 h of being opened. Multidose vials with rubber bungs are now licensed for veterinary use, but the only advantage of these over conventional ampoules is that the possibility of shards of glass entering the emulsion and subsequently being drawn up into a syringe is eliminated. Once the rubber has been penetrated, the emulsion still has to be disposed of within 8 h.

- *Central nervous effects:* Experimentally, propofol has a slightly slower onset time than thiopentone, but this is not usually particularly obvious in the clinical setting. Induction of general anaesthesia is usually smooth, although muscle twitching and tremors can occur under propofol anaesthesia, but usually diminish with time or with administration of inhalational agents. Although the drug is non-irritant with perivascular administration, pain on intravenous injection is extremely common in humans. This appears to be less problematic in animals, and occurs only rarely. Propofol appears to have both pro-convulsant and anticonvulsant effects and, although it has been suggested that the drug be avoided in epileptic patients, it has been used for the treatment of status epilepticus. Current opinion appears to be that propofol can be used safely in epileptic animals.

- *Cardiovascular effects:* The cardiovascular effects of propofol in both dogs and cats are similar to those of thiopentone; dose-related vasodilation occurs with a lesser contribution from direct myocardial depression. Unlike thiopentone, propofol does not sensitise the heart to catecholamines.
- *Respiratory effects:* The degree of respiratory depression with propofol is, again, similar to that of thiopentone, but post-induction apnoea is more common with the former. Propofol may also result in transient cyanosis at induction in a minority of patients, and this is attributed to opening up of vascular shunts within the lungs.

Propofol has a quick onset and smooth, rapid recovery, due both to redistribution and rapid metabolism. Although the latter occurs primarily in the liver, there is evidence that extrahepatic metabolism of propofol also occurs, probably in the lungs, but possibly also in the kidneys. It is useful for anaesthesia of sighthounds, since recovery is not delayed, unlike the situation with thiopentone. Due to the rapid clearance from the body, propofol is not only suitable for use as a single IV induction agent, but can also be used in dogs for maintenance of anaesthesia, either by 'top-up' injection or constant IV infusion. In addition, the drug can be delivered at subanaesthetic infusion rates to maintain sedation for prolonged periods (for instance, in dogs in intensive care). It is less suitable for maintenance of anaesthesia in cats, since the feline liver is much slower at metabolising the drug. Indeed, Heinz body formation, due to oxidative injury of red blood cells, has been reported in cats following consecutive day anaesthesia with propofol, resulting in anorexia, malaise and diarrhoea, and is due to the feline's relative inability to metabolise phenolic compounds.

Propofol is licensed for use in both dogs and cats, and has largely superseded thiopentone as the commonest induction agent in small animal practice.

The main advantage of propofol over other currently available intravenous induction agents is the rapid, smooth recovery with minimal 'hangover' – particularly useful for short procedures – while the main disadvantage is the cost and potential for contamination of the ampoule.

In no way should propofol be considered a 'safe' anaesthetic agent; in terms of its cardiovascular and respiratory effects, it is no better than many of the other agents currently available. It is certainly not the drug of choice for every sick animal!

PROPOFOL – SUMMARY

Indications

Induction of general anaesthesia
Long-term sedation in dogs

(Continued)

Side effects

Cardiovascular depression
Respiratory depression
Occasional muscle twitching or tremors
Heinz body formation (cats)
(Contamination of ampoule)

Contraindications

Inability to secure airway
Egg allergy (emulsion formulation)

Etomidate (Janssen-Cilag Ltd)

Etomidate is a carboxylated imidazole derivative used extensively in humans for anaesthesia, but which is not licensed for use in animals.

Etomidate is formulated in 35% propylene glycol and is, therefore, very hyperosmolar. As a result, it may cause pain on intravenous injection, thrombophlebitis and haemolysis. The drug is relatively expensive compared with the other commonly used induction agents.

- *Central nervous system:* Etomidate may cause retching and muscle twitching at induction, which can be minimised by prior administration of an opioid or benzodiazepine.
- *Cardiovascular effects:* The main benefit of etomidate over other intravenous induction agents is that it is *extremely cardiostable*. It has virtually no effect on cardiac output or arterial blood pressure, and this makes it very useful for high-risk patients, particularly those with cardiac disease, or those in shock.
- *Respiratory effects:* In addition, respiratory effects are minimal, causing only mild, dose-dependent respiratory depression.

Like propofol, etomidate exhibits a rapid recovery profile *via* redistribution and hepatic metabolism. The main disadvantage of etomidate is that it *inhibits adrenal steroidogenesis*, which means that the patient cannot mount an adequate 'stress response' to anaesthesia and surgery, and may develop signs of Addisonian crisis. This effect is more significant after prolonged infusions of the drug (and, for this reason, it is no longer administered in this manner), but appears to be of little concern following a single induction dose.

ETOMIDATE – SUMMARY

Indications

Induction of general anaesthesia in patients with cardiovascular compromise

Side effects

Pain on injection: thrombophlebitis
Excitatory phenomena at induction
Inhibition of cortisol production

Contraindications

Inability to secure airway
Patients unable to mount stress response (e.g. Addisonian animals)

Ketamine

Ketamine is a cyclohexamine derivative presented as a clear solution in multi-dose vials, at a concentration of 100 mg/ml. The solution has a pH of around 4, and can cause pain on injection when used by extravascular routes.

- *Central nervous system:* Ketamine produces a state of dissociative anaesthesia (superficial sleep combined with profound analgesia and amnesia), completely unlike other forms of anaesthesia. It appears to provide good somatic analgesia but poor visceral analgesia. During dissociative anaesthesia, eyelid and corneal reflexes remain intact, and the eyes remain open. Ocular lubricants should be used to prevent corneal desiccation. Ketamine stimulates the central nervous system, and may induce seizures in some patients, particularly if administered on its own. Dogs are particularly susceptible to this effect. For this reason, there is little, if any, justification for sole administration of ketamine.
- *Cardiovascular effects:* Ketamine is unique amongst anaesthetic agents in its effects on the cardiovascular system. *In vitro* it has direct negative inotropic effects, resulting in reduced myocardial contractility and cardiac output, but *in vivo* this effect is offset by concurrent stimulation of the sympathetic nervous system, usually resulting in an overall increase in cardiac output and arterial blood pressure. All other anaesthetic agents will tend to depress these physiological variables. However, the argument that ketamine may be safer for critical cases due to its cardiovascular sparing properties may be invalid, since these patients are often already exhibiting maximal sympathetic tone to maintain perfusion of vital organs, and when ketamine is administered

its direct negative inotropic effects may not be counterbalanced by a further increase in sympathetic output. This could then result in decreased cardiac output and arterial blood pressure. Ketamine appears to have minimal effects on peripheral vascular resistance. Due to the increase in arterial blood pressure, ketamine can cause elevations in intracranial pressure. This is not significant in normal patients, but may be problematic in those with intracranial pathology, e.g. brain tumours, or following head trauma.

- *Respiratory effects:* Ketamine commonly produces a characteristic respiratory pattern, termed apneustic breathing – slow inspiration, followed by a pause, followed by rapid expiration. Although this is unusual, it tends to have little effect on blood gas values, although hypoxaemia and hypercapnia may occur unpredictably in some animals. Ketamine maintains pharyngeal and laryngeal reflexes better than other anaesthetic agents, but it cannot be relied upon to provide airway protection since these reflexes are still depressed. It also increases salivation and respiratory secretions, and for this reason some authorities recommend concurrent antimuscarinic administration. This appears unnecessary when ketamine is combined with an α_2 adrenoceptor agonist.
- *Musculoskeletal effects:* Ketamine increases muscle tone and may cause rigidity if administered on its own, so is usually combined with drugs with good muscle relaxant properties (benzodiazepines; α_2 adrenoceptor agonists).

The main advantage of ketamine in small animal anaesthesia is that it can be given by either IV or IM routes, and so, is particularly useful for fractious patients, especially cats, where it may be impossible to achieve IV access. The SC route can be used but is slightly less predictable. Although 'Saffan' can also be given by the IM route, the volume required is much larger than that for ketamine, which is a major advantage of the latter. Intramuscular ketamine often provokes a pain response, however, due to the low pH of the solution. The drug is also absorbed across mucous membranes, and so can be squirted into the mouth of vicious cats, and will still work (although to a lesser extent than when administered IV or IM – an additional dose may have to be given IV or IM once the cat is manageable). However, there is little doubt that ketamine is best administered IV, as it can be titrated to effect. Prolonged recovery can occur following large doses intramuscularly.

As a highly lipid-soluble drug, ketamine provides rapid onset of anaesthesia when administered IV (although slightly slower than thiopentone or propofol). Onset is slower with IM use, but still occurs within 5–10 min.

Ketamine undergoes extensive hepatic metabolism in the dog, but is mainly excreted unchanged *via* the kidney in cats.

KETAMINE – SUMMARY

Indications

Induction of general anaesthesia
– where IV access is not possible
– ? high-risk patients
Analgesia

Side effects

Cardiovascular stimulation
CNS stimulation (seizures)
Muscle hypertonicity

Contraindications

Inability to secure airway
Raised intracranial pressure
? Arterial hypertension

Doses of injectable anaesthetic agents

Depending on the agents chosen, premedication may dramatically alter the dose of injectable anaesthetic agent required (see Table 6.1). For example, ACP will reduce the dose of thiopentone for induction of anaesthesia by about 30–50%, while medetomidine will decrease it by anything up to 90%. In addition, the state of the patient's health will also have a major bearing on the quantity of induction agent required. It has been said that: *'The dose of induction agent required is as much as the patient needs, and no more,'* i.e. anaesthetic agents should be given to effect. Thus, it is not possible to be completely prescriptive about induction doses, and the information provided in Table 6.1 should be considered only as a guideline.

Guidelines on the safe use of multidose bottles or vials in anaesthesia, and the use of glass ampoules in anaesthesia, are to be found at the end of this chapter.

MAINTENANCE OF ANAESTHESIA

In current veterinary practice, maintenance of general anaesthesia is most commonly accomplished by inhalational agents. However, there has been growing interest in the use of total intravenous anaesthesia (TIVA) in both humans and animals over the past few years, and this field is likely to develop further in the future. Consequently, both techniques will be described.

Table 6.1 Suggested drug doses for patients following 'standard premedication' with ACP ± opioid. Much lower doses will generally be required following medetomidine.

Drug	Dogs	Cats	Comments
Thiopentone	7–10 mg/kg IV	7–10 mg/kg IV	
Methohexitone	5 mg/kg IV	5 mg/kg IV	Seldom used in cats due to poor recovery
'Saffan'	Contraindicated	4–6 mg/kg IV; 12–18 mg/kg IM	
Propofol	3–4 mg/kg IV	4–6 mg/kg IV	
Etomidate	0.5–2 mg/kg IV	0.5–2 mg/kg IV	No veterinary licence
Ketamine	0.2 mg/kg diazepam + 5 mg/kg ketamine IV	0.2 mg/kg midazolam + 5–10 mg/kg ketamine IM; 80 µg/kg medetomidine + 2.5–7.5 mg/kg ketamine IM	Diazepam–ketamine combination useful for examination of laryngeal function. The two drugs can be administered in the same syringe, but should be mixed just before administration. Midazolam–ketamine can be mixed in the same syringe, and provides deep sedation in cats. Medetomidine–ketamine can be mixed in the same syringe, with potential for reversal with atipamezole (ketamine dose is so low in this combination that once medetomidine is reversed, ketamine exerts little effect). This combination is usually used without prior premedication.

Inhalational agents

Inhalational anaesthetic agents occur in one of two physical forms: liquids or gases. Volatile agents are liquids at room temperature, and require conversion in an anaesthetic vaporiser to a vapour for delivery to the patient (e.g. halothane, isoflurane). Gases can be delivered to the patient's lungs without modification by a vaporiser (e.g. nitrous oxide).

Delivery of an anaesthetic agent to the lungs is but one of a series of events that must occur before unconsciousness is achieved. In order to pass out of the lungs and reach the brain – the target site of all anaesthetic drugs – an inhalational anaesthetic must first cross the alveolar wall and the pulmonary capillary endothelium in the lungs to enter the bloodstream. The agent is then carried *via* the pulmonary circulation to the left side of the heart, from where it is distributed to all tissues of the body by arterial blood flow. The tissues of the body take up a proportion of the delivered anaesthetic agent, the amount being dependent on several factors, the most important of which is the solubility of the anaesthetic agent in that particular tissue. Upon delivery to the brain, the anaesthetic agent has to additionally cross the blood–brain barrier before a central effect (i.e. unconsciousness) can occur.

In general, passage across the alveolar pulmonary capillary membrane and the blood–brain barrier results in little delay in the agent reaching the brain, as all the commonly used inhalational anaesthetics are relatively fat-soluble (lipophilic) and cross these lipid barriers easily. The lipophilicity of each drug also correlates well with potency: the greater the lipid solubility of an inhaled anaesthetic agent, the greater the potency of the drug and the less is required to achieve an anaesthetic effect. Methoxyflurane is the most lipophilic of all the inhalational agents and is also the most potent.

More commonly, however, the potencies of different inhalational agents are described in terms of the minimum alveolar concentration (MAC). This concept describes the minimum concentration of anaesthetic agent in the alveoli, at which 50% of patients will not exhibit a gross purposeful response (movement) to a

Table 6.2 Canine minimum alveolar concentration values and blood : gas solubility coefficients for inhalational anaesthetic agents.

Inhalational agent	MAC value (%)	Blood : gas solubility coefficient
Halothane	0.87	2.5
Isoflurane	1.28	1.5
Enflurane	2.2	2.0
Methoxyflurane	0.23	15.0
Desflurane	7.2	0.42
Sevoflurane	2.36	0.68
Nitrous oxide	~200	0.47

particular surgical stimulus, usually skin incision or tail clamping (Table 6.2). It is a useful term for comparison purposes when using a new inhalational anaesthetic, but it is important to recognise that the figures relate to the concentration of agent in the alveoli, and not directly to the setting on a vaporiser. The greater the MAC value of an agent, the more is required to produce anaesthesia, and therefore, the lower its potency, i.e. MAC is inversely related to potency.

Many factors can influence the MAC value required for anaesthesia. It is reduced, for example, by premedication, concurrent delivery of nitrous oxide, hypothermia and severe hypotension. MAC also decreases with extremes of age, such that neonatal and geriatric patients require less anaesthetic, as do pregnant patients. MAC values are also species-specific, with cats generally having slightly higher values than dogs for each agent. Less commonly, MAC may be increased by hypernatraemia (high plasma sodium concentrations), hyperthermia and administration of ephedrine (a vasopressor drug, sometimes used to increase arterial blood pressure).

The rate of onset, and recovery from inhalational anaesthesia (uptake and elimination) is dependent on several factors:

(1) *Concentration of anaesthetic agent in the inspired mixture:* The greater the inspired anaesthetic concentration, the higher the concentration gradient across the alveoli, and the faster the drug will diffuse into the pulmonary blood and ultimately into the brain.

(2) *Alveolar ventilation:* As alveolar ventilation increases, more anaesthetic is delivered to the lungs, and the faster the uptake into the pulmonary capillaries will be. Thus, a patient that hyperventilates will become anaesthetised more rapidly than one who has respiratory depression.

(3) *Blood : gas solubility:* Inhalational agents that are highly soluble in blood produce a slow rise in blood concentration, or partial pressure, when they cross from the lungs into the pulmonary circulation and, consequently, a slow rise in brain concentration. This may sound illogical, as a very soluble agent could be expected to induce anaesthesia more quickly than one with very poor solubility. However, if one imagines the circulating blood to be a large sponge sitting between the alveoli (site of delivery of the anaesthetic to the blood) and the brain (site of action of the drug), it is possible to appreciate that the blood will rapidly 'soak up' very soluble agents, delaying equilibration between the alveoli and blood and prolonging the time required to exert the anaesthetic effect. For relatively insoluble agents, there is a more rapid onset of anaesthesia due to faster equilibration between the alveolar concentration and the blood concentration. The same principle is applicable to elimination of the agent from the body. Thus, for agents with high blood solubility, such as methoxyflurane, the blood acts as a reservoir, slowing the increase of partial pressure in the blood. Consequently, these agents are associated with long induction and recovery periods. In addition to promoting faster induction and recovery, low blood solubility also

facilitates more precise control of alveolar anaesthetic concentration during maintenance of anaesthesia.

Solubility of an inhalational agent in blood is described in terms of a blood : gas solubility or partition coefficient. This figure describes the proportion of agent that will dissolve in the blood compared to the portion that remains in the gaseous state, at equilibrium between the two phases. For example, the blood : gas solubility coefficient of methoxyflurane is 15; this means that 15 times as much methoxyflurane will dissolve in blood at equilibrium as will remain in the free gaseous state. In contrast, the blood : gas solubility coefficient of nitrous oxide is 0.47; therefore, this agent is very insoluble in blood, and is present in much greater amounts in the gaseous phase at equilibrium (Table 6.2).

(4) *Cardiac output:* Blood flow to the lungs is necessary for an inhaled anaesthetic to cross from the alveoli into the pulmonary capillaries. It may seem logical, therefore, that high cardiac output would facilitate uptake of anaesthetic agents. Actually, this is not the case, as high cardiac output carries the anaesthetic away from the alveoli too rapidly to allow equilibration between blood and alveolar anaesthetic concentrations. Low cardiac output, on the other hand, facilitates equilibration, and allows a faster onset of anaesthetic effect. This scenario is confirmed in the clinical setting if one attempts an inhalational induction: patients who are very excited (high cardiac output) have a prolonged time to unconsciousness, while very sick patients (low cardiac output) become anaesthetised much more rapidly.

(5) *Blood : tissue solubility:* As discussed earlier, although the brain is the target organ for anaesthetic agents, these agents are carried to all tissues of the body *via* the systemic circulation, and each tissue will absorb a proportion of the agent, dependent upon the solubility of that particular anaesthetic agent in that tissue. Thus, the blood : tissue solubility reflects the potential for a drug to be taken up by tissues, which reduces the concentration gradient between the blood and the brain and, consequently, decreases brain uptake.

Elimination of inhalation anaesthetics is by reversal of the process of uptake. Once the inspired concentration is reduced to 0%, the gradient between the alveoli and blood reverses and anaesthetic leaves the blood. This in turn reverses the blood–brain concentration gradient, anaesthetic leaves the brain and the patient begins to regain consciousness.

Although all inhalational anaesthetic agents undergo a degree of metabolism, this appears to contribute little to the speed of recovery, which is mainly dependent on similar factors to those described for uptake. However, metabolism of these agents is important in relation to patient toxicity, since this is usually associated with drug metabolites rather than the parent compound itself. Approximately 50% of inhaled methoxyflurane is metabolised, with the release of free fluoride ions, which are potentially nephrotoxic. Similarly, 20–25% of a given dose of halothane may be metabolised by hepatic microsomal enzymes. However, the hepatic metabolism of isoflurane is considerably less (< 1%). Although currently no inhalational anaesthetics are entirely eliminated from the body by exhalation, the general trend has been towards developing agents that undergo a limited degree of metabolism, to avoid toxicity to patients.

Of the factors described above, the blood : gas partition coefficient (i.e. the blood solubility) is probably the major determinant of the rate of uptake and elimination of an inhalational anaesthetic agent. Newer agents (isoflurane, sevoflurane, desflurane) have lower solubilities than older agents such as halothane and methoxyflurane, and thus, induction and recovery tend to be more rapid.

Desirable properties of an inhalational anaesthetic
Ideally, inhalational anaesthetic agents should exhibit the following characteristics:

- Easily vaporised
- Low blood : gas solubility
- MAC sufficiently low to allow delivery with high concentration of oxygen
- Non-irritant to mucous membranes
- Good analgesic
- Little effect on cardiovascular or respiratory system
- Good muscle relaxation
- Undergoes minimal or no metabolism
- Non-toxic to tissues
- Non-flammable and non-explosive
- Stable on storage
- Compatible with soda lime.

To date, no available inhalational agent fulfils all these criteria.

Halothane
Halothane is a non-flammable, non-explosive halogenated hydrocarbon, licensed for use in all domestic animal species in the UK. It is a colourless, volatile liquid at room temperature, stored in amber-coloured bottles to prevent degradation by light. In addition, halothane contains 0.01% thymol as a preservative to improve its stability. Thymol, however, accumulates within vaporisers, resulting in brown discoloration of liquid halothane, and sticking of the rotary valve. For this reason, halothane vaporisers require periodic cleaning and recalibration by the manufacturers.

Halothane is comparatively insoluble in blood, so onset of anaesthesia and adjustment of anaesthetic 'depth' is relatively fast. However, isoflurane, with a lower blood : gas solubility coefficient, provides a more rapid induction and facilitates quicker alteration of anaesthesia. In addition, recovery from isoflurane is theoretically faster than from halothane, although this is often not obvious clinically, perhaps due to other drugs, such as opioids, administered during the perioperative period.

Halothane induces dose-dependent depression of the cardiovascular system. It is a myocardial depressant, induces blockade of transmission at sympathetic ganglia and appears to have a mild effect on peripheral vasculature, causing smooth muscle to relax and vessels to dilate. Additionally, halothane sensitises the myocardium to catecholamines and, as a result, cardiac arrhythmias are not uncommon during anaesthesia with this agent. The majority of these are relatively benign, but halothane is probably best avoided in patients with pre-existing arrhythmias, or in conditions where arrhythmias are likely to occur during anaesthesia (for instance, in uncontrolled hyperthyroid cats). Halothane also slows impulse conduction through the heart and may lead to bradycardia.

Respiratory depression is dose-dependent with halothane, with many animals adopting a rapid, shallow breathing pattern.

In common with other inhalational anaesthetic agents (with the exception of nitrous oxide), halothane is a poor analgesic agent and deep levels of anaesthesia are required to obtund responses to intense surgical stimulation. Muscle relaxation is moderate with halothane, but is usually sufficient for most abdominal surgical procedures in veterinary patients.

Halothane has been associated with hepatitis in humans, but there is little evidence that a similar condition occurs in animals. However, it is usually avoided in veterinary patients with evidence of hepatic disease, not only due to the theoretical possibility of 'halothane hepatitis', but because halothane commonly reduces hepatic blood flow to a greater extent than does isoflurane.

Isoflurane

Isoflurane is a halogenated ether, licensed for use in dogs, cats and horses in the UK. Unlike halothane, it is stable in light and contains no additives. It has a higher MAC value than halothane in all species studied (i.e. is less potent), implying that a higher vaporiser setting will be required to maintain a similar depth of anaesthesia.

The low blood solubility of isoflurane indicates that uptake and elimination will be faster with this agent compared to halothane – promoting faster induction and recovery – and that the depth of anaesthesia will be easier to alter.

In common with all inhalational anaesthetic agents, isoflurane has been shown to have a direct negative inotropic effect on the myocardium, resulting in decreased contractility. Despite the consequent reduction in stroke volume, cardiac output is usually maintained, as heart rate increases to compensate. However, isoflurane causes marked peripheral vasodilation, resulting in dose-dependent arterial hypotension.

Thus, reduced blood pressure occurs with both halothane and isoflurane, but by different mechanisms: halothane reduces cardiac output through its effects on myocardial contractility and heart rate, but has relatively little effect on the peripheral vasculature, while isoflurane causes little change in cardiac output but leads to marked peripheral vasodilation.

Unlike halothane, isoflurane does not sensitise the heart to catecholamine-induced arrhythmias, and a more stable cardiac rhythm is usually observed during anaesthesia.

Isoflurane causes a dose-dependent depression of respiration which, in the absence of surgical stimulation, is greater than that induced by halothane. Under surgical conditions, some respiratory stimulation occurs, and so this side effect may be less obvious. Classically, isoflurane-anaesthetised animals breathe at slow rates but with fairly large tidal volumes.

Isoflurane appears to be a more potent muscle relaxant than halothane, and may provide improved conditions for abdominal surgical procedures. There is also some evidence that isoflurane may provide some (limited) analgesia.

Enflurane
Enflurane is a structural isomer of isoflurane with a higher blood : gas solubility. The effects of the two agents on cardiopulmonary function are similar, although enflurane causes a greater reduction in myocardial contractility. In addition, muscle twitching and seizures have been reported at deeper planes of anaesthesia with enflurane. As a consequence, this agent is seldom used in veterinary anaesthesia.

Methoxyflurane
The major advantage of methoxyflurane is analgesia at subanaesthetic concentrations. Due to the high lipid solubility of this agent, recovery tends to be slow, and thus the patient is asleep, but with adequate analgesia, for a prolonged period after anaesthesia is terminated. However, methoxyflurane is extensively metabolised, resulting in the production of free fluoride ions, which are potentially nephrotoxic. As a result, the agent has been withdrawn from the human anaesthetic market, and is no longer available.

Nitrous oxide (N_2O)
Nitrous oxide is an inorganic gas that is supplied as a liquid under pressure in cylinders. It is non-flammable and non-explosive, and is non-irritant to mucous membranes. It is a weak anaesthetic agent and cannot be used on its own to produce general anaesthesia. The predicted MAC value of nitrous oxide is around 200% in the dog, a theoretical value which is obviously impossible to achieve under normal conditions. Because of its limited potency, it is necessary to administer nitrous oxide in high concentrations to achieve any useful effect. Inspired concentrations of less than 50% are unlikely to provide any benefit to the patient, while administered concentrations should not exceed 70% to avoid delivery of a hypoxic mixture of fresh gases to the patient. Nitrous oxide is poorly soluble in blood (blood : gas coefficient 0.47) and consequently, it

undergoes rapid uptake, distribution and elimination. Nitrous oxide undergoes minimal metabolism (< 0.01%).

Due to its low blood solubility and delivery in high concentrations, nitrous oxide can promote the uptake of other, concurrently delivered, inhalational anaesthetic agents such as halothane and isoflurane. As nitrous oxide rapidly moves out of the alveoli into the pulmonary capillaries at the start of anaesthesia, the second inhalational agent becomes concentrated within a smaller lung volume, thus increasing the alveolar : pulmonary capillary concentration gradient, which enhances the rate of uptake of the second agent (**second gas effect**). Similarly, when nitrous oxide delivery is terminated at the end of anaesthesia, or during disconnection of the patient from the anaesthetic system, the gas moves rapidly from the tissues into the blood and then into the alveoli and, if the patient is breathing room air at this time, the partial pressure of oxygen in the lungs may be diluted to hypoxic levels (**diffusion hypoxia**). This is probably most significant in animals with cardiovascular or respiratory compromise. To avoid this scenario, it is recommended that animals be allowed to breathe oxygen-enriched gas (usually 100% oxygen) for 5–10 min after nitrous oxide is removed from the inspired gas.

Although poorly soluble in blood and tissues, nitrous oxide is still approximately 30 times more soluble than nitrogen, which contributes around 80% of the partial pressure of gases in tissues of animals breathing room air. Thus, when a patient is exposed to nitrous oxide, it will diffuse down its concentration gradient into any gas pocket in the body, more quickly than nitrogen can leave. Consequently, the volume of the gas pocket will expand. This may have serious consequences for animals with gaseous distension of an abdominal viscus (e.g. gastric dilatation) or pneumothorax.

Although nitrous oxide provides good analgesia in humans, it appears to be considerably less potent in this regard in animals. However, nitrous oxide has minimal effects on the cardiovascular and respiratory systems and, due to its own weak anaesthetic actions, and potential analgesic effects, it allows a reduction in the concurrently delivered, more potent, primary anaesthetic agent, whether inhalational or intravenous. Since these latter agents tend to have greater depressant effects on cardiopulmonary function, any reduction in their delivered concentration by additional administration of nitrous oxide allows an improvement in cardiovascular and respiratory performance.

Desflurane

Desflurane is a halogenated ether which has been introduced relatively recently into human anaesthetic practice. This agent has the lowest blood : gas solubility of any inhalational agent, allowing rapid alterations in anaesthetic depth and promoting fast recovery. Theoretically, it should also be extremely useful for providing rapid 'mask induction' of anaesthesia, but it causes respiratory tract irritation, which produces coughing in the conscious patient, and limits its use in this technique.

The effects of desflurane on the cardiovascular and respiratory systems are relatively similar to those of isoflurane, previously described.

Desflurane has a relatively high MAC value compared to other inhalational agents (Table 6.2), but this is not problematic as it is easily vaporised, and high concentrations are readily achieved.

The boiling point of desflurane is close to room temperature. As a result, this agent requires a special vaporiser that is electrically heated and pressurised, to ensure a constant output. Both the agent itself and the vaporiser are expensive, and this is likely to limit its use in veterinary anaesthesia.

Sevoflurane

Like desflurane and isoflurane, sevoflurane is a halogenated ether inhalational agent that is now widely used in human anaesthesia, and in veterinary anaesthesia in North America. Although its blood : gas solubility is not as low as that of desflurane, it is still significantly less than that of isoflurane, thus allowing faster alteration of anaesthetic depth and faster recovery. In addition, sevoflurane is suitable for mask induction of anaesthesia, and is widely used for this purpose in human paediatric anaesthetic practice. Recent work has confirmed that mask induction with sevoflurane produces unconsciousness significantly more rapidly than isoflurane, in cats.

The MAC value of sevoflurane is similar to that of most other inhalational agents (Table 6.2), and the agent can be delivered from a conventional vaporiser. Cardiovascular and respiratory effects are similar to those of isoflurane.

It has been demonstrated that one of the degradation products of the interaction of sevoflurane with carbon dioxide absorbents is an olefin compound known as compound A. This agent has been shown to produce renal failure in laboratory rats, but no cases have been reported to date in clinical cases. Thus, the significance of compound A production is presently unclear.

Although sevoflurane is seldom used in veterinary anaesthesia in the UK at present, it is likely that the benefits offered by its low blood : gas solubility and suitability for mask induction of anaesthesia will lead to more widespread exposure in the coming years.

Total intravenous anaesthesia (TIVA)

The concept of maintenance of general anaesthesia using only intravenous agents has developed rapidly over the past few years. Major benefits offered by this technique, when compared to inhalational agents, include improved controllability of anaesthesia, and lack of environmental contamination with waste anaesthetic gases, which may have important implications for operating room personnel. In addition, utilising a TIVA technique permits induction and maintenance of anaesthesia to become a continuum, since anaesthesia is induced with an intravenous agent that is then continued to maintain anaesthesia. This contrasts with more conventional anaesthesia, where induction is performed intravenously but the patient is then converted to an inhalational technique for maintenance. Thus, there is a 'changeover' phase where there may be inadequate anaesthesia due to dissipation of the injectable agent before the inhalational agent has achieved the necessary concentration in the brain.

Propofol has become the standard anaesthetic agent used in TIVA techniques due to rapid clearance from the body, resulting in little cumulation even after prolonged infusion. However, propofol is a poor reflex suppressant, and for major surgical procedures must be combined with a potent analgesic agent such as fentanyl. In addition, it in unsuitable for infusion in the cat, as this species is relatively slow at glucuronide conjugation, which is necessary for metabolism of the drug.

It is likely that TIVA will make a larger impact in anaesthesia in coming years, as the importance of environmental preservation becomes more pronounced.

Neuromuscular blocking drugs ('muscle relaxants')

Although most of the currently available anaesthetic agents will provide a degree of muscle relaxation, in general, most of them provide good muscle relaxation only when delivered in high concentrations. Unfortunately, these concentrations are associated with severe cardiopulmonary depression, making these agents unsuitable by themselves for situations where profound muscle relaxation is required during a surgical procedure. Two alternative groups of drugs are available to increase the degree of muscular relaxation during surgery.

Centrally acting muscle relaxants

Agents in this class provide muscle relaxation by direct effects within the central nervous system. The main drugs used in small animal anaesthesia are the benzodiazepines: diazepam and midazolam. Although these are relatively potent muscle relaxants, because of their central action they also have effects on other body systems. In addition, they cannot produce the profound degree of relaxation associated with drugs acting directly on the neuromuscular junction (NMJ).

Neuromuscular blocking drugs

Although agents such as diazepam are commonly used for their muscle relaxing effects, in general, when the term 'muscle relaxant' is used, it normally refers to drugs acting at the neuromuscular junction. These neuromuscular blocking agents (NMBAs) can provide total abolition of muscle tone, allowing complete relaxation of all skeletal muscle groups. Although widely used in veterinary patients, no NMBAs are currently licensed for use in animals.

The classical indications for NMBAs are:

(1) *To relax skeletal muscles for easier surgical access:* This can be particularly useful for dissection deep within the abdomen (e.g. when working around the kidneys or adrenal glands), but is extremely helpful even for routine abdominal procedures, such as ovariohysterectomy in the bitch.

(2) *To facilitate control of respiration during intrathoracic surgery:* Although NMBAs are not essential during thoracic procedures, they allow a smoother 'take-over' of the patient's breathing, prior to opening the chest. In general, it is fairly easy to take control of the breathing in small dogs and cats simply by hyperventilation. However, large dogs, in particular, may resist manual ventilation by attempting to continue breathing for themselves, and this can lead to stormy surgical conditions within the chest, as the dog and anaesthetist continually fight each other to control respiration. The use of NMBAs easily overcomes this situation.

(3) *To assist reduction of dislocated joints:* There has traditionally been much controversy over whether fracture reduction is similarly facilitated. However, there definitely appears to be an improvement in surgical conditions when NMBAs are administered to equine patients undergoing fracture repair, so it is reasonable to assume that these drugs may also help in small animal patients.

(4) *To facilitate endotracheal intubation in cats:* (see later, page 148).

(5) *To reduce the amount of general anaesthetic agent required:* Muscles are not usually completely flaccid, that is, they normally maintain a certain degree of tone which is held constant by a feedback control system involving the central nervous system (CNS). Afferent nerves supply information to the CNS on the degree of tone present in the muscle, and the CNS then maintains this tone by impulses delivered to the muscle, *via* the motor nerve supply. When NMBAs are administered, abolishing the normal tone of the muscle, there is a decrease in input into the CNS because of a reduction in afferent 'traffic'. Because of this decreased CNS stimulation, less anaesthetic agent is required. However, although it has traditionally been accepted that NMBAs reduce anaesthetic requirements, several studies have been published that cast doubt on this effect in humans. In addition, most veterinary anaesthetists would agree that muscle relaxants appear to have minimal effects on anaesthetic requirements.

(6) *To assist ophthalmic procedures:* NMBAs are commonly administered to animals undergoing cataract surgery to paralyse extra-ocular muscles and allow central positioning of the eye. In addition, they prevent the patient moving or coughing, which could be disastrous in the presence of an open globe.

NMBAs cause paralysis of all skeletal muscle groups in the body, including the intercostal muscles and the diaphragm. Thus, facilities for endotracheal intubation and intermittent positive pressure ventilation (IPPV) must always be available, when the use of these drugs is contemplated. In addition, NMBAs provide only muscle relaxation – they have no analgesic or anaesthetic effects – so it is possible for a patient to undergo surgery while completely awake but unable to move. For this reason, before using these drugs, one should be thoroughly competent at monitoring anaesthesia in the non-paralysed patient.

In addition, although muscle relaxants will ultimately cause paralysis of all the skeletal muscles, some groups appear more resistant than others. This is most obviously illustrated by the diaphragm, which is generally the last muscle to become paralysed when relaxant is administered, and the first to recover function, as the effect of the drug dissipates. The skeletal muscles of the upper airway are relatively sensitive to NMBAs, however, so it is not uncommon at the end of a surgical procedure utilising muscle relaxants to have a patient breathing spontaneously (due to early recovery of diaphragmatic activity), but which, when extubated, develops airway obstruction (due to the relative sensitivity of the pharyngeal muscles to the small amounts of NMBA which are still present at the NMJ). Thus, simply observing for return of spontaneous respiratory activity is not a reliable indicator of return of skeletal muscle activity throughout the body.

There are two classes of NMBA.

Depolarising (non-competitive) muscle relaxants

These agents have a similar chemical structure to acetylcholine (ACh), the neurotransmitter at the neuromuscular junction. Depolarising agents bind to the postjunctional receptor and, because of their chemical similarity to ACh, cause the muscle to contract initially, before it relaxes. This is seen clinically as widespread, short-lived, muscle fasciculations throughout the skeletal muscles of the body, followed by total flaccidity. These fasciculations can cause a significant degree of postoperative pain in humans, and also appear to induce some direct muscle damage, which may lead to potassium release from the muscle cells. This effect is exaggerated in patients with spinal cord trauma or burns, and, consequently, depolarising NMBAs should be avoided in these patients, as well as those with pre-existing hyperkalaemia.

The only depolarising NMBA used clinically is **suxamethonium** (also called succinylcholine), which has a duration of approximately 20 min in the dog, and about 3–5 min in the cat. The action of this drug is terminated by the enzyme pseudocholinesterase (or plasma cholinesterase) which is produced by the liver; thus prolonged effects may be seen in patients with liver disease. Attempts to overcome the short duration of suxamethonium by administering incremental doses are not recommended, since a phenomenon known as phase 2 block (or dual block) may occur. Phase 2 block is a poorly understood event which usually occurs after high or repeated doses of suxamethonium (although it can occur in dogs following a single, normal dose), and results in a prolonged period of neuromuscular blockade. (This is in comparison to the normal short period of neuromuscular blockade usually seen with suxamethonium – phase 1 block.) Because there are no effective drugs for reversal of depolarising relaxants, phase 2 block is important because the patient will have to be ventilated and remain anaesthetised until there is spontaneous neuromuscular function.

The only practical indication for the use of suxamethonium in present-day small animal anaesthesia is to aid endotracheal intubation in cats. The cat has an exquisitely sensitive larynx that may spasm when stimulated. Although this can be avoided by the use of local anaesthetic sprays prior to intubation, these require approximately 1–2 min to achieve peak effect, and in some situations (e.g. cats with diaphragmatic rupture), it is necessary to establish an airway in a shorter period of time. The usual technique in these cases is to pre-oxygenate the patient with 100% oxygen for several minutes by face mask, induce anaesthesia with an IV agent and then immediately administer suxamethonium intravenously. The larynx will usually relax within about 30 sec, allowing intubation to proceed. Because suxamethonium lasts about 5 min in the cat, it is necessary to continue IPPV until spontaneous respiration resumes.

Although suxamethonium can be given by the IM route, it is usually administered IV, and has the fastest onset time of all the NMBAs.

Non-depolarising (competitive) muscle relaxants

These agents are much more widely used than suxamethonium, because they are reversible and can be 'topped up' as required. They are only administered intravenously. The non-depolarising muscle relaxants compete with ACh for postjunctional binding sites (hence their name), and cause blockade of the motor endplate without the initial stimulation seen with suxamethonium, i.e. there is no initial muscle contraction with non-depolarising NMBAs. Although a number of these agents are marketed, four main ones are used clinically:

- **Pancuronium** ('Pavulon', Organon) – duration of 30–50 min in the dog and cat. Usually causes a degree of tachycardia and increased arterial blood pressure.
- **Atracurium** – duration of 20–40 min (although occasionally up to 60 min, especially with higher doses). Atracurium breaks down spontaneously in plasma by a pH- and temperature-dependent reaction (Hofmann degradation), so is not dependent on intact organ function for metabolism. As a result, it is the agent of choice for animals with renal or hepatic disease. However, hypothermia, acid–base and electrolyte abnormalities may prolong the duration. Atracurium has the potential to cause histamine release, leading to hypotension, especially if high doses are used, but this appears less common in animals than in humans.
- **Vecuronium** ('Norcuron', Organon) – duration of 20–30 min, with a more predictable and consistent duration than atracurium. Vecuronium appears to be the most cardiovascularly stable relaxant currently available. The duration may be prolonged in patients with hepatic disease.

- **Rocuronium** ('Esmeron', Organon) – fastest onset of all the non-depolarising NMBAs, although still somewhat slower than suxamethonium.

Following the initial dose of a non-depolarising relaxant, if it is necessary to prolong the period of blockade further, incremental doses of ¼ to ½ the initial dose are usually administered.

Signs of inadequate anaesthesia

It is essential that the patient remains unconscious while under the influence of NMBAs. Unlike general anaesthesia in a non-paralysed animal, if the depth of anaesthesia becomes inadequate (i.e. the patient becomes 'light'):

- the eye will *not* move, because it is already central;
- the animal will *not* develop a palpebral reflex;
- the respiratory pattern will *not* alter, since the respiratory muscles are paralysed;
- the animal will *not* exhibit gross spontaneous movement.

Thus, it is more difficult with paralysed animals to monitor depth of anaesthesia. However, signs associated with inadequate anaesthesia in patients under the influence of NMBAs include:

- increase in pulse rate (unrelated to haemorrhage);
- increase in arterial blood pressure;
- salivation;
- increased tear production;
- vasovagal syncope (bradycardia, hypotension, pallor);
- increase in end-tidal CO_2 levels (unrelated to alterations in pattern of ventilation);
- slight muscle twitching of the face, tongue or limbs, in response to surgical stimulation;
- pupillary dilation.

If any of these signs are observed, it should be assumed that anaesthesia is inadequate, and small incremental doses of a potent analgesic agent (e.g. fentanyl, morphine) or an intravenous anaesthetic agent (e.g. propofol) should be administered. Alternatively, if general anaesthesia is being maintained with volatile agents, simply increasing the vaporiser setting may be sufficient.

Reversal of neuromuscular blocking drugs

There are no reversal agents available for depolarising relaxants (suxamethonium), duration of action depending mainly on the dose administered and the circulating concentration of pseudocholinesterase. Non-depolarising NMBAs, on the other hand, can be reversed with **anticholinesterases**. These drugs inhibit the enzyme, acetylcholinesterase, which is responsible for the breakdown of acetylcholine. Thus, when an anticholinesterase is administered, ACh concentrations increase at the neuromuscular junction (NMJ), displacing the non-depolarising agent that is bound to the postjunctional receptors (remember – the non-depolarising relaxants are also called *competitive* NMBAs, because they compete with ACh for these receptors). Unfortunately, the effects of anticholinesterases are not restricted to the NMJ, and ACh concentrations increase throughout the body. This can result in unwanted effects, most notably bradycardia, salivation, bronchospasm, and diarrhoea. To offset these side effects, **anticholinergic** (antimuscarinic) drugs (atropine; glycopyrrolate) are given immediately before, or simultaneously with, anticholinesterases. (Be careful to distinguish these two groups of drugs, since they sound similar.)

There are two anticholinesterase drugs frequently used, neither of which are licensed in animals. **Neostigmine** is the commoner, while some favour **edrophonium**, since it may have fewer effects at sites out-with the NMJ.

Whichever reversal agent is chosen, ventilation must be maintained until adequate spontaneous respiration commences. Failure to restore spontaneous ventilation may occur due to relaxant overdosage (particularly with suxamethonium), hepatic or renal disease (failure to metabolise or excrete the drug), hypothermia, and acid–base or electrolyte disturbances. In addition, excessive central depression (i.e. anaesthesia which is too 'deep') will delay the return of spontaneous respiratory activity. Thus, at the end of surgery, the animal should be in a 'light' plane of anaesthesia, prior to relaxant reversal.

Peripheral nerve stimulation

Because of the relative difficulty in determining the degree of neuromuscular blockade present in a patient that has received a NMBA, it is common to utilise a nerve stimulator to help quantify the intensity of relaxation. This is a hand-held device that delivers a small electrical current through a pair of electrodes (commonly alligator clips). The electrodes are customarily attached to the skin over the ulnar nerve on the medial aspect of the elbow, the peroneal nerve at the lateral cranial tibia, or the facial nerve on the lateral aspect of the face, and the response of the muscle groups innervated by these nerves is observed when the nerve stimulator is activated.

The commonest form of stimulation in use is **train-of-four** (**TOF**), where four electrical pulses are applied to the nerve over a 2-sec period (i.e. 0.5 sec between twitches). In the non-paralysed animal, four distinct muscle twitches, each of identical strength, will occur (Fig. 6.2). If a non-depolarising relaxant is then administered, the fourth twitch in the TOF will become weaker and eventually disappear, followed by the third twitch, then the second, and eventually the first, if sufficient relaxant is given (Figs 6.3 and 6.4). This phenomenon of a gradually decreasing muscle response to nerve stimulation, with the onset of non-depolarising induced relaxation, is known as **fade.**

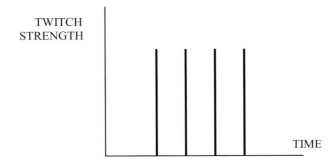

Fig. 6.2 Normal animal, no relaxant. All four twitches in the TOF are present and of equal strength.

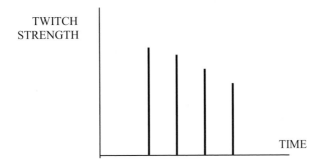

Fig 6.3 Onset of non-depolarising blockade. Fade is present in TOF but all twitches are still visible.

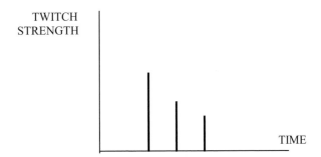

Fig 6.4 Neuromuscular blockade is now more profound; the fourth twitch in the TOF has now disappeared and the remaining three twitches are weaker.

Peripheral nerve stimulation serves two useful purposes. Firstly, it has been shown that ideal muscle relaxation for abdominal surgery is achieved when only one or two twitches remain in the TOF. This allows the anaesthetist to titrate the dose of relaxant to achieve suitable surgical conditions. Secondly, at the end of surgery, it permits an assessment of residual neuromuscular blockade. As the NMBA is reversed, the TOF should have recovered to four equal-strength twitches again, before the animal is allowed to awaken and the trachea extubated.

Suxamethonium-induced relaxation exhibits a slightly different TOF pattern to the non-depolarising type described above, in that twitch strength decreases, but fade is not observed (i.e. all four twitches become weaker, but remain equal to each other). TOF monitoring is less commonly used in monitoring of suxamethonium, due to its short duration.

Guidelines on the safe use of multidose bottles or vials in anaesthesia, and the use of glass ampoules in anaesthesia, are illustrated in Figs 6.5 and 6.6, respectively.

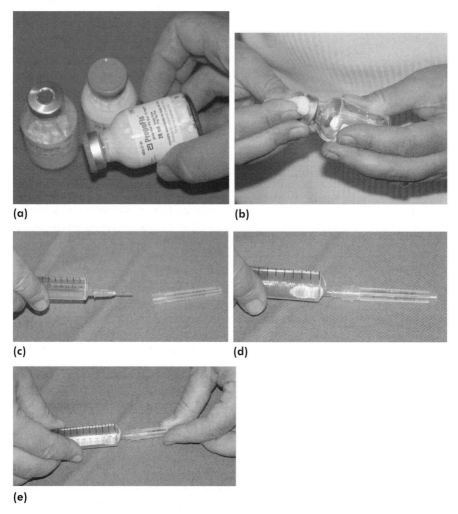

Fig 6.5 Use of multidose bottles in anaesthesia.

Fig 6.5 *(Continued)*

- Wash and dry hands.
- Select the appropriate drug and check drug concentration. If the drug has not been stored according to manufacturer's recommendations it should be discarded.
- Check that the drug is within the manufacturer's expiry period.
- Make a visual check for evidence of gross contamination or the presence of particulate matter in the solution or suspension.
- Remove any protective caps covering the rubber top (a).
- Wipe the top of the vial or bottle with a fresh cotton swab soaked with 70% alcohol, and allow it to dry (b).
- Use a new hypodermic needle *and* syringe every time fluid is withdrawn from a multidose vial.
- **Never** leave one needle inserted in the vial cap for multiple uses.
- Inject replacement air into the vial, ensuring that the needle tip is above the fluid level as injection of air into some solutions or suspensions can distort dosages.
- Invert the vial and syringe to eye level and adjust needle tip to under the fluid level.
- Rotate the syringe to allow calibrations to be viewed.
- Draw up a slight excess of fluid.
- Holding the syringe perfectly straight, tap the barrel to dislodge air bubbles, and expel both air and excess fluid back into the vial.
- Remove the needle and syringe from the vial by grasping the syringe barrel.
- Recapping needles can lead to accidental needle-stick injuries. This is of particular concern with certain drugs used for pre-anaesthetic medication, induction and maintenance of anaesthesia. If at all possible, dispose of needles immediately without recapping them. If a needle must be recapped, e.g. to avoid carrying an unprotected sharp when immediate disposal is not possible, recap the needle using the 'one-hand' technique, as follows. Place the needle cap on a flat surface and remove your hand from the cap (c). Using your dominant hand, hold the syringe and use the needle to scoop the cap onto the needle (d). When the cap covers the needle completely, use your other hand to secure the cap on the needle hub (e).
- Place a new needle onto syringe and, if the drug is not to be administered immediately, label syringe appropriately.
- Wash and dry hands.

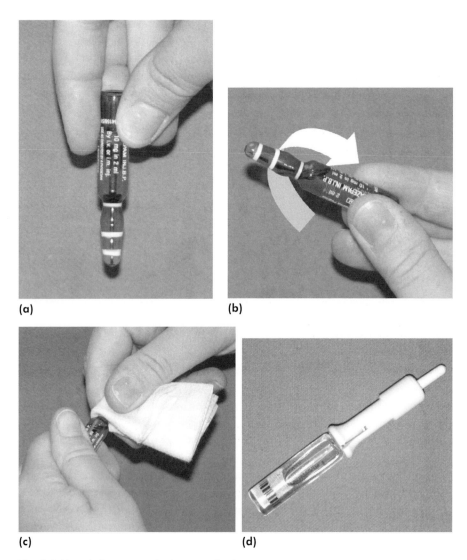

(a)   (b)

(c)   (d)

Fig 6.6 Use of glass ampoules in anaesthesia.

Fig 6.6 *(Continued)*

- Wash and dry hands.
- Select the appropriate drug and check drug concentration. If the drug has not been stored according to manufacturer's recommendations it should be discarded.
- Check that the drug is within the manufacturer's expiry period.
- Make a visual check for evidence of gross contamination or the presence of particulate matter in the solution or suspension.
- Many ampoules have coloured neckbands indicating a prestressed area to facilitate opening. Larger ampoules may not be marked in this way and the neck of these ampoules must be filed to facilitate breakage.
- Invert the selected ampoule and shake fluid into the top of the ampoule (a). Afterwards, holding the bottom of the ampoule, rotate it slowly to displace the fluid to the bottom (b).
- Clean the neck of the ampoule before opening, e.g. wipe with a clean swab and 70% alcohol solution, to reduce bacterial contamination of the medication.
- Hold the prepared ampoule in your non-dominant hand with the ampoule neck above your fingers.
- Secure the top of the ampoule between the thumb and index finger of the dominant hand. A clean swab or alcohol wipe may be used to protect the fingers of the dominant hand (c).
- Using strong steady pressure, without squeezing the top of the ampoule too tightly, the top may be snapped off.
- If any glass splinters enter the ampoule it should be discarded. Glass particle contamination of medications may occur when opening ampoules, and if such particles are injected they can cause phlebitis and granuloma formation in pulmonary, hepatic, splenic, renal and interstitial tissue. Filter needles are available to prevent aspiration of glass splinters but are rarely used in veterinary medicine.
- The ampoule top (and swab or wipe) is discarded safely.
- Reusable ampoule breakers with a built-in long-life cutter, suitable for both prestressed and unstressed ampoules, are available (d), as are disposable, single-use ampoule breakers. Such breakers reduce the chance of injury and allow for the safe disposal of the top of the ampoule.
- Draw up the medication using an appropriate needle and syringe and, if the drug is not to be administered immediately, label syringe appropriately.
- Wash and dry hands.

FURTHER READING

Thurman, J.C., Tranquilli, W.J. & Benson, G.J. (1996) *Veterinary Anaesthesia* (Lumb & Jones), 3rd edition. Williams & Wilkins, Baltimore.

Hall, L.W., Clarke, K.W. & Trim, C.M. (2001) *Veterinary Anaesthesia*, 10th edition. WB Saunders, London.

Seymour, C. & Gleed, R. (1999) *Manual of Small Animal Anaesthesia and Analgesia*. British Small Animal Veterinary Association, Cheltenham.

Flecknell, P. & Waterman-Pearson, A. (2000) *Pain Management in Animals*. WB Saunders, London.

Analgesia

7

Derek Flaherty and Janice MacGillivray

Pain is a very personal experience and even in humans, who can communicate verbally, the assessment and treatment of pain remains challenging.

Veterinary surgeons and nurses rely heavily on the interpretation of patients' behaviour to guide medical therapy of pain, and so evaluation of pain in dogs and cats remains subjective and influenced by personal bias, perception and philosophy. Indeed the recognition and management of pain in dogs and cats in both the UK and US has been shown to be suboptimal, with considerable disparity between the recognition of pain and the actions taken to treat that pain.

Veterinary surgeons and nurses must remember that their primary duty is to relieve suffering of animals in their care and so they must strive to minimise pain in their patients before, during and after anaesthesia. To this end it is important that the assessment of pain is dynamic and that veterinary surgeons and nurses expect individual patients' responses to a similar noxious insult (e.g. ovariohysterectomy) to differ.

PATHOPHYSIOLOGY OF PAIN PERCEPTION

The process by which an individual consciously perceives noxious stimuli is extremely complex. Recent advances in the understanding of the mechanisms of pain have led to many new approaches to its treatment, although the drugs available have changed little. Basically, with the onset of tissue damage, a number of inflammatory mediators are released around the traumatised site. One of the most important groups involved in this process are the prostaglandins (see later). These inflammatory mediators act in various ways to excite surrounding nociceptors, which are free nerve endings involved in detection of noxious stimuli. The nociceptive information is transmitted from the nociceptors, *via* two types of afferent sensory nerves (Aδ and C fibres), to the spinal cord, where some processing takes place. From here, there is continued transmission upwards to the brain, where further processing of the signal occurs, as well as conscious perception of the pain. In addition, the brain may attempt nociceptive suppression, by descending inhibition at the spinal cord level.

If the original tissue damage was severe enough, or if the damage is ongoing, changes occur around the traumatised area that result in a heightened response from the nociceptors, as well as an increase in the number of these nerve endings which are active in the detection and transmission of pain. This phenomenon is known as **peripheral sensitisation**.

Similarly, within the spinal cord, ongoing noxious stimulation results in an exaggerated response by the neurones in the dorsal horn. This is termed **central sensitisation**.

The main significance of peripheral and central sensitisation is that they lead to 'misinterpretation' of noxious information. For example, if one considers a cat after flank ovariohysterectomy, lightly touching the surgical site will generally elicit a pain response. Under normal circumstances, in the absence of a surgical incision in this area, light touch would not elicit pain. This altered response, wherein normally non-noxious stimuli become perceived as noxious, is called **allodynia**. Similarly, if one were brave enough to press hard against the incision – a situation which would provoke a pain response even in the absence of tissue damage at the site – the animal would exhibit an exaggerated response, i.e. would show greater pain than if there was no incision there. The condition where normally noxious stimuli are now perceived as being even more noxious is termed **hyperalgesia**.

If tissue damage and accompanying pain become chronic in nature, structural alterations occur within the spinal cord, which may contribute to a post-injury pain hypersensitivity state. Even following complete tissue healing, these spinal cord changes may facilitate ongoing chronic pain, which can long outlast tissue damage.

Two important concepts have arisen from our increased comprehension of pain processing and perception. Firstly, if analgesic therapy is instituted prior to tissue damage, peripheral and central sensitisation may be blunted, and, consequently, pain may be lessened. This phenomenon is known as **pre-emptive analgesia**. Secondly, once the complexities of the pain pathways are appreciated, it becomes less logical to attempt to provide analgesia with one drug acting at a solitary site. Wide acceptance has now been granted to the concept of **multimodal (or balanced) analgesia** – the concurrent use of analgesic drugs from several pharmacological classes, acting at different sites within the nociceptive system.

Assessment of pain

Pain may be detrimental to animals undergoing anaesthesia and surgery for a number of reasons. Pain:

- enhances fear, anxiety and the stress response leading to a catabolic state;
- delays wound healing;
- predisposes to intestinal ileus;
- impairs respiration, leading to hypoxia, hypercapnoea and acidosis;
- may increase risk of pneumonia due to a reluctance to cough;
- leads to wound interference and self-trauma;
- prolongs anaesthetic recovery, leading to an increased morbidity;
- reduces cardiovascular function;
- reduces food intake.

Consequently, it is essential that both veterinary surgeons and nurses are confident at interpreting signs and symptoms of pain in their patients.

Many subjective and objective measures of pain in companion animals have been developed. However, in recognition of the limitations of objective measurement of physiological indices, biochemical and neurohumoral factors (Table 7.1), veterinary surgeons and nurses increasingly use behavioural assessment as the most sensitive and clinically practical means of assessing pain in animals. Pain rating or scoring systems (e.g. simple descriptive scales, numerical rating scales, visual analogue scales and composite scoring systems) can be useful in tracking the response to analgesia (see chapter 10).

To assess pain subjectively from behavioural changes, it is beneficial to have some understanding of why a dog or cat shows such behavioural changes. Dogs or cats may show behavioural changes in response to pain simply as a reflex, or spinal response. Such responses are designed to protect part of or the entire animal from further damage, for example, withdrawing a limb from a painful stimulus. Animals may also modify their behaviour to minimise pain and assist

Table 7.1 Objective measurement of clinical pain.

Objective measure of pain	Classification	Comment
Blood levels of cortisol, adrenaline and noradrenaline	Neurohumoral	Invasive
		Time delay for results
		Expensive
		Non-specific
Glucose	Biochemical	Invasive
		Non-specific
Heart rate	Physiological	No direct correlation with
Respiratory rate		pain established
Blood pressure		Non-invasive
Mydriasis		Non-specific

healing, for example, by lying still or sitting hunched, and finally they may vocalise to prevent another animal (or person) from inflicting more pain.

Knowledge of the patient's normal behavioural traits can assist the veterinary surgeon and nurse when assessing severity of pain in an individual patient, and careful observation of the patient before treatment commences can be helpful in this respect. In addition, the owner may be able to provide a valuable insight into their pet's response to pain, and such information can be sought when the dog or cat is presented to the clinic.

Behavioural traits that may either indicate pain or influence the assessment of postoperative pain are detailed below.

Vocalisation

Vocalisation (whining, growling, crying, whimpering, screaming, howling, hissing, spitting) is classically one of the signs people associate with animal pain. Unfortunately, hospitalised patients may vocalise for a number of reasons (e.g. unfamiliar surroundings, presence of other dogs, separation anxiety, indicating a need to urinate or defaecate, caging, emerging from unconsciousness through a period of involuntary excitement) and not only because of pain. Indeed many patients may become uncharacteristically quiet when in pain, and may be at risk of receiving less attention from their carer. However, vocalisation in response to movement, e.g. when changing position or walking, or following gentle palpation of the wound, may provide useful information regarding the patient's pain.

Temperament or demeanour

Attention seeking, fear, quietness, depression, lack of interest, and nervous, anxious or fearful behaviour may alert veterinary surgeons or nurses that an animal requires analgesia.

Appetite

Decreased food and water intake or an altered appetite may be observed in patients that are experiencing pain.

Posture

Changes in the normal posture of the patient can be useful indicators of discomfort and pain. For example, a cat sitting hunched and immobile following surgery is likely to be in pain (Fig. 7.1a). Other abnormal postures include praying, trembling and hiding.

Mobility

Lameness may be as a consequence of mechanical abnormalities or pain. Stiffness, rigidity and a reluctance to change position may also be useful indicators of pain.

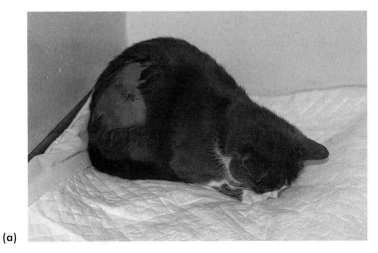

(a)

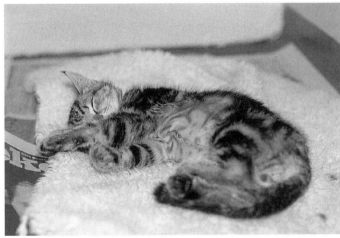

(b)

Fig. 7.1 (a) Following ovariohysterectomy this cat is depressed, quiet and sitting hunched. It resented being moved and had refused food. It was immediately given an analgesic. (b) Following major abdominal surgery and with appropriate analgesia, this cat is sleeping peacefully after eating a meal.

Self-mutilation
Allodynia and hyperalgesia may cause patients to lick, chew, rub or bite at their wound or dressings.

Interactive behaviour
An understanding of the dog or cat's normal behaviour and interaction with both humans and other animals is useful in this situation.

ANALGESIC DRUGS

A variety of drugs are available for the provision of analgesia:

- Opioids
- Non-steroidal anti-inflammatory drugs (NSAIDs)
- Local anaesthetic drugs
- Miscellaneous drugs, e.g. α_2 adrenoceptor agonists, ketamine, nitrous oxide, glucocorticoids.

Opioid analgesics

Opioid analgesics (narcotic analgesics) produce their pharmacological effects by binding to specific opioid receptors, located primarily in the central nervous system (CNS). Although a number of structurally different receptors have been identified, the most important appear to be the μ (mu), δ (delta) and κ (kappa) receptors, more recently renamed OP3, OP1 and OP2 receptors, respectively. Opioid drugs may bind to one, two or all of these receptors, although in practice the most commonly used opioid analgesics are those showing selectivity for the μ receptor. Recently it has been shown that opioid receptors may also develop at sites of inflammation in peripheral tissues, and this underlies the current trend of placing opioid drugs intra-articularly following arthrotomy.

Opioids are classified according to the magnitude of the effect that they produce. They may be **pure agonists** (full agonists), e.g. morphine, pethidine, fentanyl, methadone – drugs that can produce a maximal effect if given in a large enough dose. Alternatively, they may be **partial agonists** – drugs that are incapable of inducing a maximal response, regardless of the dose administered, e.g. buprenorphine. They may be **mixed agonist–antagonists**, indicating that they may have agonist activity at one type of opioid receptor and antagonist activity at a different receptor (e.g. nalbuphine, a μ antagonist and a κ partial agonist). The opioid **antagonists**, such as naloxone, produce no effect when injected alone, but are capable of antagonising ('reversing') the effects of drugs with agonist activity.

The clinical significance of this classification is that pure opioid agonists exhibit an almost linear dose–response curve (i.e. the dose can be increased to achieve the degree of analgesia required), whereas the partial agonists and agonist–antagonists reach an analgesic plateau, beyond which increasing doses do not achieve an increase in analgesic effect (i.e. there is a limit to the degree of analgesia which can be produced) (Fig. 7.2) Thus, these latter drugs are best limited to cases of mild to moderate pain. In addition, partial agonists and agonist–antagonists have the ability to antagonise the effects of pure agonists. Thus, if a patient has received an opioid partial agonist or agonist–antagonist but pain relief is inadequate, simply increasing the dose of the original agent is unlikely to improve the degree of analgesia due to the plateau effect (and may

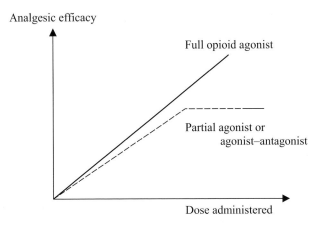

Fig. 7.2 Analgesic efficacy of pure and partial opioid agonists.

actually decrease it – see buprenorphine, below). In addition, any pure agonist subsequently administered to increase analgesia is likely to be antagonised.

Pharmacological action
Analgesia
Opioid drugs provide analgesia by acting at central (and peripheral) sites to decrease the transmission of noxious information, and by altering the affective component of pain, i.e. inducing euphoria.

Respiratory depression
Opioid drugs depress respiration – usually manifested by a reduction in respiratory rate – through a decrease in the sensitivity of the medullary respiratory centre to carbon dioxide. This is recognised as a major side effect in humans, but clinical respiratory depression is not commonly observed in animals when opioid drugs are used at recommended dose rates.

Cardiovascular effects
In general, most opioids have little effect on the cardiovascular system, although bradycardia may occur with high doses or when potent μ selective agents are administered (see page 167). Pethidine has a chemical structure similar to atropine, and may caused tachycardia. Both morphine and pethidine may cause histamine release, particularly when the intravenous route is used, and this may cause hypotension. Pethidine has also been shown to reduce myocardial contractility in dogs when used at clinical doses (> 3 mg/kg) and, consequently, is best avoided in animals with myocardial disease.

Gastrointestinal effects
Within the gastrointestinal tract, smooth muscle tone and sphincter tone tend to increase with opioid drugs, but peristalsis is decreased, reducing propulsive

activity. For this reason, some opioids, such as codeine, are commonly included in anti-diarrhoeal compounds. While most opioid drugs can induce nausea and vomiting in humans, this is much less common in animals, and is only seen with any degree of regularity with morphine. The aetiology of the vomiting is related to activation of the chemoreceptor trigger zone, and also to direct effects on the gastrointestinal tract itself. Pethidine has a spasmolytic action on the gut due to its anticholinergic activity.

Behavioural effects

In the dog and in many rodents, sedation is evident after 'clinical' doses of opioid drugs. Although morphine has been documented to cause maniacal excitement in cats, this is of little clinical consequence, as the animals in the reported study were given 100 times the normal dose for this species (Fig. 7.3). Morphine is perfectly safe in cats when administered at appropriate doses!

Antitussive activity

All μ selective opioids (with the possible exception of pethidine) depress the 'cough' centre in the medulla and therefore have antitussive activity. Butorphanol is specifically marketed for this purpose.

Tolerance and dependence

Opioids induce tolerance and dependence after prolonged administration. Tolerance and dependence are not commonly seen in animals in clinical practice, probably because long-term use does not occur. However, in patients who are maintained on opioid therapy for several days, it may be necessary to increase the administered dose to achieve an adequate effect (tolerance), and also to

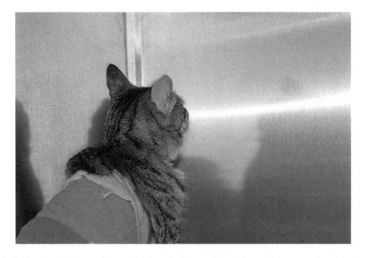

Fig. 7.3 Following repeated morphine administration this cat became dysphoric and sat staring into corners for prolonged periods. When handled its behaviour was unpredictable. The analgesic protocol was revised and the cat made an uneventful recovery.

gradually wean the patient from these drugs, rather than withdrawing them abruptly (dependence).

Contraindications
Pre-existing respiratory disease
Opioids are contraindicated in pre-existing respiratory disease, however, if an animal is not breathing well as a result of pain (e.g. due to fractured ribs), opioids will paradoxically improve ventilation.

Head injuries
Many opioids increase intracranial pressure, due to an increase in carbon dioxide concentration within the blood.

Biliary obstruction
Morphine should be avoided in animals with biliary obstruction, as its action on sphincter tone may affect the sphincter of Oddi, resulting in increased pressure within the bile duct.

Pancreatitis
Much emphasis has been placed in the past on the most suitable opioid for use in patients with pancreatitis, the general advice being that morphine is contraindicated. This was based entirely on the fact that, in humans, the bile duct and pancreatic duct are co-joined at the entrance to the duodenum, and therefore stimulation of the sphincter of Oddi by morphine could increase pressure within the pancreatic duct, leading to further damage to that organ. However, it is now recognised that the bile duct and pancreatic duct enter the duodenum separately in the vast majority of dogs, so an increase in sphincter of Oddi tone should have no effect on the pancreas and, consequently, administration of morphine should be perfectly safe. However, around 80% of cats have co-joined ducts, and morphine should therefore be avoided in cats if pancreatitis is suspected.

Route of administration
The route of choice for administration of most opioids is intramuscular, although the intravenous and subcutaneous routes may also be used for the majority of agents.

Morphine can induce histamine release, particularly when administered intravenously, but provided it is given slowly this route is safe. Continuous intravenous infusions of morphine and other opioid agonist drugs, e.g. fentanyl, alfentanil, may be used rather than intermittent intravenous or intramuscular bolus injections to provide constant plasma levels of the drug. Generally an initial 'loading dose' of the drug is given IV immediately before the infusion is started. The infusion rate may be adjusted according to the patient's response. Morphine may also be administered intra-articularly to provide analgesia following arthrotomy. Morphine is available in an oral preparation, but bio-availability is low by this route.

Pethidine may fail to achieve therapeutic blood concentrations in the dog when given by the subcutaneous route, and can cause massive histamine release when administered intravenously. Consequently, pethidine should only be administered intramuscularly in the dog, although the subcutaneous route is probably acceptable in cats.

Fentanyl is unique among opioids in that it is available as a transdermal preparation, as 'fentanyl patches' ('Durogesic', Janssen-Cilag Ltd). The patches are available in four strengths, releasing 25, 50, 75 or 100 μg of fentanyl per hour. Originally designed for the treatment of terminal pain in humans, transdermal fentanyl has now been widely used in both dogs and cats for management of severe pain. The advantage of this method of administration is that, once the patch is applied, fentanyl is continuously delivered to the patient for at least 72 h in the dog, or 108 h in the cat. Due to the delayed nature of onset of transdermal fentanyl, the patches should be applied at least 24 h before the anticipated onset of pain, if possible. In addition, the patches are expensive, and may be subject to deliberate or accidental abuse. Patients may also show signs of 'breakthrough' pain, necessitating additional treatment with further full opioid agonists.

Opioids may also be administered epidurally or intrathecally, and are extensively used in both human and veterinary medicine by these routes. The major advantage of this technique is the prolonged duration of action of the hydrophilic drugs, such as morphine, which can provide up to 24 h of analgesia following a single epidural administration.

Metabolism and excretion

Most opioids undergo biotransformation in the liver to produce metabolites with either no intrinsic activity, or much lower potency than the parent compound. Metabolites are then eliminated *via* the kidneys or excreted in bile, from where they may subsequently be reabsorbed during passage through the gastrointestinal tract (enterohepatic recirculation).

Legislation governing the use of opioid drugs

The Misuse of Drugs Act 1971 governs the purchase, storage and use of many of the opioid analgesic agents. Basically, this categorises the opioids into a number of Schedules, the most important from a veterinary point of view being those agents placed in Schedules 2 and 3.

Schedule 2 drugs have a number of specific requirements regarding their requisition and prescription. They must be detailed in a Controlled Drug (CD) Register as the practitioner receives them, their use must be strictly recorded, and they must be stored in a locked cabinet, which is fixed in position.

Legal controls over Schedule 3 drugs tend to be less stringent, although special requirements apply to their requisition and prescription. Use of Schedule 3 drugs does not need to be recorded, and, generally, they do not need to be locked away. The exception is buprenorphine, which must be retained in a locked cupboard.

Morphine (CD Schedule 2)

A full opioid agonist, morphine provides potent and reliable analgesia in all species. It has a relatively slow onset of action – around 30 min for maximal effect, even after intravenous administration. Analgesia appears to last 3–4 h in dogs, but up to 8 h in cats, as they metabolise the drug more slowly. Morphine can induce vomiting in both dogs and cats, particularly if not in pain at the time of administration. It can also induce histamine release, particularly after intravenous administration but, provided the drug is given slowly by this route, it appears to be safe. Morphine is not licensed for use in veterinary species.

Papaveretum (CD Schedule 2)

Papaveretum is a crude preparation of approximately 50% morphine and 50% other alkaloids of opium. It is similar in most respects to morphine when administered at twice the dose, but vomiting is less common. Like morphine, it is not licensed for administration to animals.

Pethidine (CD Schedule 2)

A full agonist about one-tenth as potent as morphine, pethidine is licensed for use in the dog, cat and horse. It provides reliable analgesia of rapid onset (10–15 min), but has a short duration of action, possibly only around 1 h in the dog and cat. For this reason, it has to be repeated frequently to maintain satisfactory analgesia. Pethidine does not cause vomiting, and has a spasmolytic action on the gut. It has a similar chemical structure to atropine and so may increase heart rate. Intravenous administration can induce massive histamine release, and this route is contraindicated.

Methadone (CD Schedule 2)

Methadone is a full agonist, similar in effect to morphine, but possibly of longer duration. The drug has a long half-life in humans, and cumulation may occur with multiple doses. However, the pharmacokinetics have not been well investigated in animals. Methadone does not cause vomiting, so is useful for premedication of patients where morphine-induced emesis may be undesirable or contraindicated. It is not licensed for use in animals.

Fentanyl (CD Schedule 2)

Fentanyl is a full opioid agonist, with approximately 100 times the potency of morphine. Fentanyl has a rapid onset of action following intravenous administration (~ 2 min), and a short duration of action, of approximately 20 min (dose-dependent). It is a potent respiratory depressant, and is capable of inducing severe bradycardia. Fentanyl is mainly used intra-operatively to provide profound analgesia during periods of intense surgical stimulation. It

is not licensed as a sole agent for veterinary use, but is licensed in the fentanyl–fluanisone combination, 'Hypnorm', commonly used for anaesthesia in
laboratory animals. In addition, transdermal fentanyl is now commonly used
in animals for management of severe pain (see above).

Alfentanil (CD Schedule 2)

Alfentanil is a full opioid agonist of around 10 times the potency of morphine.
It has a rapid onset following intravenous administration, and a duration of
approximately 5 min. Due to the short action, alfentanil is most commonly
used intra-operatively by infusion, although it is sometimes included as part
of an induction protocol to minimise the dose of primary anaesthetic administered. Like fentanyl, alfentanil causes respiratory depression and can induce
marked bradycardia, or occasionally cardiac arrest. It is not licensed for use in
animals.

Remifentanil (not controlled)

Remifentanil is a recently developed full opioid agonist, which is now extensively used in human anaesthesia, and has been the subject of research in veterinary anaesthesia. It is an ultra-short-acting agent of similar potency to fentanyl,
administered by intravenous infusion during surgery. The major advantage of
remifentanil over fentanyl and alfentanil is that the drug is broken down by
non-specific plasma and tissue esterases, and does not rely on metabolism and
excretion by the liver and kidneys. Thus, there should be no cumulation in patients with hepatic or renal disease. Metabolism of remifentanil is so rapid that,
even after prolonged infusion, the plasma concentration drops to subtherapeu-
tic levels within minutes.

Buprenorphine (CD Schedule 3)

Buprenorphine is a partial opioid agonist that is licensed for use in dogs, by
intramuscular injection. However, it is also commonly administered to cats.
In experimental studies, buprenorphine is a potent opioid, but clinically it may
be unreliable in terms of the analgesic effect achieved. The drug has a slow
association with, and dissociation from, opioid receptors, and this accounts
for the slow onset of action, and the prolonged duration of effect. Even after
intravenous administration, buprenorphine requires around 45 min to achieve
peak effect, and although some authorities would claim an expected duration
of approximately 12 h, more commonly analgesia starts to wane after about
6 h. There is some evidence that this agent may exhibit a 'bell-shaped' dose–response curve, which implies that efficacy starts to decrease with administration
of higher doses of buprenorphine, possibly due to the drug antagonising itself.
The clinical significance of this has recently been questioned.

Buprenorphine has been recommended as a 'reversal' agent following administration of neuroleptanalgesics in small mammals, reversing the sedative

effects of the opioid administered in the neurolepanalgesic mixture while providing analgesia in its own right.

Butorphanol (not controlled)

Butorphanol is variably classified as an agonist–antagonist or partial opioid agonist. At present, the drug is not controlled in the UK under the Misuse of Drugs Act 1971, and this accounts for its popularity in veterinary practice. The intensity of analgesia produced by butorphanol is very variable in the dog and cat, and it is probably of limited duration – possibly only around 1 h. This drug is licensed in the dog, cat and horse for use as an analgesic, and also has a separate licence as an antitussive in dogs.

Naloxone (not controlled)

Naloxone is a pure opioid antagonist, which is used to reverse the effects of both full and partial agonists. In this regard, it is much more effective in reversal of the full agonists. Buprenorphine, in particular, due to its tight binding to opioid receptors, may be particularly difficult to reverse with naloxone. The drug has a short duration of action of 30–60 min, so may need to be repeated or administered by infusion, when attempting to reverse long-acting opioid drugs. It is not licensed for animal use.

The opioid drugs are the most efficacious of the analgesic agents currently available, and are generally the treatment of choice for the management of severe pain. Side effects tend to be minimal in animals and, despite many of these drugs not being licensed for veterinary use; their safety profile is well established.

Non-steroidal anti-inflammatory drugs

Non-steroidal anti-inflammatory drugs (NSAIDs) may be classified chemically into two major groups: the carboxylic acids (e.g. carprofen, flunixin, aspirin) and the enolic acids (e.g. phenylbutazone, meloxicam). The therapeutic effects of most NSAIDs are due to inhibition of the enzyme cyclo-oxygenase (COX), which converts arachidonic acid (released from damaged cell membranes) into prostaglandins and thromboxane A_2. These eicosanoids are involved in tissue inflammation, pain production and pyrexia. In addition, thromboxane A_2 is intimately involved in platelet aggregation at sites of tissue damage, and so, by decreasing production of this eicosanoid, all NSAIDs carry the potential to increase bleeding at surgical or traumatic sites. However, this is uncommon with therapeutic doses of these agents, with the exception of aspirin, which binds irreversibly to COX inside platelets, inhibiting thromboxane A_2 for the life of the platelet. For this reason, aspirin is commonly used for antithrombotic prophylaxis, for example, in cats with hypertrophic cardiomyopathy that are prone to developing blood clots (thrombi).

Some NSAIDs, in particular flunixin, have been shown to have anti-endotoxaemic actions at doses below those which produce anti-inflammatory effects, and this drug is commonly administered to horses with colic, for this reason.

Consequently, due to the widespread effects of eicosanoids throughout the body, NSAIDs are not only anti-inflammatory, but are also analgesic, antipyretic, antithrombotic and anti-endotoxaemic.

Two forms of COX have been identified: COX-1, a constitutive enzyme, and COX-2, an inducible enzyme. Originally it was considered that COX-1 was solely involved in the production of 'housekeeping' prostaglandins, responsible for maintenance of gastrointestinal mucosal blood flow and mucus production, and renal blood flow, while COX-2 was responsible for production of prostaglandins involved in the inflammatory response. Since most available NSAIDs were relatively non-selective (i.e. inhibited both forms of COX), it was believed that cases of gastrointestinal ulceration and occasional renal failure observed in animals receiving NSAID therapy were due to unwanted suppression of COX-1. Consequently, attempts were then directed at developing a COX-2 selective NSAID, which would inhibit the inflammatory form of COX (COX-2), while sparing COX-1. Recently, it has been appreciated that the situation is not quite so clear-cut: COX-1 plays a part in inflammation, while COX-2 may have certain constitutive roles within the body. Therefore, NSAIDs that are completely COX-2 selective may not be as potent anti-inflammatory agents as those that cause inhibition of both isoforms of COX. However, there is some evidence that highly selective COX-2 NSAIDs are less likely to induce gastrointestinal side effects. Most commercially available NSAIDs inhibit both enzymes, although some, such as meloxicam, may be more selective for COX-2.

The most frequently encountered toxic side effects of the NSAIDs are gastrointestinal irritation or ulceration and nephrotoxicity. The latter may be more common in the anaesthetised patient, where hypotension may reduce renal blood flow. For this reason, most NSAIDs are not licensed in the perioperative period, with the exception of carprofen (dogs and cats) and meloxicam (dogs). Maintenance of adequate renal perfusion during anaesthesia, by using minimal amounts of cardiovascular depressant drugs and attention to fluid therapy, reduces the risk of NSAID-induced renal toxicity. NSAIDs should not be used with other potentially nephrotoxic agents and should be used with great care in animals with renal disease.

Flunixin

Flunixin is licensed for use in dogs, cats and small mammals, and available as an oral and parenteral preparation. It is a very effective analgesic, anti-inflammatory and antipyretic agent, due to its potent inhibitory effect on COX. However, side effects are not uncommon with this drug, with gastrointestinal signs such as vomiting, melaena and haemorrhagic diarrhoea frequently being the first signs of toxicity. Particular care needs to be taken when administering flunixin in the perioperative period, as acute renal failure may result.

Carprofen

Carprofen is licensed in cats (injection only) and dogs (injection and tablets). The mode of action of carprofen has not yet been established but, despite being a poor inhibitor of COX, it exhibits potent anti-inflammatory and analgesic effects. The therapeutic safety margin of carprofen appears high, and the drug is licensed for use in the perioperative period. Renal toxicity is uncommon, but gastrointestinal effects may be observed in some patients. Recent reports from North America of hepatic failure in dogs (mainly Labradors) associated with carprofen, have not been substantiated by more widespread use of the drug in Europe.

Ketoprofen

Licensed for use in dogs and cats, by injection or tablets, ketoprofen offers good anti-inflammatory and analgesic actions. This drug should be avoided in the perioperative period since it is a potent inhibitor of COX enzymes.

Meloxicam

Licensed in dogs and cats as an injectable preparation, and in dogs as an oral syrup, meloxicam is a relative COX-2 selective inhibitor. Despite its potent effects on COX, the drug has recently been licensed for perioperative administration, as toxicity studies have confirmed its high safety profile.

As the concept of pre-emptive analgesia has become widely accepted, it is now common to administer NSAIDs preoperatively to achieve maximal benefit. Consequently, carprofen and meloxicam have become the agents most commonly used, as they are licensed for use at this point.

Traditionally, NSAIDs have been thought of as drugs for the treatment of chronic, low-grade pain. However, it is now widely recognised that these agents can be potent analgesics, in some cases as powerful as opioids. They also appear to have synergistic effects with opioid drugs, improving the degree of pain control exerted by the clinician.

Until recently, it was also believed that the NSAIDs acted purely at peripheral sites in the body. However, it is now recognised that these drugs also exert their effects within the central nervous system itself.

Local anaesthetic agents

Local anaesthetics exert their effect by binding to sodium channels in the cell membrane along the nerve fibre. This stops the large transient increase in the permeability of the membrane to sodium ions (Na^+) that normally occurs when the membrane is depolarised, for example, following noxious stimulation. Thus, they prevent propagation of the action potential and consequently, inhibit the transfer of noxious information from the periphery to the CNS. In many ways, therefore, local anaesthetics can be considered the ultimate analgesic agents, as they are the only ones that are capable of completely blocking pain perception.

Local anaesthetics agents are classified as either esters or amides, based on their chemical structure. Lignocaine and bupivacaine are amides, while procaine is classed as an ester. Amides are metabolised by hepatic enzymes, while the esters are broken down by plasma cholinesterase, an enzyme produced by the liver. Consequently, the duration of both groups of drugs may be prolonged in patients with hepatic disease.

Many local anaesthetics produce vasodilation, which increases the speed of uptake of these drugs into the bloodstream, reducing their efficacy at the site of administration, and also potentially increasing their toxic side effects. Consequently, local anaesthetics are commonly combined with a vasoconstrictor – usually adrenaline – to maintain their concentration at the administration site.

Local anaesthetics may be used:

- to provide total analgesia, allowing surgical procedures to be performed in conscious or sedated animals;
- to provide analgesia intra-operatively in anaesthetised animals;
- to control postoperative pain.

In each of these situations local anaesthetic drugs may be administered by either topical application or by injection to provide analgesia.

Topical or surface application

Local analgesic agents may be applied directly into the eye (conjunctiva), onto mucous membranes (larynx, urethra, nasal passages) or onto the skin, including the external ear canal. Proxymetacaine may be used on the eye (e.g. to allow removal of a foreign body) or lignocaine gel or spray on the mucous membranes (e.g. to facilitate endotracheal intubation in cats). Local anaesthetic creams, for example, EMLA® cream, may be applied to the skin before intravenous catheterisation (Fig. 7.4).

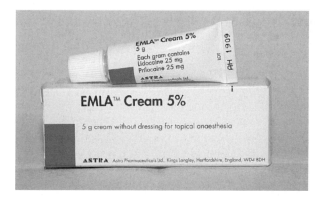

Fig. 7.4 EMLA cream.

'Splash' blocks
Local anaesthetics are flooded or dripped onto surgical sites and wounds at the end of a procedure.

Intrapleural blocks
Intrapleural administration of local anaesthetics provides analgesia following median sternotomy or intercostal thoracotomy. The drug is generally instilled into the thorax through a thoracic drain.

Intra-articular or synovial blocks
Local anaesthetics (or opioids) are instilled into the affected joint cavity following surgery. Intra-articular blocks are used commonly in horses to aid in the diagnosis of lameness.

Local infiltration
The intradermal or subdermal tissues are infiltrated by injection with a local anaesthetic agent. This is useful only for minor procedures, and normally sedation and/ or manual restraint are also required. Local toxicity may delay tissue healing.

Infiltration of local anaesthetic agents can be used to produce line blocks, ring blocks and field blocks. These techniques are more commonly used in large animals such as cattle and sheep.

If local analgesic drugs or opioids are placed either close to the spinal cord or into a major nerve plexus (brachial plexus), loss of sensation to a large part of the body can be achieved, i.e. **regional analgesia**.

Perineural infiltration
A local anaesthetic agent is injected directly around a nerve, for example, intercostal nerve block (Fig. 7.5), brachial plexus block.

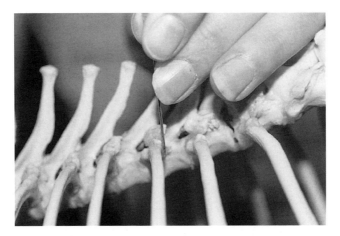

Fig. 7.5 Site of needle placement (immediately caudal to rib) for an intercostal nerve block.

Mental block

This procedure provides regional local analgesia for the rostral lower lip, post-operatively. Local anaesthetic is injected either intra-orally or percutaneously very close to the mental nerves as they emerge from the mental foraminae on the rostral lateral aspect of the mandible.

Intravenous regional anaesthesia (Bier block)

A local anaesthetic agent is injected intravenously distal to a tourniquet on a limb, providing analgesia distal to that site for the length of time the tourniquet remains in place.

Extradural analgesia

Lumbosacral extradural techniques are used to produce analgesia for all structures caudal to the umbilicus in dogs and cats (Fig. 7.6). This is an effective,

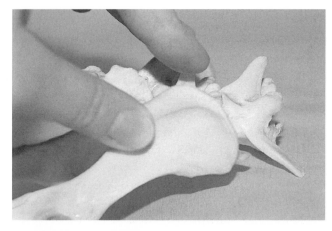

(a)

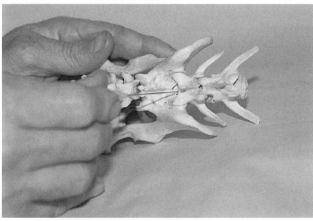

(b)

Fig. 7.6 (a) Palpating the dorsal spinous process of L7. (b) Demonstrating the position of the spinal needle in the lumbosacral space. (c) Administration of an epidural anaesthetic to a boxer dog prior to recto-anal surgery.

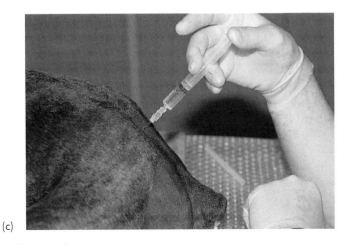

(c)

Fig. 7.6 *(Continued)*

safe and relatively easy procedure, which can be used for coeliotomies, amputation of the tail, anal sac removal, perianal surgery, urethrostomies, obstetric manipulation and hind limb surgeries.

This procedure can be performed either in lateral recumbency with the animals' legs extended and pulled forward to open up the lumbosacral space, or in sternal recumbency, again with the hindlimbs extended forward. The lumbrosacral space is a depression just caudal to the L7 dorsal spinal process, immediately cranial to the sacral crest (which feels like a series of small bumps under the skin). Strict asepsis is essential and, a 24 g to 20 g, 3.75 cm to 5 cm, spinal needle with stylet is used. The needle is introduced on the midline at 90° to the skin surface and gently advanced until a change in resistance is felt as it penetrates the interarcuate ligament. If cerebrospinal fluid is present in the needle hub, the technique may either be converted to an intrathecal block (see below) or the needle withdrawn and the process repeated (Fig. 7.7).

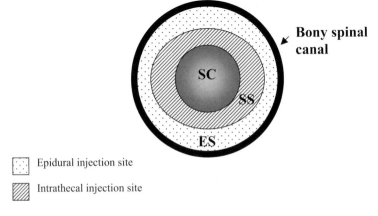

Fig. 7.7 Transverse section of the spinal canal showing the position of the spinal cord (SC), the subarachnoid space (SS) containing cerebrospinal fluid and the epidural space (ES).

This procedure desensitises the nerves that leave the spinal cord in the area of spread of the local anaesthetic. Opioid analgesics can provide prolonged analgesia without loss of motor nerve function when administered by this route, i.e. the patient retains limb function. Opioids used in this way should be free of preservatives and diluted with sterile saline to increase the volume of injection (generally to 1 ml per 5 kg). Combination blocks using both opioids and local anaesthetic drugs may also be used.

Intrathecal analgesia
An opioid or local anaesthetic drug is injected into the subarachnoid space.

Individual local anaesthetic agents
Lignocaine and bupivacaine are the agents most widely used for the provision of local analgesia, although other local anaesthetics are used to a lesser extent (Fig. 7.8).

Lignocaine
Lignocaine is a rapid onset, short-acting (1–1.5 h) local anaesthetic, commonly used as a 1% or 2% solution. It is available with or without adrenaline, and is licensed for use in small animals.

Bupivacaine
Bupivacaine is a slow onset, long duration (4–8 h, depending on route of administration) local anaesthetic agent. It is commercially available as a 0.25%, 0.5% or 0.75% solution, with or without added adrenaline. Toxicity of bupivacaine is greater than lignocaine, and inadvertent intravenous injection will normally lead to cardiac arrest. It is not licensed for veterinary use.

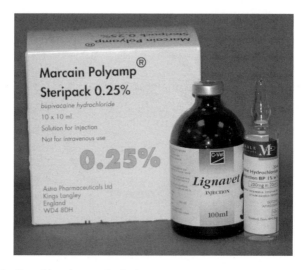

Fig. 7.8 A selection of local anaesthetic drugs.

Proxymetacaine
Proxymetacaine is available as a topical solution for the production of corneal analgesia. It has a relatively rapid onset, but a short duration of action of around 15 min.

EMLA® cream
EMLA stands for 'eutectic mixture of local anaesthetics', and is a combination of lignocaine and prilocaine as a cream formulation. It is used to provide analgesia of the skin, most commonly to facilitate pain-free placement of vascular cannulae. The cream must be applied and covered with an occlusive dressing at least 45 min before analgesia is required.

Side effects
Side effects from administration of local anaesthetic drugs are relatively uncommon, but may be seen following overdose or with inadvertent intravascular injection. Some regional anaesthetic techniques are more likely to produce toxic blood levels than others, for example, intercostal nerve block allows rapid drug absorption.

Local anaesthetic toxicity is generally manifested *via* effects on the cardiovascular and central nervous systems. Early signs are usually those of central nervous stimulation (excitement, seizures), followed by central nervous depression. Cardiovascular depression (decreased myocardial contractility, peripheral vasodilation) is a late change with lignocaine, but may occur early with bupivacaine.

Treatment of local anaesthetic toxicity relies on management of seizures, if present (diazepam/general anaesthesia, airway control), and cardiovascular support, if necessary (intravenous fluids, vasopressor drugs, inotropes).

Miscellaneous analgesic agents
A number of other drugs have analgesic effects.

Nitrous oxide
Nitrous oxide is a relatively potent analgesic in humans, but is less useful in this regard in animals. In addition, when it is turned off at the end of an anaesthetic, analgesia is completely lost within 5–10 min.

Alpha-2 adrenoceptor agonists
Drugs such as medetomidine are potent analgesics, although they are not commonly used for this purpose, due to cardiovascular side effects. However, current research would suggest that it might be possible to administer doses of these drugs that provide analgesia, without dramatic alterations in cardiac output and blood pressure. It is likely that these agents will achieve more widespread use as analgesics, over the next few years. In large animals the α_2 adrenoceptor agonists have been used successfully for epidural analgesia.

Ketamine

Ketamine provides relatively good somatic analgesia, but poor visceral analgesia. However, more importantly, ketamine is an antagonist at the NMDA (N-methyl D-aspartate) receptor in the central nervous system, which is one of the main receptor types implicated in the establishment of central sensitisation. Thus, ketamine may be able to block this effect, and there is some evidence that it may even be able to reverse central sensitisation once it is established. There is currently a huge amount of research directed towards this aspect of the pharmacology of ketamine, and, similar to the α_2 adrenoceptor agonists, it is likely that this drug will achieve more widespread use as an analgesic.

SUMMARY

As our understanding of the processes involved in the transmission of noxious information and conscious pain perception have improved over the past decade, this has led to the introduction of a number of important concepts into clinical pain management, most notably those of pre-emptive analgesia, and multimodal analgesia. Although there have been relatively few new analgesic drugs developed over this period, the manner in which we use them has changed dramatically.

The veterinary nurse carries great responsibility for the safety of patients while under the influence of general anaesthesia, and for ensuring adequate analgesia. An empathetic approach to nursing patients experiencing pain and a thorough appreciation of the actions and side effects of the drugs used during these periods will help to optimise patients' wellbeing.

FURTHER READING

Thurmon, J.C., Tranquilli, W.J. & Benson, G.J. (1996) *Veterinary Anaesthesia* (Lumb & Jones), 3rd edition. Williams & Wilkins, Baltimore.

Hilbery, A.D.R., Waterman, A.E. & Brouwer, G.J. (1989) *Manual of Anaesthesia for Small Animal Practice*. British Small Animal Veterinary Association, Cheltenham.

King, L. & Hammond, R. (1999) *Manual of Canine and Feline Emergency and Critical Care*. British Small Animal Veterinary Association, Cheltenham.

Seymour, C. & Gleed, R.(1999) *Manual of Small Animal Anaesthesia and Analgesia*. British Small Animal Veterinary Association, Cheltenham.

Flecknell, P. & Waterman-Pearson, A. (2000) *Pain Management in Animals*. W.B. Saunders, London.

McKelvey, D & Hollingshead, K.W. (2000) *Small Animal Anaesthesia and Analgesia*, 2nd edition. Mosby Inc., St Louis.

Hall, L.W., Clarke, K.W. &Trim, C.M. (2001) *Veterinary Anaesthesia*, 10th edition. W.B. Saunders, London.

Intravenous Access and Fluid Therapy

8

Kirstin Beard and Elizabeth Welsh

Fluid therapy is an essential component of veterinary care and all veterinary nurses should understand the principles of fluid balance, fluid therapy and the techniques used in fluid administration. Although a number of different routes of fluid administration are available, e.g. hypodermoclysis (subcutaneous route), and are appropriate in many situations in conscious patients and small or exotic species, rapid access to the circulation (by either intravenous or intraosseous routes) is most appropriate in anaesthetised dogs and cats. Consequently the principles of intravenous catheter and intraosseous needle placement, and maintenance of indwelling catheters and needles, are skills every nurse should become familiar with. Calculation of fluid requirements, administration rates and monitoring the response to fluid therapy are also important in patient care.

FLUID THERAPY FOR ANAESTHETISED PATIENTS

Fluids are administered during the anaesthetic period for a number of reasons:

- to maintain a patent venous access;
- to provide circulatory support to maintain oxygen delivery to body organs;
- to replace sensible fluid losses;
- to replace insensible fluid losses;
- to replace ongoing fluid losses.

Patent venous access is essential for anaesthetised patients to facilitate administration of drugs in an emergency. Effective oxygen delivery to body tissues is important to maintain aerobic metabolism, but ensuring effective delivery of oxygen to body tissues requires not only adequate cardiac output but also arterial oxygen saturation of haemoglobin. Thus providing an adequate intravascular fluid load in itself is insufficient and blood haemoglobin concentration and alveolar gas exchange must be adequate.

Anaesthetised patients have the same fluid requirements as conscious patients and similarly these may be modified by physiological status (e.g. age) and pathological conditions (e.g. cardiac disease), and thus fluid therapy should be tailored to each individual patient.

An individual patient's fluid requirement may be thought of in the following terms: maintenance fluids, replacement fluids, and ongoing losses of fluids.

Maintenance fluids

Conscious, healthy dogs and cats normally obtain fluid and electrolytes by:

- drinking water or other fluids;
- eating;
- metabolism.

The majority of fluid is acquired through drinking and eating. Metabolic water normally only contributes a small amount (10–20%).

The main methods by which conscious, healthy dogs and cats lose fluid and electrolytes from the body are:

- urination (20 ml/kg/day)
- defaecation (10 ml/kg/day)
- respiration (loss of fluid only; 20 ml/kg/day)
- sweating. Although sweating can cause significant fluid loss in some species, this is not the case in dogs and cats, that sweat from the footpads only.

These fluid losses are sometimes referred to as sensible (urination and defaecation) and insensible (respiration and sweating) fluid losses.

Fluid balance requires that fluids lost through sensible and insensible routes be matched by fluid intake. Therefore, to maintain normal water balance in a healthy dog or cat, a total of approximately 50 ml/kg/day of fluid is required (range 40–60 ml/kg/day). This calculation tends to underestimate fluid requirements in very small animals and to overestimate fluid requirements in larger animals. Fluid requirements can be calculated on the basis of lean body weight using this method to minimise overhydration, as fatty tissue contains less water than lean tissue. This would be particularly important in patients with renal disease, cardiac insufficiency, respiratory disease, hypoproteinaemia, and so on.

Obese	Body weight (kg) × 0.7 = lean body mass
Normal	Body weight (kg) × 0.8 = lean body mass
Thin	Body weight (kg) × 1.0 = lean body mass

Source: Kohn & DiBartola 2000

An alternative approach is to calculate maintenance fluid requirements using the formula 30 × body weight (kg) + 70 (Wingfield 2001).

Water intake may be decreased for a number of reasons in patients scheduled for anaesthesia. Fasting of patients prior to general anaesthesia to reduce the likelihood of regurgitation and vomiting at induction of anaesthesia, and the inability of the patient to drink and eat both under anaesthesia and in the recovery period, can lead to a significant shortfall in the daily fluid requirement. Many systemically ill patients have depressed thyroid function reducing their metabolic rate and in addition, the metabolic rate of many patients is further reduced by general anaesthesia. This will contribute to a shortfall in available water. Similarly, fluid losses may be different from normal before, during and after general anaesthesia (see replacement and ongoing fluid losses).

Replacement fluids

Many patients that require anaesthesia have physiological or pathological changes that disrupt the body's water and/or electrolyte status. Such conditions arise either through altered intake or output of water and/or electrolytes and can cause dehydration, reduced perfusion or both (Table 8.1).

Table 8.1 Causes of altered fluid intake and losses.

Altered fluid intake	Altered fluid losses
Metabolic disorders	Altered urine production (e.g. renal disease)
Systemic illness	Altered faecal losses (e.g. diarrhoea – an additional 4 ml/kg per stool or up to 200 ml/kg per day in severe cases)
Mechanical difficulty (jaw fractures)	Vomiting (e.g. an additional 4 ml/kg per incident) and regurgitation
Trauma	Transudates, modified transudates and exudates (burns, open wounds, peritonitis)
Sepsis	Blood loss
Water deprivation	Lactation
	Pyrexia – 10% increase in maintenance fluid rates should be included for every 1°C rise above normal
	Respiratory diseases causing polypnoea or tachypnoea
	Losses of body fluids to 'third spaces' (pyometra, ileus, ascites, pleural effusions, interstitial oedema)

Dehydration is the term used to describe a reduction in total body water and the signs and symptoms associated with such a loss. However, assessing an animal's hydration status alone is inadequate. The perfusion status of the patient should also be assessed. Ideally pre-existing fluid deficits causing dehydration should be corrected over a period of at least 12–24 h and preferably before patients receive pre-anaesthetic medication. Relative or absolute hypovolaemia, decreasing tissue perfusion, should also be addressed before this time. However, this is not always possible and so it is important that both hydration and perfusion status are assessed clinically during the pre-anaesthetic examination.

Body water is distributed into either the intracellular or the extracellular fluid compartments. The extracellular fluid compartment includes interstitial water and intravascular water (Fig. 8.1). However, for the purposes of estimation of fluid deficits by physical examination it is convenient to think of the body water as either intravascular or extravascular.

The intravascular space

Rapid loss of isotonic body fluid (e.g. intra-abdominal haemorrhage following rupture of a splenic neoplasm), blood loss following trauma or following relative hypovolaemia (e.g. anaphylactic shock), can deplete the volume of the intravascular space. This causes poor perfusion and inadequate tissue oxygenation, i.e. shock.

The extravascular space

The extravascular space comprises interstitial and intracellular spaces. Loss of isotonic fluid (e.g. through vomiting and diarrhoea) can deplete the volume of the extravascular space. Although initially the intracellular fluid space is not affected, the fluid loss is ultimately distributed between both the interstitial and intracellular fluid spaces and causes dehydration.

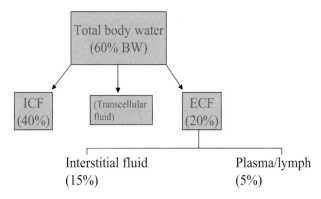

Fig. 8.1 Normal body fluid distribution.

The extravascular and intravascular space

Loss of pure water (e.g. through heatstroke) can deplete the volume of both the extravascular and intravascular space. More commonly it occurs with severe or continued (and uncorrected) loss of isotonic fluid. This causes dehydration and shock.

Physical examination for assessment of percentage dehydration is appropriate when the extravascular fluid space is dehydrated. Physical examination for assessment of perfusion is appropriate when the intravascular space is depleted. Animals examined before anaesthesia should be assessed for both hydration and perfusion. When monitoring anaesthesia the veterinary nurse should be vigilant for signs of changing hydration or perfusion status in the anaesthetised patient and alert the veterinary surgeon.

Clinical assessment of hydration

History

Questions about food and water consumption (anorexia, polydipsia), any gastrointestinal losses (vomiting, diarrhoea), urinary losses (polyuria, oliguria), abnormal discharges (open pyometra) and traumatic losses (blood loss, burns) should be sought from the owner.

Physical examination

An initial assessment of hydration status by physical examination is a useful starting point in estimating fluid deficit in many patients (Table 8.2 and Fig. 8.2). Further diagnostic tests may provide evidence of dehydration inciden-

Table 8.2 Assessing dehydration in dogs and cats by physical examination.

% Dehydration	Clinical signs
< 5%	No obvious signs
	(Concentrated urine)
5–8%	Slight tenting of skin (see Fig. 8.2)
	Slight prolonged CRT
	Tacky mucous membranes
	Third eyelid visible
8–10%	Obvious tenting of skin
	Sunken orbit
	Prolonged CRT
	Heart rate
10–12%	Tented skin stands in place
	Oliguria
	Signs of shock (see box on page 187)
>12%	Progressive shock
	Coma
	Death

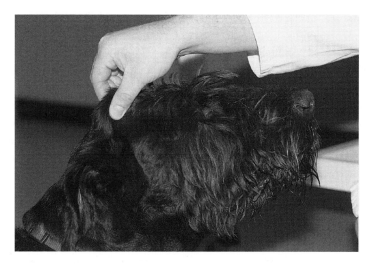

Fig. 8.2 Demonstrating skin tent in a dehydrated dog.

tally, for example, radiographic signs of dehydration such as a small vertebral heart score may be noted on thoracic radiographs.

Following physical examination the volume of fluid needed to correct the hydration deficit is calculated as follows:

$$\text{Fluid deficit (litres)} = \text{Body weight (kg)} \times \% \text{ Dehydration} \times 10$$

This calculation probably underestimates the actual fluid loss.

Laboratory analysis
See Table 8.3.

Clinical measurements
Before anaesthesia all patients are weighed. The expected daily weight loss in an anorexic animal is up to 0.1% body weight, but acute losses of weight ≥ 1% body weight per day can be presumed to represent a fluid deficit. An acute increase in body weight is nearly always caused by increased fluid content.

A number of other clinical measurements may be useful when assessing hydration, in particular urine output and central venous pressure (CVP) (see later).

Clinical assessment of perfusion
Cells within the body must receive both oxygen and nutrients to function normally. In addition, it is important that the waste products of metabolism are removed from the cells' local environment. The vascular system is responsible for carrying oxygen, nutrients and waste to and from cells. When an imbalance between the delivery of oxygen and nutrients to cells and utilisation of oxygen

Table 8.3 Laboratory investigations.

Laboratory value	Comment	Limitations
Packed cell volume (PCV)	For each 1% increase in the PCV, a fluid loss of approximately 10 ml/kg bodyweight has occurred	Relies on prior knowledge of the patient's PCV. ACP can cause a false decrease in PCV in cats
	A fall in PCV is important, as the haemoglobin within red blood cells is essential for the transport of oxygen*	Unsuitable following acute blood loss
Haemoglobin	Dehydration will also result in an increase in the haemoglobin concentration of the blood	Care in interpretation is required in anaemic patients
Total plasma protein (TPP)	Dehydration will cause a rise in TPP. It is useful to assess both the TPP and PCV in an animal that has been diagnosed clinically as dehydrated because only rarely will pre-existing disease result in an elevation of both these parameters	Care in interpretation is required in hypoproteinaemic patients
Blood urea and creatinine	Blood urea and creatinine levels will rise in dehydrated animals (pre-renal azotaemia)	Interpretation of azotaemia should follow determination of the urine specific gravity
Electrolytes	Electrolyte status may need to be modified prior to anaesthesia, e.g. hyperkalaemia	Estimation of the plasma electrolyte level, e.g. Na^+, K^+, Cl^- is possible but is frequently of limited value in determining the degree of dehydration as recorded values are not always an accurate reflection of the total body content of the individual ion
Plasma lactate	Lactate is produced during anaerobic metabolism. Increases in plasma lactate levels (> 2 mmol/l) may be indicative of poor perfusion	
Arterial blood gases	Provides information about acid–base balance in addition to respiratory function including PaO_2 and $PaCO_2$	Handheld patient-side analysers now readily available, e.g. i-STAT® (Fig. 8.3)

*Packed cell volume and haemoglobin (Hb) concentration alone do not determine oxygen delivery. Other factors such as cardiac output are important. However, acute blood loss with a PCV ≤ 20 may necessitate administration of whole blood before or during anaesthesia and target pre-anaesthetic PCVs of 30–34% in dogs and 25–29% in cats have been suggested (Moon 1991). Whether or not an individual patient with a PCV or Hb concentration below the normal or pre-anaesthetic target range actually requires a transfusion before anaesthesia depends on several factors: type of procedure and expected blood loss, age of patient, presence of cardiac disease that may affect cardiac output and pre-existing disease, e.g. animals in chronic renal failure may tolerate a lower than normal Hb better than healthy patients.

and nutrients by cells occurs, the patient is said to be suffering from 'shock'.

Clinical assessment of perfusion allows an estimate of the severity of shock. In particular heart rate, mucous membrane colour (Fig. 8.4), capillary refill time, pulse quality and the ability to palpate a peripheral pulse should be evaluated (see box, page 187).

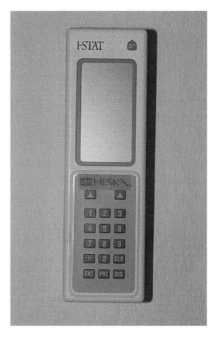

Fig. 8.3 i-STAT® bedside biochemistry, haematology and blood gas analyser.

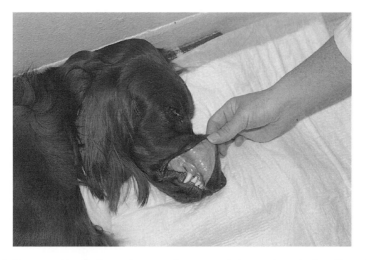

Fig. 8.4 Depressed level of consciousness in a severely hypovolaemic dog. The colour of the mucous membrane is abnormal.

CLINICAL SIGNS OF POOR PERFUSION (SHOCK)
Weak rapid pulse with reduced pulse pressure and duration
Increased heart rate (tachycardia) with quiet heart sounds
Pale mucous membranes
Prolonged capillary refill time (≥ 2 seconds)
Increased ventilation
Slow jugular refill and collapsed peripheral veins
Hypothermia and cold extremities
Depressed level of consciousness (Fig. 8.4)
Muscle weakness

Ongoing losses

Anaesthetised patients may have losses in excess of those normally expected in conscious patients. Under general anaesthesia both sensible and insensible losses continue. Generally, these losses are at least matched if maintenance fluids are administered during anaesthesia. However, relative or absolute volume depletion can occur as a direct result of either the general anaesthetic protocol or the surgical procedure performed. Potential causes of increased fluid loss or circulatory compromise under general anaesthesia include the following.

Anaesthetic drugs

Many anaesthetic drugs can cause vasodilation and thus relative hypovolaemia (see Table 8.4). This means that the patient may have a normal circulating blood volume but the capacity (volume) of the vessels is increased. Anaesthetic drugs may also decrease cardiac output. This can cause a perfusion deficit.

Anaesthetic techniques

Intermittent positive pressure ventilation can reduce venous return to the heart and thus cardiac output. IPPV also increases central venous pressure and the consequent increase in renal venous pressure can decrease renal interstitial pressure and urine production. IPPV may also increase production of antidiuretic hormone (ADH).

Regional anaesthetic techniques can cause hypotension (see above).

Respiratory losses

Delivery of dry gases from non-rebreathing systems directly to the respiratory tract increases evaporative losses of fluid. This can contribute to dehydration.

Evaporative losses from the surgical site

This is particularly important during intra-abdominal and intrathoracic surgery because the peritoneum and pleura, respectively, present extremely large evaporative surface areas. Prolonged surgery and high ambient temperatures in the theatre can further increase evaporative losses. This can contribute to dehydration.

Table 8.4 Anaesthetic drugs: mechanism of action and effects on fluid balance.

Drug	Mechanism of action	Effects on fluid balance
Acetylpromazine	α_1 antagonist	Hypotension
	Dopamine antagonist	? Inhibit effects of dopamine on renal blood flow
Xylazine, medetomidine	α_2 agonist	↓ Cardiac output / hypotension Diuresis
Opioids	OP3 agonists	Antidiuretic effect (?ADH release)
	OP2 agonists	Diuretic effect
Ketamine	↓ Baroreceptor responses	Diminished response to relative hypovolaemia
Propofol, thiopentone	Hypotension	Relative hypovolaemia due to vasodilation
Halothane		Dose-dependent depression of cardiovascular system (↓CO) with hypotension
Isoflurane		Relative hypovolaemia due to vasodilation
Local anaesthetics	Extradural techniques for thoracotomy when sympathetic outflow tracts are blocked	Relative hypovolaemia due to vasodilation

Operative blood loss

Loss of whole blood during surgery can occur (Fig. 8.5). These losses can be estimated in a number of ways:

10×10 cm swab (dry initially) – 5–10 ml blood
12×12 inch laparotomy swab – Approx. 50 ml blood
Weigh swabs (assume negligible dry weight) – 1 g = 1 ml blood
Blood in suction apparatus – Volume in container

ESTIMATION OF AMOUNT OF BLOOD IN LAVAGE FLUID

$$X = \frac{L \times V}{P - L}$$

where
X = amount of blood lost
L = PCV of the returned lavage fluid
V = volume of lavage fluid infused
P = PCV of the peripheral blood before IV infusion of fluids

Operative blood loss can cause a perfusion deficit.

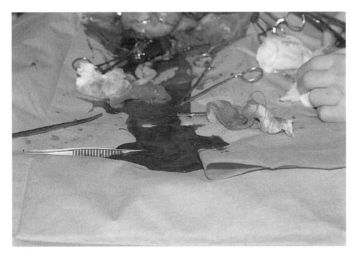

Fig. 8.5 Loss of whole blood during a caesarean operation.

Loss of transudates, modified transudates or exudates from surgical wounds

It may be possible to estimate such losses either by weighing soaked dressings, measuring the volume of fluid recovered from surgical drains or by simply measuring the weight of the patient on a regular basis. Such losses can cause a perfusion deficit.

Third spacing of fluids

The normal body spaces containing fluids are the intracellular space and extracellular space, i.e. the intravascular and interstitial spaces. Third spacing occurs when fluid moves into the interstitial space, as with oedema, inflammation and burns, or into body cavities (e.g. ascites; Fig. 8.6) and with intestinal ileus. Consequently, although there may be enough total fluid in the body, the fluid may not be able to return readily to the circulation and contribute to normal fluid dynamics. Third spacing creates the potential for hypovolaemia and decreased urine output. A patient with significant uncorrected third spacing will have a high urine specific gravity. This can contribute to dehydration and reduce perfusion if severe.

Increased salivary losses

Patients with postoperative nausea may salivate excessively (ptyalism), which may also be observed in animals in pain. This can contribute to dehydration.

Hyperthermia

Large patients with long hair coats can become overheated during anaesthesia, particularly if supplemental heating is provided, e.g. thermostatically controlled heat pad or table. This can lead to an increased insensible fluid loss as in

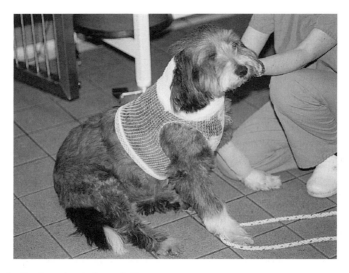

Fig. 8.6 Ascites in a dog in heart failure.

pyrexic patients. This can contribute to dehydration and reduce perfusion if severe.

Ongoing losses as a consequence of pre-existing disease
During and following anaesthesia compromised patients may continue to lose excess body fluid through pathological processes, e.g. urine, vomit, diarrhoea, pyrexia, and so on. This can contribute to dehydration and reduce perfusion if severe.

> Volume of fluid required =
> Fluid deficit + Maintenance fluid requirement + Ongoing losses

In addition to deficits in the circulating volume, general anaesthesia and surgery may cause acid–base disturbances. Metabolic acidosis (reduced tissue perfusion) and respiratory acidosis (hypoventilation) are most frequently encountered.

INTRAVENOUS FLUID SELECTION

Colloids and crystalloids are the two fluid types available for intravenous or intraosseous administration. Colloids are fluids that contain large molecules that remain within the circulation and increase the plasma effective oncotic pressure and expand plasma volume. Both natural and synthetic colloids are available. Crystalloids are non-colloidal fluids that contain ions or solutes and pass readily through cell membranes. They do not remain within the extracellular fluid compartment but equilibrate with the intracellular fluid compartment.

An isotonic balanced crystalloid is an appropriate choice of fluid in most circumstances for healthy anaesthetised patients and may also be administered to correct pre-existing dehydration. Crystalloids also provide adequate circulatory support in hypotensive patients if appropriate volumes are administered.

Hartmann's solution (lactated Ringer's solution)

This crystalloid is an isotonic, balanced electrolyte solution. A balanced electrolyte solution is one that closely resembles plasma electrolyte concentrations. In addition to water, Hartmann's contains sodium, potassium, chloride, calcium and also lactate. Lactate is metabolised by the liver to form bicarbonate. Some clinicians are concerned about the ability of patients with hepatic disease to metabolise lactate to bicarbonate, thus causing or exacerbating pre-existing acidosis. This does not appear to happen as lactate can be metabolised by peripheral tissues (Pascoe 2000). However, the patient must be adequately perfused to facilitate this! Similar balanced electrolyte solutions containing different buffers, e.g. acetate, are available. They do not rely on hepatic function for metabolism to bicarbonate and so may be useful in patients with impaired hepatic function.

Hartmann's solution contains calcium and so it should not be administered through the same fluid administration set as blood products as clot formation may rapidly occur.

Sodium chloride 0.9% (normal saline)

This crystalloid is an isotonic electrolyte solution but is not balanced. Normal saline contains sodium and chloride and water. It is considered an acidifying solution as administration dilutes plasma bicarbonate concentrations.

Ringer's solution

This crystalloid is an isotonic, balanced electrolyte solution. In addition to water, Ringer's solution contains sodium, potassium, chloride and calcium. It is considered an acidifying solution as administration dilutes plasma bicarbonate concentrations.

Following intravenous administration of Hartmann's, Ringer's or normal saline solutions, only approximately 20% of the administered volume will remain within the intravascular space after 1 h. The remaining fluid will redistribute to the interstitial fluid compartment, but not to the intracellular fluid compartment because these fluids are isotonic and no concentration gradient exists. If these fluids are administered to improve perfusion, e.g. following haemorrhage, at least three times the volume of blood lost must be administered to replace intravascular volume because of the redistribution that occurs.

Glucose 5% (dextrose 5%)

This crystalloid is an isotonic solution of glucose in water. Following administration of this solution the glucose is rapidly taken up by the cells and metabolised.

Consequently, the glucose molecules only exert a transient osmotic effect, and so 5% glucose solutions are used to deliver free water in an osmotically acceptable form to patients. Glucose 5% is not suitable for intravascular volume expansion because the free water provided will distribute equally between all body fluid compartments and this is only rarely indicated for anaesthetised patients.

Sodium chloride 0.18%–glucose 4% (glucose saline)

This crystalloid is an isotonic electrolyte solution but is not balanced. It contains sodium, chloride and glucose in addition to water. This crystalloid is often used to provide maintenance fluid requirements and must be supplemented with potassium if administered for a prolonged period. Glucose saline is not suitable for intravascular volume expansion because the free water provided will distribute equally between all body fluid compartments.

Sodium chloride 7.2% (hypertonic saline)

This crystalloid is a hypertonic electrolyte solution and is not balanced. Hypertonic saline contains sodium and chloride and water. This solution is used for rapid intravascular volume replacement and has been shown to increase cardiac contractility and output.

A dose of 4–7 ml/kg (dogs) and 2–4 ml/kg (cats) is administered. Because the solution is hypertonic, fluid is drawn into the intravascular space from the interstitial and intracellular fluid compartments. However, the effects are short-lived (30–60 min) as the sodium diffuses out of the vascular space. The effects may be prolonged by concurrent administration of a colloid. Although hypertonic saline is a good resuscitation fluid, ultimately the fluid deficit must be replaced with either an isotonic crystalloid or a colloidal solution.

Hypertonic saline is useful to correct perfusion deficits but it is contraindicated in dehydration because the interstitial and intracellular spaces will not have an adequate fluid load to provide water for the intravascular space. It is also contraindicated where there is uncontrolled haemorrhage as the rapid volume expansion achieved can precipitate further haemorrhage, and should also be used with caution in patients with cardiorespiratory disease (Hughes 1999).

Intravenous fluid supplements

Potassium chloride

This crystalloid is available in various strengths and is used to supplement potassium levels (Table 8.5). Hypokalaemia can cause muscle weakness and cardiac arrythmias. The maximum infusion rate for potassium is 0.5 mEq/kg/h and it is important not to exceed this level (Fig. 8.7).

Sodium bicarbonate 8.4% (equivalent to 1 mmol/ml)

Sodium bicarbonate may be administered to correct severe acidosis following estimation of arterial or venous blood gas values. This drug can also be used in the management of hyperkalaemia.

Table 8.5 Use of potassium chloride in fluid supplements.

Serum potassium (mEq/l)	mEq/l KCl added to 250 ml of fluids
< 2	20
2.1–2.5	15
2.6–3.0	10
3.1–3.5	7

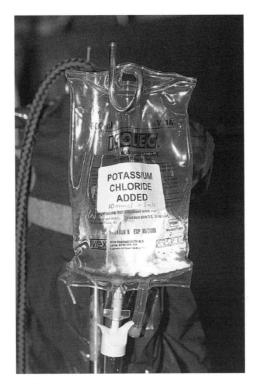

Fig. 8.7 It is important to label intravenous fluid bags to alert clinicians and nurses when drugs or other medications are added to the fluid bag.

Calcium

Hypocalcaemia causes increased neuromuscular excitability and calcium gluconate may be administered to correct such deficits. Calcium gluconate or chloride solutions can also be used in the management of hyperkalaemia.

Glucose

Glucose supplementation may be required in a number of anaesthetised patients including neonates and those that are septic, those with diabetes mellitus, Addison's disease, hepatic disorders, insulinomas, portosystemic shunts and neoplasia. Close monitoring of blood glucose levels every 30–120 min both during anaesthesia and in the postoperative period is essential, as the normal clinical signs of hypoglycaemia will either not be apparent under anaesthesia or may be missed in the recovering patient.

If hypoglycaemia is detected, glucose may be added to a balanced electrolyte solution and administered to the patient, for example, 2.5–5% glucose in Hartmann's solution at a rate of 3–5 ml/kg/h. (Adding 31.25 ml of 40% glucose solution to 468.75 ml of Hartmann's solution provides 2.5% glucose solution in Hartmann's.) The administration rate should be adjusted according to the blood glucose estimation.

Many clinicians debate whether crystalloids or colloids are the most suitable fluid for resuscitation of patients with perfusion deficits (shock). Typically, an excess of colloid leads to circulatory overload with right-sided heart failure and ultimately congestive cardiac failure. Too much crystalloid, on the other hand, will initially stimulate diuresis (*via* inhibition of antidiuretic hormone (ADH) release) in patients with normal renal function, but as the electrolyte solution moves from the circulation into the remainder of the extracellular space, signs of oedema may develop, i.e. fluid will accumulate in the interstitial fluid space. Most seriously, pulmonary oedema may develop which will initially impair oxygenation; however, ultimately it can result in the death of the patient. Some clinicians may prefer a combination of crystalloid and colloid if the patient has signs of both dehydration and poor perfusion, but for patients with known or expected perfusion problems and in patients with hypoalbuminaemia colloids are useful because smaller volumes may be administered to achieve expansion of the intravascular space and colloids can supplement plasma oncotic pressure in the face of low plasma protein levels.

Gelatins (Haemaccel®, Gelofusine®)

The gelatins are synthetic colloids produced from animal collagen. They are delivered in fluids containing sodium and chloride, although some (e.g. Haemaccel®) also contain potassium and calcium. These fluids are hyperoncotic.

Dextrans (Dextran 70, 6% solution; Dextran 40, 10% solution)

The dextrans are synthetic colloids. They are polysaccharides produced by bacterial fermentation of sucrose. They are delivered in fluids containing either 0.9% sodium chloride or 5% glucose. These fluids are hyperoncotic.

Starches (e.g. Hespan 6%®)

A range of synthetic colloids based on hydroxyethyl starch (HES) is available. They are made from amylopectin derived from corn wax. They are delivered in fluids containing sodium and chloride. These fluids are either iso- or hyperoncotic.

Oxyglobin®

Oxyglobin® is a synthetic colloid produced from purified bovine haemoglobin.

It does not contain red blood cells and it is delivered in lactated Ringer's solution. This synthetic colloid is novel as it not only provides oncotic support but also oxygen-carrying capacity. This fluid is hyperoncotic.

Whole blood

Whole blood is a natural colloid and when administered fresh provides oncotic support, red blood cells, and platelets and clotting factors. Before infusion, cross-matching and/or blood typing should be performed to ensure the blood is compatible for transfusion. The A antigen is the most important factor in canine blood typing and ideally donor dogs should be A negative (DEA 1.1 negative). However, initial transfusion reactions are unusual in dogs. Most cats are type A and the chance of an incompatible reaction occurring if the blood is not typed prior to transfusion can be as high as 60%. In-house blood typing kits for both dogs and cats are now available and should be used before transfusion whenever possible (Fig. 8.8).

In addition to transfusion reactions (immediate immune and non-immune-mediated and delayed immune-mediated) other complications may occur following blood transfusion: pyrogenic reactions, acidosis, over-administration, air emboli, citrate toxicity and hypothermia.

Plasma

Plasma is a natural colloid and in addition to providing oncotic support it is suitable for animals that are hypoproteinaemic as it provides albumin. Fresh and fresh frozen plasma contains albumin and clotting factors; frozen plasma contains albumin.

Table 8.6 summarises the fluids discussed.

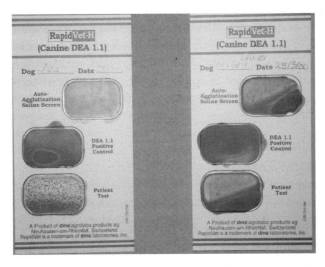

Fig. 8.8 Rapid-H® blood typing card. Cards are available for in-house blood typing of dogs and cats. Photograph courtesy of Alison Ridyard.

Table 8.6 Fluids and indications for use.

Fluid	Fluid type	Indications	Specific indications
Hartmann's	Crystalloid	Fluid replacement	Acidosis
		Intravascular volume resuscitation	Hypernatraemia
Normal saline	Crystalloid	Fluid replacement	Alkalosis
		Intravascular volume resuscitation	Hypochloraemic alkalosis (pre-pyloric vomiting)
			Hypercalcaemia
			Hyperkalaemia
			Hyponatraemia
			Addison's disease
Ringer's	Crystalloid	Fluid replacement	Alkalosis
		Intravascular volume resuscitation	
5% glucose	Crystalloid	Fluid replacement	Loss of pure water
Glucose saline	Crystalloid	Maintenance fluid	
Hypertonic saline	Crystalloid	Rapid intravascular volume resuscitation	
Gelatins	Synthetic colloid	Rapid intravascular volume resuscitation	
Dextrans	Synthetic colloid	Rapid intravascular volume resuscitation	
Starches	Synthetic colloid	Rapid intravascular volume resuscitation	Septic inflammatory response syndrome
Oxyglobin	Synthetic colloid	Oxygen-carrying capacity	Anaemia (dogs)
Fresh whole blood (0–6 h)	Natural colloid	Rapid intravascular volume resuscitation	Acute haemorrhage
			Anaemia with hypoalbuminaemia
			Thrombocytopenia
			Coagulopathy
Stored whole blood	Natural colloid	Rapid intravascular volume resuscitation	Acute haemorrhage
			Anaemia with hypoalbuminaemia
Fresh / fresh frozen plasma (0-6 h)	Natural colloid	Rapid intravascular volume resuscitation	Hypoalbuminaemia
			Coagulopathy
Frozen plasma (collected from stored blood)	Natural colloid	Rapid intravascular volume resuscitation	Hypoalbuminaemia

Calculation of fluid requirements during anaesthesia

The majority of patients that undergo general anaesthesia will be clinically healthy and have had free access to water until the time of administration of pre-anaesthetic medication. They may have no requirement for replacement fluids and have few ongoing losses under anaesthesia. It could be assumed that these patients will compensate for any minor fluid deficits by increasing their oral fluid intake following a rapid recovery from general anaesthesia. Unfortunately, for a variety of reasons (patients are not anaesthetised when anticipated or are anaesthetised longer than anticipated; water is not made available in the recovery area, and so on) this scenario probably occurs for very few animals. Moreover, regardless of the health of the patient before induction of anaesthesia, the drugs used for pre-anaesthetic medication and induction and maintenance of anaesthesia can have significant effects on the circulation that the animal's normal physiological homeostatic mechanisms are unable to compensate for. Furthermore, many anaesthetic agents are metabolised by the liver and excreted by the kidneys, and adequate perfusion is essential to facilitate these processes. Thus, ideally, all patients should be provided with circulatory support both during anaesthesia and in the recovery period.

Fluid administration rates of 5–10 ml/kg/h for balanced isotonic crystalloids are routinely used for such patients. This 'maintenance' rate for anaesthetised animals is greater than that used in conscious healthy patients (~2 ml/kg/h) to provide not only for sensible and insensible fluid losses (which may be increased) but also to support the circulation in the face of the possible haemodynamic effects of the anaesthetic drugs.

Some authors recommend normal maintenance fluid rates of 2 ml/kg/h under anaesthesia initially, increasing the administration rate intra-operatively by an additional 5, 10 or 15 ml/kg/h depending on the perceived severity of surgery, i.e. mild, moderate and severe surgical trauma, respectively (Muir *et al.* 2000). However, the patient's clinical response to the fluid load provided must always be closely monitored and the fluid administration rate adjusted accordingly, regardless of the initial approach adopted.

The anaesthetic maintenance rate may be increased, for example, in patients with significant pre-existing fluid deficits and/or ongoing losses that have not been corrected prior to anaesthesia, or in response to increased fluid losses or haemodynamic changes causing hypotension during anaesthesia. It is important to remember that rapid replacement of chronic fluid losses in this way may lead to haemodilution and dilution of plasma proteins and electrolytes, and that by preference such deficits are replaced over a period of at least 4–6 h (if not over 24 h) prior to anaesthesia.

Administration of 3 ml of a balanced electrolyte solution for each 1 ml blood loss will provide adequate circulatory support until the total protein levels fall below 35 g/l. After this a colloidal fluid such as a gelatin may be more suitable. Similarly, when the PCV falls acutely below 20% whole blood may be the fluid of choice to ensure adequate oxygen-carrying capacity. However, these guidelines are just that – guidelines: some individuals may require more aggressive circulatory support at either an earlier or a later stage.

Patients anaesthetised for minor procedures with minimal expected fluid loss or non-surgical investigations and those with cardiac disease, oliguric or anuric renal failure, pulmonary oedema, pulmonary contusions, head trauma and closed cavity haemorrhage (e.g. haemothorax) may require significantly lower fluid administration rates under general anaesthesia, and when anaesthetising these patients it is particularly important to be alert to the clinical signs associated with over-hydration:

- serous nasal discharge;
- subcutaneous oedema;
- increased urinary output with normal renal function;
- chemosis;
- exophthalmos;
- increased respiration rate.

Additional signs that can be observed in response to over-hydration in the postoperative period include shivering, nausea, vomiting, restlessness, coughing and ascites.

Constant rate infusions

The veterinary surgeon may wish to administer certain drugs to anaesthetised patients by constant rate infusion (CRI), e.g. morphine, dobutamine.

Dosages for most drugs given by CRI are expressed in micrograms, but the drugs are available in concentrations of milligrams per ml. The following formulae allow conversion from micrograms to milligrams.

Quantity of drug (mg) to be added to fluids for infusion for µg/kg/min infusion

$$\frac{\text{Dose rate of drug (µg/kg/min)} \times \text{body weight (kg)} \times \text{volume of fluid (ml)}}{\text{Delivery rate (ml/h)} \times 16.67 \text{ (conversion factor)}}$$

Delivery rate (ml/h) of the infusion

$$\frac{\text{Dose rate of drug (µg/kg/min)} \times \text{body weight (kg)} \times \text{volume of fluid (ml)}}{\text{Quantity of drug (mg) added to fluids} \times 16.67}$$

(Continued)

> ## Quantity of drug (mg) to be added to fluids for infusion for mg/kg/min infusion
>
> Dose rate of drug (mg/kg/h) $\times$ body weight (kg) $\times \dfrac{\text{volume of fluid (ml)}}{\text{Delivery rate (ml/h)}}$

FLUID ADMINISTRATION

Access to the circulation is important in any anaesthetised animal, whether anaesthetised for short or longer periods or anaesthetised using intramuscular, intravenous or inhalational methods. It is especially important should an emergency occur under anaesthesia, e.g. cardiopulmonary arrest. Intravenous access allows circulatory system support, administration of drugs and collection of blood samples. Intraosseous access may be used in preference in certain situations, e.g. neonates, small and exotic species.

The fluid line should be checked before surgical drapes are placed to ensure fluids can run freely, e.g. the animal's leg may need to be extended. Regardless of the route of administration, it is essential that the veterinary nurse monitoring anaesthesia has access to the fluid administration line, allowing additional drugs to be administered through injection ports either on the administration line itself or at the T-port. If necessary the fluid administration line should be labelled, allowing easy identification in an emergency. This is particularly important when intra-arterial lines are being used in addition to intravenous lines.

Although parenteral fluids must be stored according to manufacturers' instructions, they should be warmed to normal body temperature before administration. The overwrap should be left in place while the fluids are warmed to ensure the integrity of the solution. A number of methods are available to warm fluids including forced warm air ovens (controlled by a calibrated thermometer) and warm water baths. A standard warming procedure cannot be recommended for microwave ovens because of variations in wattage and performance from oven to oven. Once warmed, the fluid bag may be insulated with wheat, cherry stone or gel-filled bags that can be heated in a microwave oven. Warmed fluids should either be used within 24 h of removing from the heat source or discarded and not returned to stock.

Unfortunately, the problem lies, not in heating the fluid bag initially, but in keeping the fluids warm as they travel down the administration line. This is particularly difficult when small rates of administration are required, and this will tend to be in smaller patients who are already at greater risk of hypothermia. Parenteral fluids may be run through coiled administration tubing placed in a warm water bath close to the patient. This technique has several disadvantages including poor regulation of temperature and the ease with which such water baths may be spilled!

Although body heat losses by radiation, conduction, convection and evaporation are much greater than those caused by administering fluids at room temperature (or lower) the effect may well be more significant if rapid infusion of large fluid volumes is required.

Intravenous catheters

There are various types of intravenous catheters available. The choice of catheter is dependent on several factors including operator experience, availability, cost and patient requirements.

Over-the-needle catheters

Over-the-needle catheters (Fig. 8.9) are usually placed in peripheral vessels, but can be used in the jugular veins of smaller patients and neonates. They are available in a range of sizes (10–24 gauge) and varying lengths (1.9–13 cm). They are made of Teflon, polypropylene or polyurethane. The latter is believed to be less thrombogenic than other materials. They are generally used for short-term intravenous therapy of up to 72 h but may be maintained for longer in the absence of signs of thrombophlebitis or local infection. If rapid administration of fluid is required a short, a large-gauge catheter should be chosen to allow maximal flow rates.

Through-the-needle catheters

Through-the-needle catheters (Fig. 8.10) tend to be longer catheters (20–30 cm), available in a range of sizes (14–22 gauge) that are used to gain central venous access. They are commonly placed in the external jugular vein so that the catheter tip lies within the cranial vena cava. Placing the catheter in the medial saphenous vessel can also access the caudal vena cava.

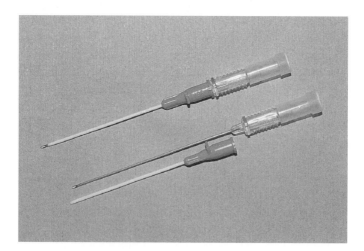

Fig. 8.9 An over-the-needle catheter.

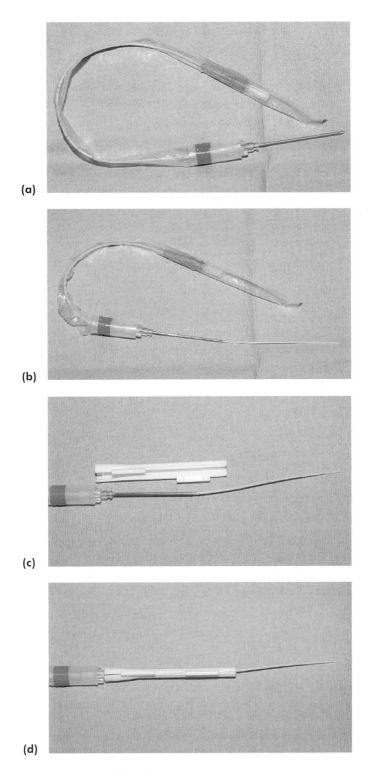

(a)

(b)

(c)

(d)

Fig. 8.10 A through-the-needle catheter.

Central venous access allows for easy removal of blood samples, which reduces the distress of patients requiring multiple blood sampling. Additional advantages include the facility for central venous pressure measurement, administration of hypertonic solutions, rapid administration of drugs used in cardiopulmonary resuscitation and administration of other agents and parenteral nutrition. Furthermore, the catheters are easy to secure and the flow of fluids is not affected by patient positioning.

Multilumen catheters

Multilumen catheters are available for delivering multiple fluid or drug therapies. They have separate entrance and exit ports, and therefore incompatible solutions can be administered simultaneously. Double- or triple-lumen catheters are available in a large selection of lengths and sizes. They are commonly placed using a guidewire or an introducer that peels away.

SITES SUITABLE FOR VENOUS CATHETERISATION IN DOGS AND CATS

Peripheral veins

Cephalic
Accessory cephalic
Medial saphenous
Lateral saphenous
Auricular

Central veins

Jugular
Medial saphenous
Femoral

EQUIPMENT REQUIRED FOR INTRAVENOUS CATHETER PLACEMENT

Appropriate catheter
Scalpel
T-connector or injection bung
Clippers
2 ml heparinised saline
Chlorhexidine surgical scrub
Cohesive bandage
Isopropyl alcohol

(Continued)

Gloves
Swabs
Adhesive tape
Semi-occlusive dressing
Padding bandage
Assistant

Additional equipment required for central venous catheter placement

Sterile fenestrated drape
Sterile gloves
Suture material
± Antibiotic ointment

Preparation for catheter placement

Strict aseptic technique should be observed for skin preparation and catheter insertion to reduce the incidence of catheter-related infections. A generous clip centred on the intended venipuncture site should be performed. No hair should be in contact with the catheter during or following placement.

Hands should be washed with a detergent or antiseptic solution, dried using disposable papers towels or an air drier, and disposable gloves donned. The patient's skin is cleaned with a suitable surgical scrub, e.g. chlorhexidine, using gauze swabs or cotton balls. This will remove surface debris. Do not scrub the skin aggressively as this will increase the bacteria rising to the skin surface from the deeper skin layers and hair follicles. Residual scrub solution is removed by wiping with isopropyl alcohol.

Techniques for catheter placement

The techniques used for placement of the different catheter types are described in the boxes below.

PLACEMENT OF AN OVER-THE-NEEDLE CATHETER
(see Fig. 8.11)
- Collect equipment and flush T-connector/injection bung with heparinised saline.
- An assistant restrains the patient.
- Clip a generous patch of hair over the injection site.
- Prepare the site with surgical scrub, followed by wiping with alcohol (a).
- An assistant raises the vein.

(Continued)

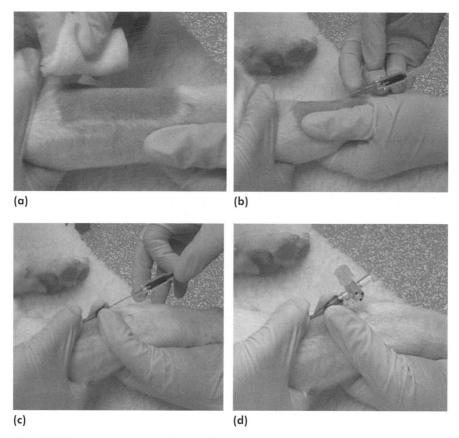

(a)   (b)

(c)   (d)

Fig. 8.11 Placement of an over-the-needle catheter.

- The skin is held taut with one hand to stabilise the vein. The catheter is held firmly at the junction of the needle and catheter hub and inserted through the skin and into the vein. (Occasionally a small nick with a no. 11 scalpel blade may be required. This will allow the catheter to pass through without damage to the catheter tip.)
- Once the vein is penetrated, blood will flush back into the hub of the catheter. The catheter is advanced a few millimetres to ensure the catheter tip is within the lumen of the vein (b).
- The stylet should be immobilised with one hand, while the outer catheter is advanced into the vein (c).
- The assistant now occludes the vein at the level of the tip of the catheter while the stylet is removed. This prevents spillage of blood.
- An injection bung, T-connector or 3-way tap is attached (d).
- The catheter and connector are secured in place using adhesive tapes.
- Flush the catheter with heparinised saline to ensure correct placement and maintain patency.
- The catheter site is covered with a sterile dressing to maintain asepsis and bandaged in place using padding bandage followed by cohesive bandage.

PLACEMENT OF THROUGH-THE-NEEDLE CATHETER (See Fig. 8.10)

- Collect equipment required and flush T-connector/injection bung with heparinised saline.
- An assistant restrains the patient in lateral recumbency, with the head extended and the forelimbs drawn caudally.
- The site over the jugular vein is clipped and prepared aseptically as for surgery.
- Sterile gloves are donned and a fenestrated drape is placed over the site.
- An assistant raises the jugular vein.
- The needle is inserted through the skin and into the jugular vein distally (a).
- When blood has flowed back into the hub, the catheter is threaded through the needle into the vein (b).
- The needle is withdrawn from the vein lumen and the skin.
- The protective needle guard is placed over the needle and all sections are connected tightly (c, d).
- Attach the pre-flushed T-connector and flush the catheter with heparinised saline.
- The protective guard can be sutured to the skin to secure the unit in place.
- Antibiotic ointment may be applied to the catheter entry site and a sterile dressing is applied.
- The neck is bandaged with a layer of padding bandage, followed by cohesive or stockinette bandage. Ensure the bandage is not too tight around the neck as this may restrict breathing.

PLACEMENT OF PEEL-AWAY-SHEATH CATHETER

- Collect equipment required and flush T-connector/injection bung with heparinised saline.
- Restraint and aseptic preparation is carried out as described previously for through-the-needle catheters.
- A small skin incision is made with a no. 11 scalpel blade.
- Insert the sheathed catheter through the small nick in the skin and into the vessel.
- Once within the vessel, the needle is stabilised and the sheath is advanced into the vessel.
- The needle is removed and a gloved finger is placed over the opening to prevent excessive haemorrhage or inadvertent air embolisation.
- The catheter is inserted through the sheath's lumen and advanced into position.
- The two knobs of the sheath are grasped and pulled outwards and upwards at the same time, to peel away the sheath from the catheter. Care must be taken to avoid displacing the catheter (see Fig. 8.12).
- The catheter is flushed, capped and sutured to the skin.
- The site is dressed as described previously.

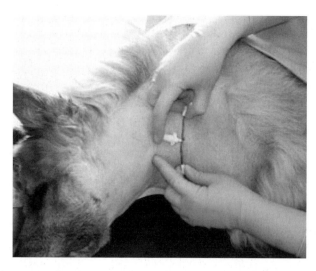

Fig. 8.12 Placement of peel-away sheath catheter.

SELDINGER TECHNIQUE FOR INTRODUCING CATHETERS
(see Fig. 8.13)
- Collect equipment required and flush T-connector/injection bung with heparinised saline.
- Restraint and aseptic preparation is described previously for through-the-needle catheters.
- Insert a percutaneous entry needle into the vessel (a).
- Pass the guidewire through the needle and advance a portion of the wire into the vessel (b).
- Withdraw the needle from the vessel and off the wire (c).
- Enlarge the puncture hole into the vessel wall by passing a dilator down the guidewire and rotate it to facilitate insertion (optional on some occasions). The dilator is removed, leaving the wire in place.
- The catheter is advanced over the guidewire and into the vessel (d).
- Remove the wire, cap the catheter and flush with heparinised saline (e).
- Suture catheter to the skin and dress as described previously.

Intraosseous needles

Intraosseous needles provide an alternative direct route into the circulation. Intraosseous access is particularly useful in an emergency when intravenous access is difficult due to collapse of the vascular system. They also are often used in paediatric patients and small mammals where venous cannulation is difficult due to the small size of the patient. Various needles can be used for intraosseous injection, but most commonly needles with central stylet, e.g. spinal needles, or

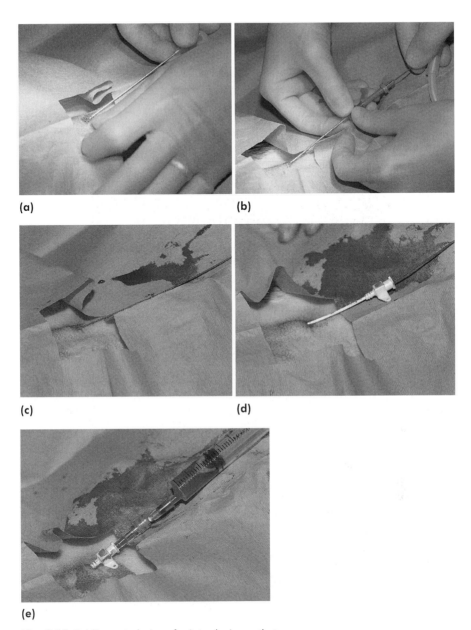

(a)   (b)

(c)   (d)

(e)

Fig. 8.13 Seldinger technique for introducing catheters.

commercial intraosseous needles are used (14–20 gauge). Hypodermic needles
are occasionally used in paediatric patients and small mammals.

The system can be managed in a similar manner to an intravenous catheter
and they can remain *in situ* for up to 72 h, though they are more difficult to
secure in ambulatory patients.

SITES FOR INTRAOSSEOUS NEEDLE PLACEMENT
Greater tubercle humerus
Intertrochanteric fossa femur
Medial surface of proximal tibia
Wing of ileum
Tibial tuberosity

Technique for intraosseous needle placement
The technique used for placement of intraosseous needles is described in the box below.

PLACEMENT OF AN INTRAOSSEOUS NEEDLE
(see Fig. 8.14)
- Collect equipment required and flush T-connector/injection bung with heparinised saline.
- An assistant restrains the patient in lateral recumbency.
- The skin over the proposed needle placement site is clipped and prepared aseptically as for surgery.
- Sterile gloves are donned and a fenestrated drape may be used.
- A small skin incision is made with a no. 11 scalpel blade over the site of needle placement.
- The needle is inserted through the skin incision and seated firmly into the cortex of the selected bone using gentle rotation.
- Once the needle has penetrated the cortex of the bone it will advance easily into the medullary cavity.
- The stylet (if present) is removed from the needle and gentle suction applied with a sterile syringe. If the needle is correctly positioned bone marrow will be aspirated.
- Cap the needle and flush with heparinised saline to main patency.
- Secure the needle to the skin and dress the area with a sterile dressing appropriate to the site selected.

Maintaining intravenous catheters
It is extremely important to maintain aseptic technique during both placement and subsequent handling of intravenous (IV) catheters and intraosseous (IO) needles. A number of simple steps can be taken to ensure this happens:

- Wash and dry hands and don disposable gloves before and after handling IV catheters and IO needles.

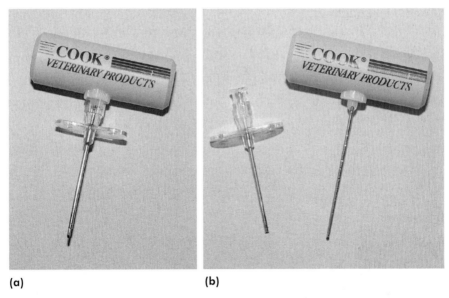

(a)   (b)

Fig. 8.14 (a) An intraosseous needle; (b) with stylet removed.

- Maintain a closed system at all times with the use of injection caps or stop-cocks.
- Flush indwelling catheters and needles regularly with heparinised saline to maintain patency when not in use (every 4–6 h).
- Ensure the protective dressing is kept dry and clean and the catheter or needle is assessed at least daily.
- Replace the dressing promptly if it becomes contaminated with urine, faeces, vomit, saliva, or other exudates.
- The catheter should be removed and an alternative vein catheterised if any signs of redness, swelling, pain or fever are present which might indicate thrombophlebitis. The catheter tip can be cultured if a catheter-related septicaemia is suspected.

FLUID DELIVERY SYSTEMS

There are various methods available to administer intravenous fluids at a set rate per minute or per hour.

Giving sets
Giving sets can be categorised into three types: standard, paediatric and blood sets. It is important to remember that, if infusion pumps are to be used, the brand of infusion set must be compatible with the equipment.

Standard giving sets
Standard giving sets deliver 15 or 20 drops/ml, but can vary with the manufacturer, therefore the package must be checked prior to calculating the drip rate.

Paediatric sets
Paediatric sets deliver 60 drops/ml. This allows more accurate administration
of smaller flow rates.

Blood sets
Blood sets incorporate a nylon net filter to remove any coagulation debris during blood transfusion. They generally deliver 15 or 20 drops/ml.

Burettes
A burette is a graduated chamber that holds a small amount of fluid, e.g. 150 ml
(Fig. 8.15). They are incorporated into the fluid system as either part of the giving set itself, or as a separate attachment which is connected to a standard giving set. They are designed for precise measurement and control of small volume
infusions in animals. They are also useful in drug therapy, when the agent must
be administered over a set period of time.

Fluid infusion pumps
Fluids are commonly administered by gravity flow with manual adjustment
of a roller clamp to select the appropriate number of drops per minute. The

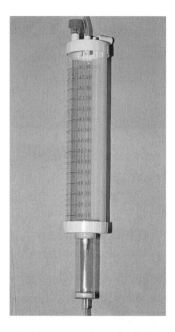

Fig. 8.15 A burette. This may be incorporated into the fluid system as either part of the giving set itself, or as a separate attachment which is connected to a standard giving set.

fluid bag must be placed above the level of the patient to ensure fluid flows into the patient and to prevent the backflow of blood from the patient. Problems encountered using this system include difficulty in maintaining constant flow, high dependency on patient position to maintain flow, and inaccurate visual selection of drip rate.

$$\text{Drops per minute} = \frac{\text{Body weight (kg)} \times \text{Infusion rate (ml/h)} \times \text{Infusion set calibration (drops/ml)}}{60 \text{ (minutes in 1 h)}}$$

Infusion pumps and drip rate counters may be used to regulate and monitor fluid administration rate and overcome some of the problems encountered using the manual gravity flow system.

Infusion pumps operate either by applying peristaltic pressures to the outside of the giving set and measuring the rate of flow by counting the drops passing through an optical gate clipped on to the drip chamber (peristaltic or rate consistent pump), or by drawing in measured quantities of fluid from the fluid bag according to the required infusion rate (volumetric pump) (Fig. 8.16).

Depending on the pump a variety of settings are available: fluid infusion rate (ml/h), volume to be infused, volume delivered, and so on. Most pumps incorporate alarm systems that detect air within the fluid line, obstructions to fluid flow, selected volume to be infused delivered, and so on. Some pumps will continue to deliver a small volume of fluid to keep the intravenous catheter patent once the total volume to be delivered has been achieved.

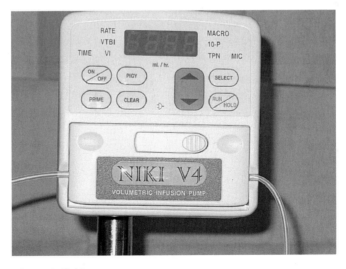

Fig. 8.16 Volumetric fluid pump.

Syringe drivers (see Fig. 8.17)

Syringe drivers are useful for infusion of small volumes of fluid or for controlled intravenous delivery of drugs, e.g. metronidazole. Syringe drivers normally take standard disposable syringes on a rack that is driven by a worm drive coupled to a gearbox and motor, or directly to a stepping motor. These usually work from the mains electricity supply but may also be battery operated or clockwork.

The springfusor (Go Medical Industries Pty Ltd) is a reusable spring driven syringe pump, but flow control tubing; available in a range of different flow rates, controls infusion rates.

Accessories

Various other pieces of equipment are available for use in fluid administration.

Injection caps and stopcocks

These assist in maintaining a closed system by plugging catheters or fluid lines when fluids are not being administered. This minimises contamination of the catheter. Additionally it allows easy administration of heparin and other drugs.

Extension sets

Tubing with male and female luer connections at both ends are available. They attach to the catheter or T-connector and giving set, providing extra length to

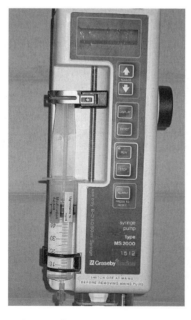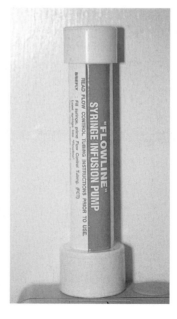

Fig. 8.17 Syringe drivers.

the giving set, and allow disconnection from the fluid system when moving the patient. Additionally, extension sets are more lightweight than standard giving sets and can help to reduce the drag on the patient connection. This is especially important in cats and small dogs.

T-connector

A T-connector consists of an injection bung, tubing and slide clamp (Fig. 8.18). It is attached between the catheter and extension set or giving set. It allows direct venous access for intravenous medications that are administered *via* the injection port, rather than necessitating the removal of the giving set or injection of the drug through one of the injection ports on the giving set at a site distant to the patient. This is particularly important when drugs need to be administered as a bolus, e.g. cardiopulmonary arrest.

Intravenous stylets

Stylets are used to maintain catheter patency without the need for intermittent heparinisation. The IV stylet seals the catheter throughout its entire length and removes the risk of clot formation within the catheter lumen and around its tip. These are of particular value in smaller patients that may be at risk of over-heparinisation following repeated administration of heparinised saline.

Y-type set

Y-type connectors allow administration of two separate fluid types into the same catheter. These are more practical in larger patients.

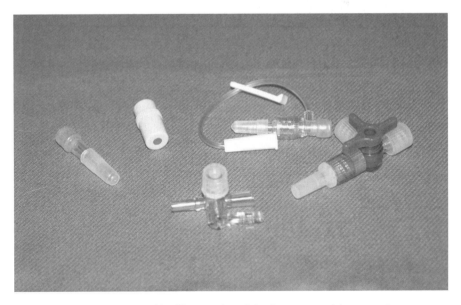

Fig. 8.18 T-port connector. Also illustrated are injection caps and three-way taps.

MONITORING THE CLINICAL RESPONSE TO FLUID THERAPY

A variety of physiological parameters are routinely monitored in anaesthetised patients (see chapter 9). These measurements provide critical information about the central nervous, cardiovascular and respiratory systems that is essential to judge the effect anaesthetic drugs are having on the patient and to assess the depth of anaesthesia. However, the same measurements can provide useful information about the patient's fluid balance:

- Mucous membrane colour, e.g. pale, ashen or hyperaemic (or 'injected') rather than pink.
- Mucous membrane status, e.g. tacky or dry rather than moist.
- Capillary refill time (CRT). Although CRT is frequently used as an indicator of volume status it may be changed as a result of vasoconstriction, e.g. in response to hypovolaemia, heart failure or endotoxaemia. Changes in body temperature can also change CRT.
- Heart rate. Heart rate may increase in response to hypovolaemia. However, heart rate may also increase in response to an inadequate depth of anaesthesia, pain, and so on.
- Peripheral pulse rate, rhythm quality (pressure and duration). The labial, lingual, coccygeal, auricular or dorsal metatarsal arteries should be assessed in preference to the central arteries as this provides a better assessment of peripheral perfusion.
- The temperature of the peripheral extremities is a reflection of the quality of the circulation. Cold extremities suggest poor perfusion.
- Respiratory rate, rhythm and character.
- Skin turgor.
- Subcutaneous oedema.
- Arterial blood pressure; invasive or non-invasive methods. Hypotension may be indicative of a decrease in effective circulating blood volume (see chapter 9).
- Urine output; minimum production of 1–2 ml/kg/h. Oliguria (< 0.5 ml/kg/h) may indicate decreased renal perfusion in anaesthetised patients.
- Central venous pressure (CVP).
- Blood analysis. Blood samples may be required from anaesthetised patients. If this is anticipated, a dedicated intravenous catheter may be placed or samples collected from the CVP catheter. The range of values that may be required and can be measured will largely depend on the practice laboratory facilities, but all of the following may be measured and used to assess changes in the fluid therapy protocol: urea, creatinine, sodium, potassium, chloride, calcium, bicarbonate, total protein, albumin, glucose, lactate, PaO_2, $PaCO_2$, pH and PCV.

Measurement of urine output and CVP are particularly useful tools when assessing the adequacy of the fluid load in anaesthetised patients.

Measurement of urinary output

Accurate measurement of urinary output in anaesthetised patients requires an indwelling or temporary urinary catheter. Intermittent catheterisation is unsuitable in anaesthetised patients.

There are a variety of suitable catheter types available (Foley, PVC dog, Jackson cat, and silicone rubber catheters) and most may be attached to closed urine collection systems (Fig. 8.19). The catheter should be placed using aseptic technique to minimise the chances of the patient developing a urinary tract infection, and the collection bag should be secured below the level of the patient to avoid urine reflux into the urethra and bladder. Closed collection systems ensure that the patient remains clean, dry and comfortable. This is particularly important as excessive wetting of the hair coat can lead to hypothermia. In addition the veterinary nurse can access the fluid collection bag easily to record urine volume without compromising surgical asepsis. Alternatively, intermittent drainage may be used, although in many cases the position of the animal and the use of surgical drapes can make this difficult.

Central venous pressure

Monitoring CVP in patients undergoing intensive fluid therapy is very useful. The CVP measures the pressure of the blood in the right atrium, and can give an indication of the ability of the heart to pump the blood returned to the heart. Measurement of CVP will allow an estimation of the animal's intravascular fluid status and fluid requirements and will allow accurate monitoring of the

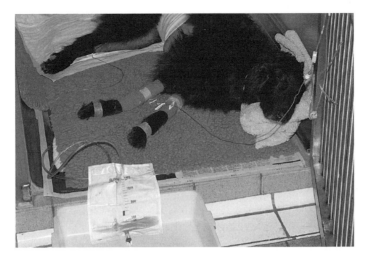

Fig. 8.19 Closed urine collection system attached to an indwelling urinary catheter. Photograph courtesy of Donald Yool.

effects of fluid replacement. In patients with renal or cardiac failure who are prone to developing hypertension, it is advisable that the CVP is monitored.

One or all of the following can affect CVP:

- circulating blood volume
- venous tone
- heart rate
- right ventricular function
- intrathoracic pressure
- intrapericardial pressure.

Measurement of CVP

A long catheter is inserted aseptically into the jugular vein, and advanced until the tip of the catheter lies within the anterior vena cava. The catheter is connected by an extension set to a three-way tap. Also connected to the three-way tap is a bag of crystalloids *via* a giving set. A water manometer tube (marked in centimetres) is connected to the remaining opening of the three-way tap. The zero point of the scale should be level with the right atrium, i.e. at the level of the manubrium if the patient is in lateral recumbency, or the level of the fourth costochondral junction if the patient is in sternal recumbency. The crystalloids may be used to provide fluids to the patient during the anaesthetic procedure (Fig. 8.20).

To measure CVP the three-way tap is turned to allow fluid from the fluid bag to fill the manometer line. This prevents fluids being administered to the patient. The three-way tap is then turned to open the filled manometer tube to the extension set and jugular catheter. The fluid level in the manometer will fall and equilibrate until it stabilises at the patient's CVP. If the tip of the catheter is in the correct place, the meniscus in the manometer will fluctuate a few millimetres during respiration.

Changing trends in CVP are much more significant than an individual reading. Thus, it is important to measure CVP in as technically precise a manner as possible and to obtain consecutive measurements with the patient in the same position each time.

Normal CVP range (dog): 0–10 cmH$_2$O
Normal CVP range (cat): 0–5 cmH$_2$O

A central venous pressure reading of less than 0 indicates that fluid therapy is required. If the CVP reading is at the high end of the normal range or 2–5 cmH$_2$O above that level, fluid therapy should be conservative, i.e. normal maintenance rate. Above this level, fluid therapy should be discontinued or reduced because the patient may be in heart failure or volume overload.

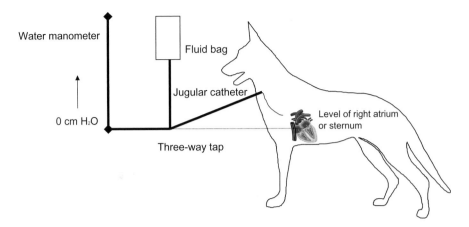

Fig. 8.20 Measurement of central venous pressure.

SUMMARY

The veterinary nurse plays a key role in the management of patients receiving fluid therapy.

Understanding body fluid dynamics and recognition of the clinical signs associated with dehydration and poor perfusion are critical, both to establish the need for fluid therapy and to monitor the patient's response to administration of fluids.

Knowledge of catheter types and sizes available, and experience with different placement techniques, allows a more diverse choice in vascular access; all intravenous catheters must be properly placed and well maintained to reduce the incidence of phlebitis and extravasation of intravenous fluids. Similarly, selection of an appropriate administration system is important, as is the correct calculation of flow rates because overinfusion of fluids can endanger the patient, and to this end constant re-evaluation of the fluid therapy regime is essential for optimal patient care.

REFERENCES AND FURTHER READING

Battaglia, A.M. (2001) Fluid therapy. In: *Small Animal Emergency and Critical Care*, WB Saunders.

Battaglia, A.M. (2001) Patient's lifeline: the intravenous catheter. In: *Small Animal Emergency and Critical Care*, WB Saunders.

DiBartola, S.P. (1992) Introduction to fluid therapy. In: *Fluid Therapy in Small Animal Practice*, WB Saunders, London.

DiBartola, S.P. (2000) Introduction to fluid therapy. In: *Fluid Therapy in Small Animal Practice* 2nd edition (ed. S.P. DiBartola). pp 265–280. WB Saunders, London.

Hansen, B. (1992) Technical aspects of fluid therapy. In: *Fluid Therapy in Small Animal Practice* (ed. S.P. DiBartola). WB Saunders, London.

Hughes, D. (1999) Fluid therapy. In: *Manual of Canine and Feline Emergency and Critical Care*. British Small Animal Veterinary Association, Cheltenham.

Kohn, C.W. & DiBartola, S.P. (2000) Composition and distribution of body fluids in dogs and cats. In: *Fluid Therapy in Small Animal Practice,* 2nd edition (ed. S.P. DiBartola). pp 3–25. WB Saunders, London.

Macintyre, D.K. (1995) The practical use of constant-rate infusions. In: *Kirk's Current Veterinary Therapy* XII, 184.

Moon, P. (1999) Fluid therapy. In: *Manual of Small Animal Anaesthesia and Analgesia*. British Small Animal Veterinary Association, Cheltenham.

Muir, W.W., Hubbell, J.A.E., Skarda, R.T. & Bednarski, R.M. (2000) *Handbook of Veterinary Anesthesia,* 3rd edition. Mosby Inc., London.

Oxley, L. *et al.* (2000) Nursing the emergency patient. In: *Manual of Veterinary Nursing*. British Small Animal Veterinary Association, Cheltenham.

Pascoe, P.J. (2000) Perioperative management of fluid therapy. In: *Fluid Therapy in Small Animal Practice,* 2nd edition (ed. S.P. DiBartola). pp 307–329. WB Saunders, London.

Stanway, G. & Morgan, A. (2000) Anaesthesia and analgesia. In: *Manual of Veterinary Nursing*. British Small Animal Veterinary Association, Cheltenham.

Welsh, E. (1999) Fluid therapy and shock. In: *Veterinary Nursing,* 2nd edition. Butterworth Heinemann.

White, R.N. (1999) Emergency techniques. In: *Manual of Canine and Feline Emergency and Critical Care*. British Small Animal Veterinary Association, Cheltenham.

Wingfield, W.E. (2001) *Veterinary Emergency Medicine Secrets,* 2nd edition. Hanley & Belfus.

Monitoring the Anaesthetised Patient

Louise Clark

General anaesthesia is a controlled reversible loss of consciousness accompanied by analgesia, amnesia, and narcosis and depressed reflex responses. In removing consciousness, anaesthesia also changes the function of other body systems, especially and critically the cardiovascular and the respiratory systems. Anaesthetic monitoring is performed to recognise any harmful trends in the function of these systems and to allow timely and appropriate action to be taken.

The level of sophistication of monitoring technology available in general practice has increased markedly in recent years. The choice of any particular monitoring technique may be governed by availability but should also take into account the patient status and the nature of the procedure being performed. *Expensive and complex equipment is no substitute for good observation and sound clinical judgement.* All available information must be assimilated and interpreted to allow appropriate decisions to be made.

Monitoring should be continual, although it is usual to record data in chart form every 5 minutes. This serves as a pictorial record of the anaesthetic and allows early appreciation of developing trends. A written record is also a medico-legal document.

Whilst the majority of this chapter is concerned with intra-operative patient monitoring, all animals should be observed once pre-anaesthetic medication has been administered. This is mandatory in any animal with respiratory problems and in brachycephalic breeds. Adverse or excessive reactions to sedatives administered will also be noted promptly.

Many of the techniques described are also applicable during the recovery period (see chapter 10).

CENTRAL NERVOUS SYSTEM FUNCTION

Monitoring the depth of anaesthesia is largely based upon assessment of the degree of neuraxial depression. Patients should be anaesthetised to a depth just adequate to prevent obvious responses to surgery. The procedure being performed and the skill of the surgeon will influence the appropriate depth.

Classically, descriptions of the stages of anaesthesia describe the responses of humans undergoing mask induction with an inhalational agent, traditionally ether (Guedel 1974). These descriptions discuss four stages of anaesthesia:

Stage I (Voluntary excitement or analgesia)
- From induction until unconsciousness is present.
- May resist induction and show fear and apprehension, then disorientation.

Stage II (Involuntary excitement)
- From unconsciousness until rhythmic breathing is present.
- All cranial nerve reflexes are present and may be hyperactive.

Stage III (Surgical anaesthesia)
- Divided into four planes.
- Anaesthesia progressively deeper with increasing plane.
- Planes 2 and 3 satisfactory for most surgical procedures.
- Plane 4 – very deep surgical anaesthesia – not usually required clinically.

Stage IV (Overdose)
- Respiratory paralysis.
- Pulse impalpable.
- Ashen pale mucous membranes.
- Beware: agonal gasping can mimic light anaesthesia.

This system is no longer widely taught and to some extent is no longer valid because of the widespread use of injectable induction agents where Stages I and II are not observed, and the use of newer inhalational agents administered after preanaesthetic medication where induction of anaesthesia is generally very smooth. However, the progression of signs described generally represents the transition from light to deep anaesthesia and then to overdose and finally death.

Recovery from general anaesthesia and a return to consciousness involves the reverse of the stages described above, i.e. Stage III plane 3, plane 2, through Stage I.

Cranial nerve reflexes

Deepening anaesthesia reduces cranial nerve reflexes. The most useful indicators of anaesthetic depth and usually the most accessible are the ocular reflexes.

- Palpebral reflex becomes sluggish with increasing depth of anaesthesia and is usually lost at a surgical plane. This is tested by gently running a finger along the edge of the eyelid. Repeated testing reduces the presence of the reflex.
- Eye position in dogs and cats becomes ventromedial, a return to a central eye position occurring with deep anaesthesia (Fig. 9.1).
- Ketamine anaesthesia is associated with a brisk palpebral reflex and a central eye position.
- Corneal reflex is not a good indicator of depth of anaesthesia; it can be present after cardiac arrest. It is usually tested with a damp cotton bud wiped over the cornea; the patient blinks and withdraws; the eye retracts into the orbit. It is easy to cause trauma in attempting to elicit it and is rarely used.
- Palpebral fissure is wide during very light or deep anaesthesia.
- Lacrimation may be seen during light anaesthesia, as may nystagmus (particularly in horses). Lacrimation slows dramatically in deeply anaesthetised patients and a sterile ophthalmic ointment should be instilled into the conjunctival sac following induction of general anaesthesia to minimise corneal dessication.
- Pupillary light reflex is active under anaesthesia.
- Mydriasis or miosis may be present, depending upon the anaesthetic technique used. For example, buprenorphine causes mydriasis in cats, ketamine causes mydriasis in many species.
- Pharyngeal and laryngeal tone diminishes with increasing anaesthetic depth.
- Electroencephalography (EEG) has been used in both humans and animals to provide a direct measure of neural activity. It is a technique with significant limitations and is only widely used in research work.

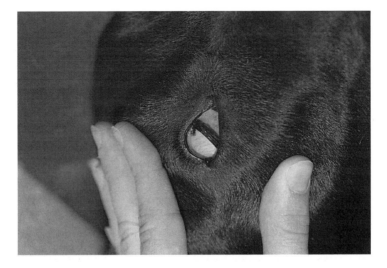

Fig. 9.1 The eye in this anaesthetised dog is rotated ventromedially.

Other reflexes
- Muscle tone is progressively diminished as the depth of anaesthesia increases.
- Loss of jaw tone and tongue curl is indicative of deepening anaesthesia. This is useful in determining whether a sufficient 'depth' has been reached to allow endotracheal intubation.
- A pedal withdrawal reflex is elicited by pinching the skin between the toes. It is lost at surgical planes of anaesthesia.
- Some anaesthetic agents used in isolation, e.g. ketamine, are poor muscle relaxants and muscle tone is lost only once the degree of neuraxial depression is excessive.
- Muscle tone cannot be used to evaluate anaesthetic depth when neuromuscular blocking agents are used.

Cardiovascular responses to surgery
- Surgical stimulation and anaesthetic depth influence heart rate and blood pressure.
- Heart rate and blood pressure are lowered with deep anaesthesia.
- Horses tend to have a stable heart rate uninfluenced by anaesthetic depth.

Respiratory responses to surgery
- Rate, tidal volume and pattern alter with anaesthetic depth.
- Generally, as anaesthesia deepens, minute volume decreases.

Skeletomuscular responses to surgery
- Remember that paralysed animals are unable to move in response to inadequate anaesthesia.
- Movement may be the first sign of lightening anaesthesia in the horse.

CARDIOVASCULAR FUNCTION

The cardiovascular system provides tissue perfusion by maintaining a driving force for blood flow through blood vessels. This driving force (mean arterial pressure; MAP) is dependent upon cardiac output (CO) and systemic vascular resistance (SVR).

$$MAP = CO \times SVR$$

Cardiac output is determined by heart rate (HR) and stroke volume (SV).

$$CO = HR \times SV$$

Since stroke volume depends on preload and afterload, the function of the heart and vascular system are interdependent and evaluation of the overall cardiovascular status of the patient requires assessment of several pieces of information.

Control of heart rate (HR)

- Autonomic nervous system: parasympathetic tone predominates at rest
- Local factors, e.g. temperature, pH and tissue stretch
- Drug administration, e.g. atropine
- Disease

Control of stroke volume (SV)

- Change in preload
- Change in afterload
- Change in HR
- Change in myocardial contractility
- Cardiac arrhythmias

Control of systemic vascular resistance

- Autonomic nervous system
- Central venous pressure
- Cardiac output
- Mean arterial blood pressure
- Humoral mechanisms, e.g. adrenaline, noradrenaline, renin–angiotensin, vasopressin
- Local factors, e.g. accumulation of metabolic byproducts, tissue oxygen demand, electrolytes, prostaglandin release, etc.
- Drugs, e.g. ACP, barbiturates, volatile agents all decrease SV

Preload

- Venous blood volume
- The force acting on a muscle just before contraction
- Frank–Starling Law of the Heart: 'the energy of contraction is proportional to the initial length of the cardiac muscle fibre', i.e. as end diastolic volume increases as a result of increased venous return, cardiac muscle fibre length increases and stroke volume increases
- Hypovolaemia, vasodilation and venous occlusion decrease preload

Afterload

- The tension that a muscle must develop before it can begin to shorten (contract)
- The afterload of the left ventricle depends on aortic pressure, systemic vascular resistance, the capacitance of the vascular system and the viscoelastic properties of blood
- Increases in afterload decrease stroke volume
- High sympathetic tone, diseases such as hyperthyroidism, cardiac outflow disorders and drugs, e.g. ketamine, increase afterload

Heart

Rate and rhythm

Palpation of the apex beat is used in very small animals but gives no indication of cardiac output. Auscultation with a normal stethoscope will allow measurement of rate and rhythm and appreciation of mechanical activity but is often difficult to use under drapes. Instead, an oesophageal stethoscope (Fig. 9.2) can be used, either connected to earpieces or to amplifier and loudspeaker. It consists of a hollow tube and a cuff with multiple holes that is placed in the oesophagus to the level of the heart base. It is placed by measuring from the mouth to about the fifth intercostal space and advancing it dorsally to the endotracheal tube until the heart and breath sounds can be heard. Lubrication with water or K-Y™ jelly allows it to be placed more easily.

Cardiac output cannot be appreciated so it should be used in conjunction with palpation of a pulse as a minimum.

Electrocardiography

Electrocardiographs (ECGs) record electrical activity within the heart and allow the accurate diagnosis and treatment of cardiac arrhythmias. They do not, however, supply any information regarding the mechanical activity or cardiac output of the heart. *It is quite possible for an ECG to appear normal when mechanical activity has ceased, and the ECG should never be used as the sole indicator of cardiac function.*

Standard lead configuration (for anaesthetic monitoring) consists of three electrodes, placed on the two forelimbs and the left hindlimb. Good contact with the animal is essential and can be provided with surgical spirit or electrode gel. Gel tends to be longer lasting. ECG pads are better than crocodile clips but are more expensive (Fig. 9.3). The usual placement of leads is red on right forelimb, yellow on left forelimb, green on left hindlimb. A lead II trace

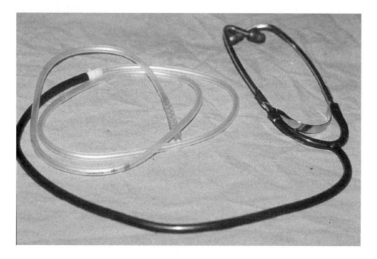

Fig. 9.2 An oesophageal stethoscope.

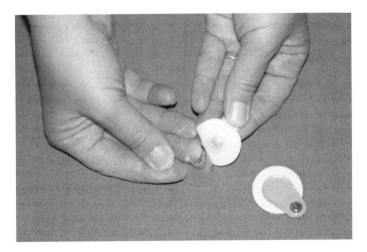

Fig. 9.3 ECG pads are less traumatic than crocodile clips.

comparing right forelimb and left hindlimb can then be obtained. This most closely follows the axis of the heart and therefore gives the largest trace. Alteration of electrodes may be required due to positioning or surgery. A base apex configuration can be used in this situation, with one lead at the heart base, one at the apex and a third acting as earth. It should be noted that this results in a change in ECG morphology, but is useful for arrhythmia detection.

In some cases, placing the ECG lead before induction of anaesthesia is worthwhile, especially in critically ill patients or those known to be at risk of developing arrythmias, e.g. following trauma, gastric dilation or volvulus.

Problems with ECGs are often associated with either poor contact or electrical interference. This may cause frustration and discourage their routine use, but with practice the ECG is a non-invasive easy-to-use monitor that provides information not readily obtainable by other methods. Figure 9.4 shows a normal ECG.

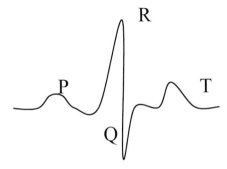

Fig 9.4 Normal ECG. P wave – depolarisation from the sino-atrial node across the atria. QRS complex – depolarisation of the ventricular myocardial mass. T wave – repolarisation of the ventricular myocardium. (Not to scale)

ELECTROCARDIOGRAPHY – IMPORTANT POINTS
- Electrocardiographs (ECGs) record electrical activity within the heart and allow the accurate diagnosis and treatment of cardiac arrhythmias
- ECGs do not supply any information regarding the mechanical activity of the heart or cardiac output
- ECG can appear normal when mechanical activity has ceased
- ECGs should never be used as the sole indicator of cardiac function
- An ECG is a non-invasive easy to use monitor that provides information not readily obtainable by other means

Common intra-operative problems and their management
Bradycardia
At very low heart rates, cardiac output may be insufficient to maintain adequate blood pressure. Causes of intra-operative bradycardia include:

- anaesthetic agent overdose
- hyperkalaemia
- drugs
- vagal stimulation
- hypothermia
- terminal hypoxia
- hypoglycaemia
- heart failure.

The underlying cause must be determined to establish the appropriate treatment.

Tachycardia
High heart rates increase the heart's demand for oxygen and can lead to myocardial hypoxia. Very high rates also compromise cardiac output because the time available for the ventricles to fill with blood is reduced. Myocardial hypoxia can lead to arrhythmias. Causes of intra-operative tachycardia include:

- inadequate anaesthesia or analgesia
- hypoxia
- hypercapnia
- hypotension
- parasympatholytic drugs
- β_1 agonist drugs
- hypothermia
- hyperthermia
- catecholamine-secreting adrenal tumours (unusual).

Arrhythmias

While the presence of arrhythmias may be indicative of myocardial or systemic disease, in the anaesthetised patient they may be a result of:

- myocardial trauma
- myocardial hypoxia
- hypercapnia
- electrolyte disturbances.

Good anaesthetic management will minimise the development of arrhythmias.

Cardiac arrhythmias require treatment when: (1) they cannot be corrected by removing the underlying cause, or (2) they are haemodynamically relevant, or (3) they may potentially deteriorate into a life-threatening arrythmia.

'R-wave monitors'

'R wave monitors' are designed to count QRS complexes. They have a tendency to also count T-waves in domestic species leading to inaccurate heart rates and do not allow diagnosis of arrhythmias.

Blood pressure

Blood pressure provides the driving force for tissue perfusion. Normal blood pressures are shown in Table 9.1. When the mean arterial blood pressure is maintained in the range of about 60–120 mmHg, blood flow to the major organs is autoregulated. In other words, there are local mechanisms that ensure that blood flow to the vital organs is adequate. When mean arterial pressure falls below about 60 mmHg, it is said that tissue perfusion is reduced. This results in the accumulation of lactic acid, leading to acidosis. Hypoxia due to a failure of perfusion can also result in ischaemic damage to tissues. The canine and feline kidneys are vulnerable to such damage, which is the reason why poorly managed anaesthesia can precipitate or hasten the onset of renal failure.

In addition, monitoring of blood pressure over time can indicate changes in anaesthetic depth (mean arterial pressure tends to increase with inadequate anaesthesia and decrease if anaesthesia is too deep) and also supply information regarding the vascular volume status of the animal.

Table 9.1 Normal blood pressure in conscious animals.

	Dog	Cat
Systolic pressure (mmHg)	110–190	120–170
Diastolic pressure (mmHg)	55–110	70–120

Mean arterial blood pressure = Diastolic pressure + (systolic – diastolic pressure)/3

Assessment of blood pressure

Palpation

The palpable pulse pressure is the difference between systolic and diastolic blood pressure. A difference of 30 mmHg between the systolic and diastolic pulse pressures is necessary to palpate a strong pulse. It is difficult to accurately assess mean arterial pressure in small animals, although some assessment may be possible in horses by occluding the artery.

It is usual to palpate peripheral arteries (e.g. metatarsal, lingual) (see Fig. 9.5), because palpable peripheral pulses are lost at a higher mean arterial pressure than in central arteries such as the femoral artery. The femoral artery may be the only palpable artery in very small animals.

PALPATION OF PERIPHERAL ARTERIES
(see Fig. 9.5)
- Lingual: near midline, ventral surface of proximal tongue
- Dorsal metatarsal: dorso-medially on the metatarsus
- Carpal: medial to midline, palmar aspect of metacarpus
- Auricular: middle of the pinna of the ear
- Labial: upper lip caudal to canine
- Coccygeal: ventral surface near the top of the tail

Direct blood pressure monitoring (invasive)

This is the 'gold standard' for blood pressure monitoring because of its accuracy. An intra-arterial catheter is placed and connected to a strain gauge or transducer *via* saline-filled non-compliant tubing. Normally the dorsal metatarsal artery is cannulated in the dog (Fig. 9.6) and the femoral artery in the cat, though auricular arteries may be useful in some breeds of dog. Arterial catheterisation has the risks of introducing infection and of haematoma formation, but using aseptic technique and the application of pressure over the artery when cannulae are removed can reduce these. It is also reported to be quite painful.

All arterial lines must be clearly labelled, as the consequences of accidental intra-arterial injection can be disastrous. Frequent flushing of these catheters is required as thrombus formation can dampen the signal obtained.

Connection of the catheter to a *calibrated* electronic transducer allows the arterial pressure waveform to be displayed on an oscilloscope screen. This allows continuous monitoring of blood pressure and the morphology can provide further useful information.

A cheaper alternative is to connect the arterial line to an aneroid manometer. This utilises a 'Pressureveil' system to convert the pressure exerted by the column of saline to a value on a pressure gauge. This system measures only mean arterial pressure.

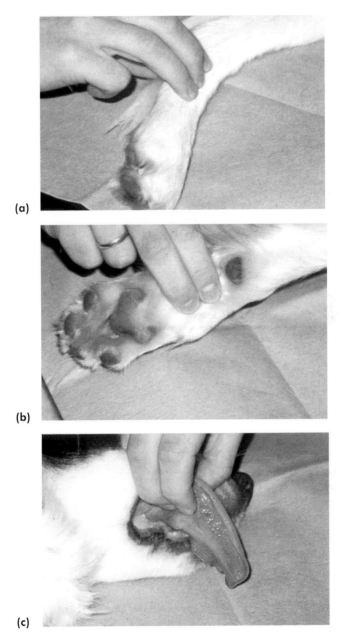

(a)

(b)

(c)

Fig. 9.5 Location of peripheral arteries. (a) Palpating the dorsal metatarsal artery dorso-medially on the metatarsus. (b) Palpating the carpal artery, medial to midline, on the palmar aspect of the metacarpus. (c) Palpating the lingual artery, near midline on the ventral surface of the tongue.

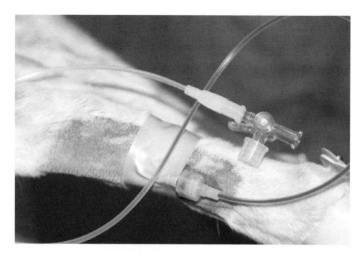

Fig. 9.6 An arterial catheter in the dorsal metatarsal artery.

Direct arterial blood pressure measurement is rarely used in general practice and is reserved for cardiovascularly compromised patients.

Indirect blood pressure monitoring (non-invasive)

These systems are quicker and easier to use than direct methods and are becoming more widely available in practice.

Indirect blood pressure monitors use an occlusive pneumatic cuff placed over a peripheral artery. The cuff is inflated to a pressure greater than systolic blood pressure and blood flow distal to the cuff stops.

The selection of the correct cuff and the way it is applied are important to minimise errors in the technique. The correct cuff width is usually described as 40% of the circumference of the limb to be measured, or sometimes as 20% wider than the limb diameter. These measurements are approximately equal. Cuffs should be applied firmly but not tightly on either the distal fore- or hind-limb. The cuffs may also be used on the tail.

Oscillometric technique

This measures mean arterial pressure.

Oscillometry relies on the repeated inflation and deflation of an occlusive cuff. As the cuff deflates the arterial pulse in the limb causes oscillation within the cuff that is detected by a transducer. The maximal amplitude of these oscillations occurs at the mean arterial pressure. The machines (e.g. Dinamap®, Arteriosonde®) can be programmed to cycle automatically and measure the blood pressure at given intervals. The frequency of these measurements should not exceed more than one every 3 minutes for a prolonged period; otherwise distal limb swelling can develop. This method is useful and fairly accurate for mean arterial pressure in normotensive moderate-sized dogs. Accuracy is lower in small, tachycardic, bradycardic or hypotensive animals and in the presence of ventricular arrhythmias – cases where it could be argued that blood pressure measurement is most valuable!

Doppler probe

This measures systolic arterial pressure and involves the use of a piezoelectric crystal (a 10 MHz ultrasound probe) and relies on 'Doppler shift' whereby the frequency of the sound reflected from moving tissues, i.e. arterial blood, differs from that transmitted from the crystal. This shift in frequency is converted into an audible signal.

The Doppler probe is positioned over a peripheral artery distal to the cuff and the cuff is inflated until the arterial signal is no longer audible (Fig. 9.7). The hair should be clipped from this area and ultrasound gel applied over the artery to improve the signal. As the cuff is slowly deflated the probe detects the return of arterial blood flow, i.e. the systolic blood pressure.

Doppler instruments have been shown to be accurate for systolic blood pressure measurement even in small animals. Their main disadvantages are an inability to measure mean arterial pressure and susceptibility to operator error.

Intra-operative hypotension

Hypotension can be classified as a mean arterial blood pressure of < 60 mmHg. Hypotension can reduce the perfusion of vital body organs, leading to postoperative organ failure. Severe hypotension can reduce coronary artery blood flow and even lead to cardiac arrest. There are three underlying causes of hypotension: (1) decreased cardiac output; (2) decreased systemic vascular resistance; (3) a combination of the above.

Decreased cardiac output can be caused by a fall in stroke volume, either due to a reduced contractility of the myocardium or due to a decreased preload (see above, page 223). It can also result from a very low heart rate or from severe

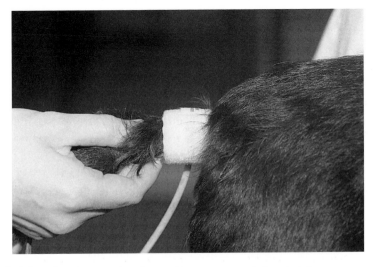

Fig. 9.7 A Doppler ultrasound probe used to measure systolic arterial pressure.

cardiac arrhythmias. A reduction in contractility can be seen in myocardial disease and also in toxaemia or sepsis. Anaesthetic overdose may also decrease contractility. Preload is reduced if venous return is compromised. Causes of decreased venous return include:

- hypovolaemia;
- drug administration, e.g. acetylpromazine;
- surgical packing of the vena cava;
- gastric dilation;
- positive pressure ventilation;
- dorsal recumbency in gravid females, gross ascites, diaphragmatic hernia, abdominal masses, etc., causing pressure on the caudal vena cava;
- pericardial tamponade;
- sepsis and toxaemia.

Decreased systemic vascular resistance can result from:

- anaesthetic overdose;
- extradural local anaesthesia;
- drugs (particularly α_1 antagonists);
- sepsis.

In order to establish the correct treatment for the hypotension, the cause must first be established. Hypovolaemia is reportedly the most common cause of hypotension and should be resolved by rapidly infusing appropriate intravenous fluids. In addition the surgeon should be alerted in case of unobserved ongoing haemorrhage. Steps should also be taken either to reduce the depth of anaesthesia or to change the anaesthetic technique.

Inotropes such as the β_1 agonist dobutamine, or α_1 agonists, e.g. methoxamine, may be required.

Cardiac output

Direct measurement of cardiac output in anaesthetised animals is normally only performed as a research technique. It is invasive and requires the placement of a Swan-Ganz catheter. This is a specialised balloon-tipped catheter that is passed from the jugular vein, through the right atrium into the pulmonary artery. It can temporarily occlude the pulmonary artery and is used for the instillation of iced saline when a thermodilution technique is being used to measure cardiac output. It can also be used to measure pulmonary capillary wedge pressure. This is equivalent to the mean ventricular filling pressure. This measurement is used in human cardiac intensive care patients.

Perfusion

Blood must flow through the capillary beds for red cells to deliver oxygen to their associated tissues. While the importance of maintaining arterial blood pressure has been discussed, subjective assessment still forms the basis of monitoring of perfusion at the level of the capillaries in practice. The following provide a subjective assessment of the flow of blood through the peripheral tissues. Individual parameters are inaccurate if considered in isolation. A clinical picture must be assimilated from all the visible signs.

Capillary refill time

Removing blood from the mucous membranes by direct pressure, then allowing the capillaries to refill, allows some assessment of perfusion.

Blanching oral membranes should give a capillary refill time of < 2 seconds. Intense vasoconstriction or hypotension leads to delay.

Beware – recently dead animals can have a normal capillary refill time.

Mucous membrane colour

Changes in mucous membrane colour can be indicative of disease processes, but may not be directly indicative of changes in perfusion. The colour should be salmon pink although it is often paler in cows and cats.

ABNORMAL MUCOUS MEMBRANE COLOURS
- Bright pink: indicates vasodilation, often due to hypercapnia
- Pale: profound vasoconstriction or anaemia can look similar
- Blue: cyanosis (haemoglobin desaturation), can be hard to see if also anaemic
- Yellow (icteric): liver disease/obstructed biliary flow/red cell destruction
- Red/brown/congested: often associated with toxaemia or sepsis (SIRS) (see Fig. 9.8)

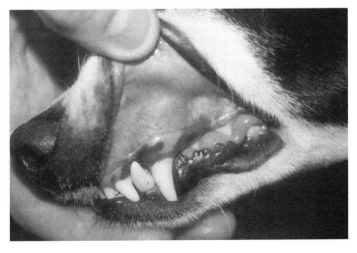

Fig. 9.8 Congested dry mucous membranes in a toxaemic dog.

Examination of surgical site
Brightly coloured blood should be visible at the surgical site in animals attached to a breathing system and breathing oxygen-enriched gases. This is capillary blood and it should not be dark or slowly oozing.

Urinary output
Catheterising the bladder and collecting the urine produced intra-operatively provides information on the adequacy of renal perfusion. This assumes that decreased urine production is associated with decreased renal perfusion. Many non-renal factors including anaesthetic drugs may directly or indirectly affect urine production. Generally speaking, urine production of 1–2 ml/kg/h or more is considered adequate in an animal with normal renal function. The specific gravity of urine collected will be increased in dehydrated or hypovolaemic animals that have normal kidney function. This is due to water and sodium conservation.

Core–periphery temperature difference
Core temperature is a measure of central body temperature unaffected by the vasoconstrictor effects of peripheral vasculature. Rectal temperature is simple to measure but not indicative of core temperature if the thermometer is located within a faecal ball, for example. Core temperature is best measured by a flexible thermistor placed in the oesophagus or nasopharynx. Peripheral temperature can be measured from the lip, for example. The core–periphery temperature difference provides an indication of the degree of peripheral vasoconstriction present. Profound peripheral vasoconstriction is associated with poor peripheral perfusion.

A subjective assessment of the degree of peripheral vasoconstriction can be made if ears and other extremities are cold. (See section on monitoring temperature, pages 241–242.)

Volume status
Central venous pressure
Central venous pressure is the blood pressure within the intrathoracic portion of the cranial or caudal vena cava. It is almost equivalent to right atrial pressure and the terms tend to be used interchangeably. It is measured clinically for two reasons: (1) to gain information about intravascular blood volume; (2) to gain information about cardiac function.

A complex relationship exists between central venous pressure (CVP), cardiac output and the vascular system. CVP reflects venous blood volume and venous return to the heart. Changes in vascular volume can be accommodated with only small changes in intravascular pressure. A single measurement of CVP yields little information, but serial measurements are useful.

When intravenous fluids are administered to the normovolaemic patient, the intravascular blood volume is increased; venous return and CVP begin to rise, returning to normal as vasomotor tone accommodates the increased fluid volume.

Rapidly infusing 20 ml/kg of crystalloid into a normovolaemic patient will lead to a modest (2–4 cmH$_2$O) and transient (approximately 15 min) increase in CVP. If CVP does not increase, this implies a reduced vascular volume and that the fluid bolus has been accommodated. A large increase in CVP can be seen with volume overload and with animals with failing right heart function. CVP can be useful in differentiating low arterial blood pressure due to hypovolaemia from low arterial blood pressure due to cardiac failure.

In a practical situation and in conjunction with other clinical signs, fluids may be administered to maintain CVP at 5–10 cmH$_2$O.

RESPIRATORY FUNCTION

The function of the respiratory system is to deliver inspired gas to the alveoli, facilitate gas exchange and then remove the expired gases. Monitoring the respiratory system in the anaesthetised patient involves an assessment of ventilatory adequacy and gas exchange.

Monitoring ventilation

Ventilation is assessed in terms of rate, rhythm and tidal volume.

Observation of the reservoir bag can be used to measure respiratory rate and to estimate tidal volume; this method is very subjective.

Minute volume is the term used to describe the amount of gas expired by the patient per minute and is approximately 150–250 ml/kg/min. The normal tidal volume for mammals is 10–20 ml/kg/min.

$$\text{Minute volume (MV)} = \text{tidal volume (TV)} \times \text{respiratory rate (RR)}$$

It is however the alveolar minute volume that is important in gas exchange. Animals with high respiratory rates, e.g. panting, may have low effective alveolar minute volumes because they are breathing a lot of dead space gas and therefore may be ventilating very inefficiently. Slower deeper breaths are generally more efficient. With deepening anaesthesia, minute volume decreases and carbon dioxide is retained. This is important because hypercapnia leads to acidosis and can also promote cardiac arrhythmia formation. Animals that are hypoventilating should be supported with frequent 'sighing'. This is when the anaesthetist delivers supra-maximal lung inflation by closing the valve on the breathing system, squeezing the reservoir bag, and then opening the valve again. Sighing will help prevent carbon dioxide retention and therefore hypercapnia if facilities for mechanical ventilation do not exist. Subjective assessment of ventilatory adequacy has been supplemented by a number of mechanical methods of differing complexities, that can provide further useful information.

Respirometers (Wright's respirometer)

These are not widely used in practice; they are more often used a research tool. They consist of a mechanism through which the expired gases pass that moves a pointer along a calibrated scale. They can be used to measure tidal and minute volume although inertia makes them inaccurate in very small animals.

Apnoea monitors

Apnoea or respiratory monitors detect the movement of warm gases through the breathing system at the proximal end of the endotracheal tube. They can be activated by cardiac oscillations that cause gas movement in the trachea. They provide no information on tidal volume and, although popular in practice, they yield no useful information about the physiological status of the patient.

Apnoea or respiratory monitors should not be relied on as a sole measure of ventilatory adequacy.

Capnography

Capnography measures the carbon dioxide concentration in expired gas. The data is usually displayed as a waveform (the capnogram; Fig. 9.9) and the CO_2 concentration at the end of expiration is displayed. This is called the end-tidal CO_2 (F_ECO_2). It is useful because in patients with stable cardiac function and normal lung function it closely approximates the arterial partial pressure of CO_2 (P_aCO_2).

Capnography is easy to use and non-invasive as well as providing a continuous although slightly delayed measurement (due to the time taken to aspirate the sample). It provides information on the adequacy of ventilation, airway obstruction, and disconnection from the breathing system and severe circulatory problems.

Most capnographs utilise infrared absorption spectroscopy. Gas is drawn from the breathing system by a narrow tube connected to an adapter at the proximal end of the endotracheal tube. Typical gas sampling rates are 50–150 ml/min. The tip of the sampling tube should be as near as possible to the trachea in order to sample alveolar gas.

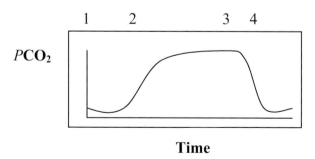

Fig. 9.9 The normal capnogram. 1 Inspiratory baseline. 2 Expiratory upstroke. 3 Expiratory plateau end-tidal CO_2 (F_ECO_2). 4 Inspiratory downstroke.

Table 9.2 Measuring end-tidal carbon dioxide.

mmHg	kPa	Interpretation
< 35	< 4.6	Hypocapnia
35–45	4.6–6.0	Normocapnia
> 45	> 6.0	Hypercapnia

Table 9.2 shows some typical values.

The significance of these values depends upon the clinical situation. For example, mild hypercapnia may or may not require artificial ventilation. Table 9.3 explains the significance of abnormal traces and Table 9.4 classifies changes in respiratory rate in anaesthetised patients.

Gas exchange
Pulse oximetry
The adequacy of oxygen transport can be assessed by pulse oximetry. This also gives some measure of the adequacy of gas exchange. Pulse oximeters measure the percentage of arterial oxygen saturation of haemoglobin. They do not directly measure tissue oxygen delivery, as this is also dependent upon cardiac output and haematocrit (available haemoglobin).

The technology involved is quite complicated and involves two basic physical principles. First, the absorption of red and infrared light (each with different wavelengths) differs depending upon the degree of oxygenation of

Table 9.3 Interpretation of abnormal traces.

Trace abnormality	Symptom of	Reason
Elevated baseline	Rebreathing	Gas flow too low
		Exhausted soda lime
Oscillations on trace	Cardiac trace	Cardiac movement moves gas in airways
Extra peak at end	Additional ventilation	Reversal of neuromuscular block 'Fighting' the ventilator
Sloped plateau	Delayed expiration	Obstructed endotracheal tube Obstructive airway disease
High F_ECO_2	Hypercapnia	Hypoventilation
Low F_ECO_2	Not full expiration	High ventilation rate
	Decreased cardiac output	Fresh gas contamination
Sudden decrease in F_ECO_2	Decreased pulmonary perfusion	Cardiopulmonary crisis
No trace	No gas to analyse	Apnoea
		Airway obstruction
		Disconnection
		Ventilator failure

Table 9.4 Common causes of changes in respiratory rate in anaesthetised patients.

Hypoventilation	Hyperventilation	Apnoea
Absolute drug overdose	Light anaesthesia	Drug effects, e.g. post-induction propofol apnoea
Relative drug overdose	Pain	Administration of neuromuscular blocking drugs
Administration of drugs that depress respiration, e.g. opioids	Surgical stimulation	Overzealous assisted ventilation
Deep anaesthesia	Hypoxia	Cardiac arrest
	Hypotension	Pressure build-up within breathing system, e.g. pressure relief valve closed
	Pyrexia or hyperthermia	

haemoglobin. Second, the light signal following transmission through the tissues has a pulsatile component, resulting from the changes in volume of arterial blood with each pulse. This is distinguished by the microprocessor from the non-pulsatile component resulting from tissue, venous and capillary light absorption. Thus the percentage of arterial oxygen saturation of haemoglobin is calculated.

The signal is obtained from the animal by placing a probe containing the light sources across any well-perfused area of tissue. The most commonly used sites include tongue, pinna, prepuce, toe web and vulva (Fig. 9.10). The suitability of each site may depend upon the conformation of the patient and the

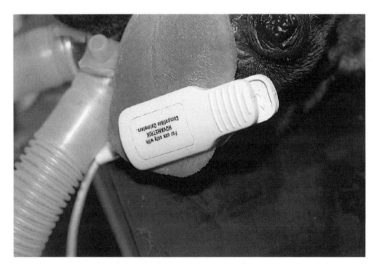

Fig. 9.10 A pulse oximeter probe attached to the tongue.

type of surgery being undertaken. Rectal probes that measure the reflected component of the light emitted have recently become available.

The pulse oximeter displays a continuous waveform or signal together with a numerical oxygen saturation value written as SaO_2. Most pulse oximeters also display pulse rate. Pulse oximeters have become widely used in practice as their price has fallen. They are non-invasive, easy to use and provide continuous immediate monitoring. In order to optimise their use, the limitations and pitfalls in their use must be appreciated.

- Pulse oximetry measures the arterial oxygen saturation of haemoglobin. It gives no indication of available haemoglobin. Therefore anaemic patients may have a high SaO_2 but a markedly reduced oxygen-carrying capacity.
- Pulse oximetry cannot distinguish between different forms of haemoglobin. Carboxyhaemoglobin (haemoglobin combined with carbon monoxide) is registered as about 90% oxygenated haemoglobin and 10% desaturated. The oximeter therefore overestimates the functional haemoglobin. Methaemoglobinaemia prevents accurate measurement and the saturation will tend towards 85%, regardless of the true value. Foetal haemoglobin does not affect the readings obtained by the pulse oximeter.
- Polymerised bovine haemoglobin (e.g. Oxyglobin) used as a blood substitute does not interfere with pulse oximetry readings.
- SaO_2 is related to PaO_2 by a sigmoid relationship (the oxyhaemoglobin dissociation curve). This means that the SaO_2 will remain high as the PaO_2 falls and the SaO_2 will only fall when the PaO_2 has reached low levels. In this respect the pulse oximeter has been described as a 'cliff-edge monitor' because by the time SaO_2 falls (below about 90%) the actual PaO_2 has already fallen markedly (see Table 9.5).
- Lack of perfusion will prevent a signal being obtained. This can occur naturally in areas such as the distal pinna, or may be a result of the use of α_2 agonists in the anaesthetic technique. It also occurs due to tissue compression by the probe, necessitating repositioning. However peripheral vasoconstriction

Table 9.5 Interpretation of pulse oximeter data.

SaO_2	PaO_2	Action required
100%	~ 100 mmHg or more	Normal monitoring and actions appropriate
90%	~ 60 mmHg	Inform veterinary surgeon
75%	~ 40 mmHg	Ensure adequate ventilation (Airway, RR, TV, O_2
50%	~27 mmHg	supply, CO_2 clearance)
		Increase FiO_2 to 100%
		Assess cardiac function
		Consider patient positioning, surgical effects, medical disorders

may be due to underlying problems (e.g. hypovolaemia, severe hypotension, cold, cardiac failure or arrhythmias) and this must always be considered.

- Movement artefact will reduce accuracy and may prevent an adequate signal being obtained. This problem is most often encountered in recovery when shivering occurs.
- Ambient light interference from surgical lights can be a problem. Diathermy can also interfere with the signal obtained.

Blood gas analysis

The analysis of carbon dioxide and oxygen tensions in an arterial blood gas sample provides information on (i.e. defines) pulmonary function. In addition, blood gas analysers can provide information on the acid–base status of the patient. Whilst not widely used (or required) in small animal practice, benchtop portable analysers are becoming more widespread.

Heparinised arterial blood samples drawn anaerobically (all the air must be expelled before use) are required for analysis. Commercial 'blood gas' syringes are available containing lyophilised heparin. Alternatively, undiluted heparin is drawn into the needle and syringe to be used and then all the heparin is discarded from the syringe, the needle changed and the blood sample collected. Arterial blood gas analysis may be carried out on a single occasion by puncture of a peripheral artery, taking care to apply pressure afterwards. If multiple samples are to be taken, placement of an arterial catheter is advised. This also facilitates blood pressure monitoring. Arteries usually used for blood collection include the dorsal metatarsal or tibial arteries in dogs and the femoral artery in cats.

Handling of the sample is very important in order to prevent errors in the analysis. The sample must not contain excess heparin (see above), therefore if taken from a catheter some blood should be discarded or withdrawn and replaced (in small animals) before the blood for analysis is taken. Exposure to room air must be prevented and, if prompt analysis is not possible, the blood samples must be stored on ice to prevent ongoing cell metabolism. The data must be corrected for the patient's body temperature to ensure accuracy of the results.

Most blood gas analysers will measure or calculate PaO_2, $PaCO_2$, pH, BE, HCO^{3-}, K^+, Na^+ and often other electrolytes. They are therefore useful in the assessment of acid–base status as well as gas exchange.

In animals breathing room air and with normal lung function, PaO_2 would be expected to be greater than 85 mmHg. Hyperventilation can result in values as high as 120 mmHg. Increases in inspired oxygen concentration lead to increases in PaO_2. As a general rule, PaO_2 should be five times the inspired oxygen concentration. Therefore an animal on 100% oxygen would have a PaO_2 of greater than 500 mmHg.

$PaCO_2$ is influenced by the rate of production and elimination of carbon dioxide from the body. Since production is fairly constant, $PaCO_2$ is determined primarily by ventilation. The normal range is about 35–45 mmHg in the dog (see section on capnography, pages 236–237).

MONITORING TEMPERATURE

The ability of patients to thermoregulate is depressed by anaesthesia. Anaesthetic agents depress the central nervous system, reducing its sensitivity to changes in body temperature. In addition, anaesthetised animals are unable to adapt their behaviour in order to maintain body temperature, for example, move to a warmer environment, huddle, or shiver. They may have been starved preoperatively and have reduced gut activity. Core body temperature is best measured by a thermistor placed in the oesophagus or nasopharynx (not next to inspired gases). Rectal temperature is easy to measure but at best can only provide information about trends, as it does not measure core temperature accurately.

Hypothermia is significant during anaesthesia because:

- it causes a general central depressant effect. It reduces MAC, thus reducing the amount of volatile anaesthetic agent required. This may result in prolonged recoveries from anaesthesia;
- it releases catecholamines;
- blood viscosity increases;
- it interferes with normal haemostasis;
- cardiac output decreases;
- arrhythmias are more common, e.g. atrial fibrillation;
- there is a slowing of electrical conduction through the heart.

The methods of heat loss are evaporation, conduction, convection and radiation.

Evaporation

Evaporative losses are increased when patients breathe cold unhumidified air through breathing systems. Rebreathing systems can minimise evaporative losses in larger patients, while heat and moisture exchangers may be added (at the expense of increasing mechanical dead space) to the end of the endotracheal tube.

Exposure of tissues to the atmosphere during surgery also increases evaporative losses – especially where there are open cavities, e.g. during exploratory laparotomy.

Measures should be taken to limit patient wetting during surgery, surgical lavage and as a consequence of urination, e.g. water-impermeable drapes, double draping, suction, use of incontinence pads, urinary catheterisation.

Conduction

Patients should not be placed directly onto metal tables. Bubble wrap provides a suitable insulating material against conductive losses. Heated operating tables are available. Care must be exercised to avoid hyperthermia when heavy patients are placed on heated tables for prolonged periods of time.

Convection

Convection heat losses occur by the transfer of heat through the movement of gases. Patients should not be positioned in draughty areas e.g. corridors.

Radiation

In conscious mobile patients, radiation (i.e. the exchange of heat between objects that are not in direct contact) accounts for the majority of heat loss. This illustrates the importance of appropriate ambient temperature within the induction area, surgical theatre, diagnostic imaging areas and the recovery area.

Small animals with large surface area to volume ratios undergoing surgery where there are open body cavities lose heat fastest.

Reducing heat loss requires insulation and may necessitate adaptations to the anaesthetic technique. Heat loss can be reduced by:

- reducing the anaesthetic time;
- maintaining a high ambient air temperature;
- avoiding alcohol-based surgical scrubs;
- warming inspired gases (using heat and moisture exchangers);
- warming fluids.

Heated tables and 'BAIR huggers' (circulating warm air blankets) are very useful but expensive. Heat pads and hot water bottles also have their uses. Patients should not be placed in direct contact with these, to limit the possibility of thermal burns. Warm fluids for abdominal lavage are also useful. Warm enemas or bladder lavage can also be performed. These are useful central warming techniques and avoid the risk that heat applied to the body surface will cause peripheral vasodilation and possibly a further decrease in core temperature.

MONITORING SURGERY AND FLUID THERAPY (see chapter 8)

Liaison with the surgeon helps the veterinary nurse monitoring the patient to anticipate critical events and to act accordingly.

Regular assessment of ongoing haemorrhage helps to determine changes to fluid therapy and avoid hypovolaemia developing. Table 9.6 lists ways in which blood loss can be estimated.

Table 9.6 Methods for estimating blood loss.

Method	Estimated volume
4 × 4 inch swab (dry initially)	5–10 ml
Weigh swabs (assume negligible dry wt)	1 g = 1 ml
Blood in suction apparatus	Volume in container
Blood in suction apparatus + lavage fluid	Compare fluid PCV with animal's PCV
12 × 12 inch laparotomy swab	Approx. 50 ml

MONITORING BLOOD GLUCOSE

Hypoglycaemia can be a complication of anaesthesia in animals with certain disease states (e.g. insulinoma, diabetes mellitus, severe hepatic disease), in neonates and in very small animals. It may manifest itself as a very slow recovery, postoperative depression or even seizures. Blood glucose samples can be taken every 30 minutes during anaesthesia through a preplaced venous catheter (preferably not one with IV fluids being infused). Where there is concern over intra-operative hypoglycaemia, supplementation with glucose-containing fluids (e.g. 5% dextrose in water) in addition to the normal perioperative fluid therapy, may be required.

MONITORING NEUROMUSCULAR BLOCKADE

It is desirable to monitor the onset, duration and depth of neuromuscular blockade to allow drug doses to be adjusted for the individual animal. Monitoring is performed using a peripheral nerve stimulator (Fig. 9.11). This allows the assessment of the response of a muscle following electrical stimulation of its

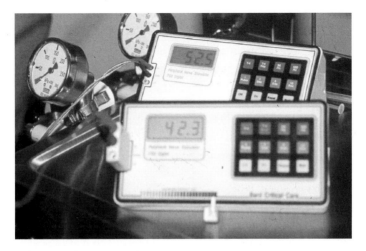

Fig. 9.11 A peripheral nerve stimulator.

motor nerve. The response of the muscle is usually judged visually. A number of different stimuli patterns and duration have been developed in order to maximise the amount of information that can be obtained about the quality of the neuromuscular blockade.

The most commonly used nerve stimulator pattern is the 'train of four', where four stimuli are administered at a frequency of 2 Hz. The number of twitches obtained from the stimulated muscle is then counted and the relative strength of the twitches assessed. The fourth twitch is compared to the first to give the 'train of four' ratio. A ratio of at least 0.8 is usually required before animals are considered to have acceptable enough muscle function to withdraw ventilatory support (see chapter 6).

Where a peripheral nerve stimulator is not available, the first sign of fading neuromuscular blockade is the return of diaphragmatic twitching. This would be an indication that the neuromuscular blocking agent should be re-administered if continued paralysis was required.

Neuromuscular blocking drugs must *never* be used if adequate anaesthesia cannot be ensured. The following are clinical signs of inadequate anaesthesia where neuromuscular blocking drugs have been used:

- paradoxical jaw tone or tongue twitching
- salivation
- mydriasis
- lacrimation
- tachycardia
- hypertension
- arrhythmias.

MONITORING THE ANAESTHETIC EQUIPMENT AND GENERAL MANAGEMENT

There are several pieces of monitoring equipment that have been designed to help alert the anaesthetist to anaesthetic equipment problems, but their use does not preclude good observation. Therefore, in addition to observing the patient, regular checks should be made on the associated anaesthetic equipment. This should all have been checked thoroughly before undertaking the case, but there are certain problems that may occur during the course of an anaesthetic (see chapter 4).

The endotracheal tube may become obstructed, particularly if the neck is ventroflexed (e.g. when performing a CSF tap), or the tube laterally deviated due to intra-oral surgery. Polyethylene type tubes become softer as warm air flows through them and obstruction may develop. Consider the use of armoured tubes if this complication is likely to occur. Endotracheal tube cuffs should always be checked preoperatively, but consider a leaking cuff as a cause of an inability to apply effective positive pressure ventilation.

The breathing system must be checked for misconnection, particularly if the patient and system are moved to another machine, e.g. when moving from the induction area to theatre.

Valve function and any soda lime should also be periodically checked. If the colour indicator on the soda lime canister shows that 50% of it is exhausted, the soda lime should be replaced as soon as possible.

Sighing the patient (i.e. delivering supramaximal lung inflation at 5-min intervals) prevents atelectasis, minimises hypoxia and hypercapnia and allows an appraisal of pulmonary compliance. Low compliance (lungs feel difficult to inflate) may be caused by pressure on chest, pneumothorax or airway obstruction. High compliance indicates disconnection of the breathing system or endotracheal cuff leak.

Flowmeter and vaporiser settings should be regularly checked, especially if the machine has no oxygen alarm, as should the gauges on the oxygen cylinders. Cylinders that will not be used, e.g. carbon dioxide, must be turned off for safety.

Fluid administration rates, particularly in small patients, need periodic checking.

Respiratory gas monitors

While the primary reason for the use of capnography is to assess the cardiovascular and, in particular, the respiratory function of the patient, the primary reason for monitoring other gases is for anaesthetic safety.

Many machines can measure oxygen, nitrous oxide and anaesthetic gas concentrations as well as carbon dioxide.

- *Oxygen:* The measurement of inspired oxygen concentration is useful to ensure that the patient does not breathe a hypoxic mixture. This is particularly relevant with rebreathing systems where nitrous oxide is used, especially where 'low flow' anaesthesia is practised. The inspired oxygen concentration is useful for patients where arterial blood gas analysis is being performed. It allows the calculation of the alveolar–arterial oxygen tension difference. This is a useful measurement of pulmonary function.
- *Nitrous oxide:* The measurement of nitrous oxide is also used to prevent the delivery of an inappropriate gas mixture to the patient. Expired nitrous oxide concentration can be monitored at the end of anaesthesia when delivery has been discontinued and the patient is breathing oxygen alone. The nitrous oxide rapidly leaves the blood, diffusing into the patient's alveoli, and can cause hypoxia unless the inspired oxygen concentration is supplemented until most of the nitrous oxide has been exhaled (see the second gas effect, page 143).
- *Anaesthetic gases:* Anaesthetic gas monitoring is usually performed as a research technique. It measures the end-tidal carbon dioxide and the inspired volatile agent concentration, and sometimes relates these to the minimum alveolar concentration (MAC).

SUMMARY

In order to safely and effectively monitor anaesthesia in animals, the nurse must rely heavily on clinical skills and observation of the animal. While new technology has made complex monitoring equipment more widely available, this cannot possibly replace clinical judgement. If monitoring equipment is to be used successfully, an appreciation of its limitations is essential.

Monitoring should be carried out regularly and information accurately and concisely recorded.

REFERENCES AND FURTHER READING

Guedel, A.E. (1974) Third stage ether anaesthesia. In: *Signs and Stages of Anaesthesia* (Wood Library, Museum of Anesthesia). Park Ridge, IL.

Haskins, S.C. (1996) Monitoring the Anaesthetised Patient. In: *Lumb & Jones' Veterinary Anaesthesia*, 3rd edition (eds J.C. Thurmon, W.J. Tranquilli & G.J. Benson G.J.), pp 409–423. Williams & Wilkins, Baltimore.

Haskins, S.C. (1999) Perioperative monitoring. In: *Manual of Small Animal Anaesthesia*, 2nd edition (ed. R.R. Paddleford), pp 123–146. WB Saunders, Philadelphia.

Johnson, C. (1999) Patient monitoring. In: *BSAVA Manual of Small Animal Anaesthesia and Analgesia* (eds C. Seymour & R.D. Gleed), pp 43–55. British Small Animal Veterinary Association, Cheltenham.

Hall, L.W., Clarke, K.W. & Trim, C.M. (2000) Patient monitoring and clinical measurement. In: *Veterinary Anaesthesia*. pp 29–59. WB Saunders, Philadelphia.

Martin, M.W.S. & Corcoran, B.M. (1997) Electrocardiography. In: *Cardiorespiratory Diseases of the Dog and Cat*. Blackwell Science, Oxford.

Murison, P.J. (2001) Prevention and treatment of perioperative hypothermia in animals under 5 kg bodyweight. *In Practice*, July/August, 412–418.

10

Nursing the Patient in Recovery

Janis Hamilton

Before induction of anaesthesia, plans should have been made for the recovery period. This is a very important stage in patient care, and one that is often overlooked until the last minute. The speed of recovery from general anaesthesia depends on many factors including:

- *Breed:* Sighthounds such as greyhounds may have prolonged recovery periods following barbiturate anaesthesia.
- *Systemic illness:* Hepatic, renal and endocrine diseases, amongst others may cause prolonged recovery periods because of altered metabolism and excretion of drugs.
- *Temperature:* Hypothermia increases morbidity and mortality of patients, in particular in critically ill patients. It can prolong recovery times by reducing clearance of anaesthetic drugs from the body, while shivering – a normal physiological response to hypothermia – significantly increases oxygen consumption.
- *Duration of general anaesthetic*
- *Anaesthetic drugs administered*
- *Route of administration of anaesthesia.*

Every patient recovering from a general anaesthetic has a requirement for a certain amount of care and monitoring, and some patients will require intensive care. There are certain general monitoring requirements which will apply to most patients and some which are more specialised for patients who have either undergone a specific procedure or are affected by systemic disease.

RECOVERY AREA

Recovery from anaesthesia is essentially the reverse of induction of anaesthesia. The patient goes from an unconscious state to a conscious state with all the associated planes in between (see chapter 9).

The recovery area should be situated close to the theatre or preparation room, and be easily accessible. It is essential that staff members can observe recovering patients. It should also be quiet. Separate recovery areas for dogs, cats and exotic species are desirable, but not always achievable. This removes some of the stress associated with interaction of the different species.

Ideally patients will not be spending too long in the recovery area before returning to the hospital kennels or transferring to an intensive care unit. Consequently the kennels in the recovery area need only be large enough to allow patients to recover in comfort and safety, and to allow turning of the patient if and when required. Cats often prefer to recover in small kennels where they feel safer. Kennels which are easy to clean are an asset, especially if there is a high caseload passing through the recovery area. It is very important to ensure kennels are cleaned thoroughly between patients, so this should be borne in mind if purchasing kennels for this purpose. Ideally a sink should be available with access to the necessary cleaning equipment.

It is important to ensure the lighting is adequate for observation of patients. An additional directable light is a great asset for those patients who insist on recovering in the corners of the kennels or for closer inspection of a patient.

A sharps bin should be available for correct disposal of intravenous cannula stylets, needles and scalpel blades.

An enclosure or area of recovery for exotic patients will be required. A heated vivarium is an excellent purchase for the practice that has a large caseload of exotic patients. A secondhand incubator would be a good substitute. This would also be useful for juvenile and neonatal patients.

Bedding plays an important role in the comfort and heat conservation of recovering patients. 'Vet Beds' can be used for most patients. They provide comfort, conserve heat and will keep patients dry in case of urination, exudates from wounds and drains or fluid spillage. Incontinence pads with soft absorbent material backed with a waterproof layer are invaluable in the immediate postoperative period to collect voided urine and faeces as they may be simply disposed of into clinical waste once soiled. Hay may be used for rodents and rabbits, as it provides heat, a place to hide and food on recovery.

The type of equipment in a recovery room depends on available funds, space and the number of patients passing through the area, but some items should always be available.

Thermometer

The most common cause of prolonged recovery from anaesthesia is hypothermia and every precaution should be taken to avoid it. These precautions may be simply reducing the time patients are anaesthetised by careful planning of the theatre list or avoiding excessive wetting of the patient during aseptic preparation of the surgical field.

A simple digital or mercury thermometer to record the temperature of patients is essential. Digital thermometers are more robust and avoid the health and safety implications of containing a mercury spill in the recovery area following breakages. Aural thermometers with single-use protective sheets applied to the probe are now widely available. These thermometers are minimally invasive and easy to use in the recovery area.

A room thermometer to record the temperature of the surrounding environment is a useful tool. This is especially important for small and exotic patients, which can prove difficult to obtain a core temperature from.

Means of maintaining or raising body temperature
Means of maintaining or raising body temperature should be available.

- *Heat lamps:* Care must be taken to avoid thermal injury if lamps are placed too close to the patient. Infra-red lamps should be at least 100 cm from the surface of the patient.
- *Electric heat pads:* The patient should not be placed directly onto these pads, to avoid accidental thermal injury.
- *Circulating warm air blankets ('BAIR huggers'):* These blankets circulate warm air through fenestrated, disposable, sterile blankets. They minimise the risk of localised thermal necrosis of the skin because there is no direct heat contact with the skin.
- *Recirculating water-filled thermostatically controlled pads.*
- *Simple hot water bottles, heated intravenous fluid bags and water-filled gloves:* It is important that that the patient is protected from direct contact with the bottle, bag or glove, which should be wrapped in either bubble-wrap or fabric. These devices are one of the most frequent causes of thermal injury in anaesthetised human patients.
- *Reusable wheat or cherry-stone filled bags:* These can be heated in a microwave and retain their heat for several hours.
- *Incubators.*
- *Heated intravenous fluids:* High flow rates are required to avoid the fluid cooling before it reaches the patient. High flow rates are not always indicated (see chapter 8).
- *Reflective aluminium space blankets and plastic bubble-wrap* are good insulators for small patients, and can be disposed of if they become soiled. Remember that a patient recovering from anaesthesia may not be able to move away from the heat source if it becomes too hot, and close monitoring of the patient's temperature and regular repositioning are essential when using external heat sources.

Care must be taken that blankets or insulating materials such as those mentioned previously do not limit the nurse's view of the patient.

Oxygen

An oxygen supply to supplement patients who are suffering from respiratory depression, dyspnoea or shock should be available. This may be delivered by a pipeline supply directly to a flowmeter, as in larger hospitals, or *via* a simple free-standing oxygen cylinder which will require a pressure-reducing valve connected to a flowmeter.

The following equipment should be readily accessible:

> Oxygen masks
> Endotracheal tubes
> Oral gags
> Laryngoscope
> Flexible stylet to aid intubation
> Cuff inflator
> Endotracheal tube ties
> Water-soluble lubricant
> Local anaesthetic spray

A *pulse oximeter* to measure oxygen saturation of the blood would be useful. The probe should not be attached to the tongue or lip of a recovering animal, as it is likely to be bitten and destroyed. A preferable site would be the ear, prepuce or vulva. Rectal probes are available for some instruments.

Suction

Suction should be available to remove excess oral secretions or vomit.

Pen torch

A pen torch to test the pupillary light reflex is useful.

Fluid pumps or syringe drivers

Useful for delivering exact amounts of fluid or drugs. An audible alarm will alert the nurse to any interruptions in delivery.

Miscellaneous supplies

Dressing materials, disposable gloves and paper towels should be on hand.

Safety of both staff and patients is an issue that must never be overlooked. Patients weighing more than 25 kg will require two or more people to lift them. *Trolleys and stretchers* should always be used to move anaesthetised patients in and around the theatre and recovery area. This is for the safety of the patient as much as the theatre staff. Even small patients are less likely to be dropped if transported on a trolley or stretcher, and it also ensures the trachea remains extended. Adequate ventilation should be provided as patients may be exhaling volatile anaesthetic gases in the recovery period. *Monitors* are available for staff to wear, which measure the amount of halothane and/or nitrous oxide present in the surrounding atmosphere (see chapter 1). If required a health and safety specialist will visit the workplace and suggest improvements to working practice which should lower staff exposure. Care must also be taken when moving or turning large patients. Assistance should always be sought to avoid back injury to personnel. *Mechanical hoists* are available for lifting the larger patient.

The comfort and requirements of staff in the recovery area should be considered. There should be a place to sit, from where all patients can be easily observed. A method of calling for assistance is desirable, perhaps a panic alarm which would bring assistance without the nurse having to leave the recovery area.

It is important to record events in the patient's records, even if recovery is uneventful with no obvious problems.

EXTUBATION

At the end of the surgical procedure or period of investigation, the patient is recovered from anaesthesia. It is important not to anticipate the end of the procedure and create a situation where the animal is recovering consciousness before procedures such as suturing or bandaging are complete.

Recovery from anaesthesia begins with termination of delivery of the anaesthetic agent, whether an inhalational agent or an intravenous agent, and removal of the patient from the oxygen supply. If nitrous oxide has been used, it should be removed from the inspired gases before the oxygen, and the patient allowed to breathe 100% oxygen to minimise the effects of diffusion hypoxia. Nitrous oxide can contribute as much as 66% of the volume of the inspired gases and it is essential that the flow rate of oxygen is adjusted to maintain an adequate fresh gas flow to the breathing circuit and patient when the nitrous oxide has been switched off. To minimise atmospheric pollution in the recovery area, the breathing system should be flushed with oxygen to remove any residual traces of gaseous or volatile anaesthetic agents into the scavenging system.

Once disconnected from the breathing system, the patient is breathing room air, initially through an endotracheal tube, and should not be left unattended. The tie, which has been used to secure the tube in place, can be loosened although the cuff, if present, should remain inflated until just before extubation, when it may be fully deflated. Failure to deflate the cuff of the endotracheal tube before extubation can traumatise the tracheal and/or laryngeal mucosa. An exception to fully deflating the cuff would be if the patient has undergone a dental procedure or oral surgery, which may have left blood or fluids in the oral cavity. In such patients it may be wise to leave the cuff partially inflated during extubation, to prevent any fluids entering the trachea. Following extubation in these patients the oral cavity should be inspected with the aid of a laryngoscope to ensure no debris such as loose teeth remain within the oropharynx, which could lodge in the airway during recovery.

Generally speaking, in dogs, the endotracheal tube should be left *in situ* until the gag reflex has returned. This generally indicates that the patient is able to protect their own airway in the event of regurgitation or vomiting. In brachycephalic breeds the tube is often left in slightly longer, until the patient is almost fully conscious. Because these dogs usually have very long soft palates, this can lead to some respiratory distress on extubation, and re-intubation should be performed if these patients become distressed or dyspnoeic on extubation. The patient may need to be re-anaesthetised to secure a patent airway.

It is often more difficult in cats to decide when to remove the endotracheal tube. Return to consciousness is indicated by signs such as tail, limb and ear movement and a swallowing reflex. Care must be taken not to delay extubation too long as this can lead to laryngospasm.

Following extubation all patients should be positioned with the head and neck extended to help maintain the patency of the airway.

MONITORING OF THE PATIENT

There are certain parameters that should be monitored in every patient recovering from a general anaesthetic. All measurements taken or observations made should be noted on the patient's records along with the time and the initials of the person responsible for the observation. The veterinary nurse also should alert the veterinary surgeon in the event of unexpected observations.

Position of the patient

When presented to the recovery area the patient must be positioned according to the procedure that has just been performed. For patients that have not undergone a major surgical procedure, lateral recumbency is appropriate in most cases until it is possible to prop the patient up into sternal recumbency. If a patient has not moved voluntarily for 30 min, they should be turned over to minimise the risk of hypostatic congestion developing in the dependent lung. Often the stimulation of turning the patient can be sufficient to accelerate the recovery process.

For surgical patients, it is generally better to have the wound uppermost. This is usually more comfortable for the patient and allows the wound to be monitored or attended to more easily.

Pulse

The pulse and heart rate should be recorded every 5 min in the early stages of recovery. A peripheral pulse such as the carpal or tarsal pulse is preferable to a central pulse such as the femoral. The peripheral pulses give a more accurate indication of the condition of the circulatory system, as these pulses would be among the first to disappear should the patient develop circulatory shock. The character of the pulse should also be noted, e.g. strong, weak, thready, bounding or regularly irregular as in sinus arrhythmia. The patient should be monitored for the presence of pulse deficits. This occurs when a heart beat does not generate a peripheral arterial pulse and the heart rate is therefore greater than the pulse rate.

Respiration

Respiratory rate and effort should be recorded every 5 minutes in the early stages of recovery. It should be noted and reported if the breathing is abdominal rather than thoracic, or if it becomes laboured at any time during the recovery period. In these situations the patient should be placed in lateral recumbency and the head and neck extended.

Temperature

Any patient who enters the recovery area wet due to fluid spillage or urine soiling should be thoroughly dried before being placed in a recovery kennel. The rectal temperature should be taken as soon as possible after the patient is settled in the recovery area. This provides a baseline value to which any subsequent values can be compared. The temperature should be checked every 30 min in a patient that has a normal temperature initially, and every 15 min in a patient that is showing signs of hypothermia or hyperthermia or is having a protracted recovery. In patients showing mild hypothermia, care must be taken not to overheat with artificial means. Usually all that is required is some insulation in the form of blankets or bubble-wrap, to conserve heat and prevent further loss. Hyperthermia may cause patients in recovery to become agitated and pant, and this simple cause of distress during the recovery period should not be overlooked.

Temperature probes affixed to ears and tails can give unreliable readings. Aural thermometers are now available. They sit in the ear canal of cats and dogs and give a core temperature reading.

Mucous membrane colour and CRT

The colour of the mucous membranes and the capillary refill time (CRT) gives an indication of the peripheral circulation. A pale colour may indicate shock, anaemia or haemorrhage. A blue tinge (cyanosis) indicates severe hypoxia and brick-red membranes can indicate infection or septic shock.

Additional or advanced patient monitoring may be indicated during unexpectedly prolonged recoveries, following individual abnormal or unexpected observations or to investigate trends such as a continuing decline in body temperature (see chapter 9).

Analgesia

On humane grounds it is necessary to provide analgesia when required. In the patient who is having a stormy recovery or who is vocalising during the recovery period, it may be difficult to tell if the reaction is due to pain or excitement or is just part of the recovery process (Stage II). On the other hand some patients are very stoical and show little response to pain, even when severe pain is expected, so how does one tell which patients need analgesia? The answer is simple: if the patient has undergone a procedure, which would be expected to produce pain in people, it should be assumed it will be painful in animals, and analgesia should be provided. If, after giving analgesics, the patient still appears to be in pain, a more potent analgesic or a top-up dose of the original analgesic may be required.

A useful way of gauging whether or not the analgesic has had the desired effect is to use a pain score. This is a simple technique which involves the use of a scale from 0 to 10, with 0 being comfortable, resting quietly and pain-free, and 10 being severe agonising pain. A line is drawn with 0 at one end and 10 at the other. A cross is made on the line at the point where it is thought the patient is in terms of pain. This is then reassessed after giving analgesics and another cross made. This allows a judgement to be made about the effect the analgesic is having on the patient (Fig. 10.1).

Hydration status

Many patients undergoing general anaesthesia receive intravenous fluid therapy to support the circulation. It is good practice to continue fluid therapy into the recovery period until the patient is able to drink unaided. This is especially important for patients who experience a protracted recovery. Most isotonic intravenous fluids will be adequate for short-term circulatory support.

The only acceptable method of delivering intravenous fluids during anaesthesia is through an aseptically placed intravenous catheter; taping a hypodermic needle into a vein is not acceptable. It can be useful to place the intravenous catheter after the pre-anaesthetic medication has taken effect and then it may be used to induce anaesthesia. Once the patient has been intubated and is maintained on inhalational anaesthetic gases, the intravenous catheter can be used to administer intravenous fluids. This system also ensures patent venous access both during the anaesthetic procedure and in the recovery period.

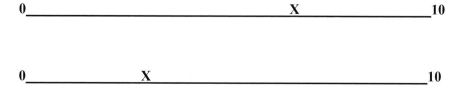

Fig. 10.1 The pain score of a patient (top) before administration of analgesics and (bottom) one hour later, demonstrating a decrease in the level of pain noted by the observer.

The jugular veins should not be overlooked when considering a vein suitable for catheterisation. These veins are particularly useful when multiple blood samples are required, as in the case of an animal with diabetes mellitus, when blood glucose levels will be monitored both during the period of general anaesthesia and in the recovery period, or if peripheral venous access has proved difficult in small or dehydrated patients. The technique is similar to catheterisation of the peripheral veins, with a longer, larger gauge catheter, e.g. 16G (Vygon), although placement in the conscious patient may be slightly more demanding. Care should be taken to ensure the intravenous catheter is held securely in the vein and, with jugular catheters, this may mean suturing them in place. Frequent checks should be performed to ensure and maintain patency of intravenous catheters. This will involve 4-hourly flushing of the catheter with heparinised saline when not being used to administer fluids or drugs. A dressing should always cover the catheter and the dressing should be renewed at least daily, allowing inspection of the catheter entry site for signs of infection and so on. The use of a T-connector instead of a bung can be a time-saving and more aseptic means of ensuring good catheter hygiene. It removes the necessity for removing and replacing catheter bungs, whose sterility is often questionable; each time venous access is required (see chapter 8).

A simple way of assessing the hydration status of patients in the postoperative period is to monitor their urinary output. Simply noting and recording when a patient passes urine voluntarily is one way. This method does not allow the amount of urine to be measured. A more accurate method of monitoring urinary output would be to insert a urinary catheter aseptically into the bladder and either drain the bladder intermittently or attach it to a closed collection system. Dog urinary catheters and cat catheters may be occluded with a catheter bung or injection cap, while spigots (Portex) are available to occlude the end of Foley catheters. Purpose-made urine collection bags can be purchased, or a system using an empty intravenous fluid bag with a giving set attached to the urinary catheter works just as well. A closed system of collection should be used by preference, as there is less chance of introducing infection into the urinary tract. This system is suitable not only for male dogs, but also for bitches and tomcats. Catheterising queens is not routinely performed and is generally only undertaken with critically ill patients.

Routine urinary catheterisation of patients who have undergone a long surgical procedure and who may be in the recovery unit for some time is a simple way to make these patients more comfortable by relieving the pressure of a full bladder.

Wound management

Any patient with a surgical wound should have it attended to before settling them in recovery. This may be as simple as removing ultrasound gel or cleaning blood from around the wound, to ensuring appropriate dressing materials have been applied to the wound. Surgical wounds should be carefully observed for any excessive swelling or discharge in the postoperative period.

If a wound has had a dressing applied postoperatively, dressing checks should be performed every 30 min for the first 2–3 h to ensure that the dressing has not become too tight due to postoperative swelling, or that there is not excessive bleeding or discharge. If a dressing does need to be changed, it is important that a note is made in the records, as frequent dressing changes, due to strikethrough, may be a sign there is a problem with either haemostasis or excessive discharge of exudates, both of which can have serious implications on the patient's fluid balance. Weighing the dressing materials before application and after removal can give an indication of the amount of fluid being lost. Even simple wound dressings, e.g. Primapore (Smith & Nephew), can soak up a large amount of fluid if they are changed often. Dressing changes, and the reason for the change, should always be noted on the patient's records. This ensures that following personnel changeover the wound management history is available. Patients who attack their dressings on recovery may be responding to pain, or the dressing may be genuinely uncomfortable. If the patient has previously ignored the dressing, a sudden interest may indicate either a dressing or an underlying problem. Try to ensure the dressing is not too tight and, if there is any doubt, remove the dressing and reapply.

It is good practice to cover any surgical wound with a light dressing postoperatively. This can be in the form of a simple adhesive strip with a centrally placed non-adherent dressing such as Primapore (Smith & Nephew), which will cover the incision site and protect it from contamination until the wound edges have formed a seal, which usually happens within 6–10 h.

Drug therapy

It is important to ensure that patients who are already on drug therapy regimes receive their drugs at appropriate times. This can sometimes prove difficult if the patient is still in the early stages of recovery and unable to receive oral medications. Alternative routes of administration should be considered. This may mean using a different form of the drug, e.g. an injectable form rather than an oral form. Care should always be taken to check the dose rate of the different drug form, as it may have to be altered.

Nutrition

The willingness of a patient to eat is usually a good sign that the patient is comfortable. Most animals will sleep peacefully on a full stomach. Food and water should be offered as soon as the patient is sufficiently recovered from the anaesthetic to eat and drink without risk of aspiration, if their medical condition permits it. A diet which is palatable, energy dense and easily digestible is required. Commercial diets are useful as the nutritional information is readily available and energy requirements can be easily calculated using the formula for basal energy requirements (BER). This can be calculated using the formula:

$$\text{BER (kcal/day)} = 70 \times (\text{weight in kg} \times 0.75)$$

This gives the number of kcal per day for a healthy animal doing nothing more than sitting in a kennel. A 'disease factor' is introduced to take into account the increase in calorific requirements necessary to assist healing.

Total kcal required per day = BER × disease factor

Disease factors are generally accepted as:
Cage rest = 1.25
After surgery = 1.25–1.35
Trauma or cancer = 1.35–1.5
Sepsis = 1.5–1.7
Major burn = 1.7–2

Some patients benefit more than others from early nutrition after anaesthesia or surgery, including neonates, geriatrics and patients who fall under the heading of 'exotic'. These patients have lower reserves than normal adult patients and this should be borne in mind in the recovery phase.

Environment
A vivarium is an ideal environment for the recovery of exotic patients, and an incubator is a good substitute. Thought should be given about the area in which to site the enclosure. Many exotic species have a very advanced sense of sight, smell and hearing, and the close proximity of cats and dogs can be very distressing for them. This is especially true for small rodents, who can become very stressed if there are cats, which are their natural predators, in the area – even if they cannot see them. Lighting should be dim, which will be less stressful to the patient, but should allow the recovery nurse to make observations without shining a bright light into the enclosure. Ultraviolet lighting, a source of heat and a means of increasing the humidity for the reptilian species in the enclosure are desirable. A simple spray bottle containing water is all that is required to increase humidity. A hide area, which still allows the patient to be seen, is also desirable.

Monitoring after ophthalmic procedures
Protection
Many of these patients will have undergone delicate surgical procedures and protection of the surgical site is very important. This may require the use of an Elizabethan collar to prevent rubbing of the eyes and surrounding tissues. The sight of these patients may be temporarily or permanently impaired, and they must be protected from blunt trauma, which can occur if the patient walks into kennel walls or doors because they are disorientated. Allowances must be made

for this reduction or loss of sight when considering basic needs such as finding their water or food bowls.

Medication

This may be in the form of topical eye drops. Some procedures, such as cataract removal, require several different medications in drop form, both before and after the surgery, and it is important to space the drops out equally. This may require the compilation of a specific eye drop chart with times clearly marked when medications should be applied (Fig. 10.2). Analgesia should not be overlooked in these patients, and local anaesthetic drops can be useful if they are not detrimental to the condition being treated.

Complications

Intraocular haemorrhage can be a complication with some surgical procedures like cataract removal, so care must be taken not to increase intracranial pressure (ICP), which can precipitate haemorrhage. To reduce the chances of this happening, raise the head by 15° using a blanket, if the patient is in lateral recumbency.

Intracranial pressure can increase with hypercapnia and patients should be monitored to ensure adequate respiratory function in the postoperative period. Opioids in themselves do not increase ICP, however, opioid administration that causes respiratory depression and thus an increase in the partial pressure of carbon dioxide can raise ICP, and care should be taken to adhere to the dosage intervals prescribed by the veterinary surgeon.

Intracranial pressure can be raised when a patient pulls tightly on a collar round the neck, therefore the use of a body harness is recommended in patients who may be at risk. The normal effort expended when patients pass a bowel movement can be enough to raise ICP, so steps should be taken to reduce this effort as much as possible by supplying the patient with a bowel regulator such as Isogel, both before and after the surgery.

MEDICATION RIGHT EYE	1000	1200	1400	1600
Atropine 1 drop	✓			
Viscotears® 2 drops				
Tiacil® 1 drop		✓		

Fig. 10.2 Partially completed eye drop chart.

Monitoring after abdominal procedures

Wound management

Most patients recovering from abdominal surgery will have large incision sites that should be monitored every 30 min in the early postoperative period for haemorrhage and swelling. If a body bandage is not required, the wound should be covered with a simple postoperative dressing for protection.

Surgical drains, such as Penrose drains, may be in place, and must be kept clean to prevent ascending infection. Sterile disposable gloves should be worn when dealing with surgical drains and a sterile absorbent dressing, without exception, should cover drains. This may be difficult, depending on the position of the drains, and bolus or 'tie-over' dressings may be required. The dressing should be changed and the drain site cleaned using either sterile saline or 0.05% chlorohexidene at least twice daily, or more frequently if strikethrough of exudates occurs. A barrier cream or ointment such as soft paraffin can be smeared around the drain exit wound to protect the skin from excoriation.

Analgesia

Human patients report that abdominal surgery is among the most painful surgery. There is no reason to believe animals are any different, so the recovery nurse should be vigilant concerning analgesia, even in the quiet, apparently comfortable patient. If the analgesic protocol states that the patient should receive analgesia every 4 h, then it should be adhered to, in the absence of signs of overdosage, even if the patient appears comfortable. Administration of analgesics should not be postponed until the patient shows signs of pain.

Fluid therapy

Many abdominal surgical procedures are lengthy, with abdominal organs exposed to the air for long periods of time. This allows a great deal of heat and fluid to evaporate. Fluid lost in this manner may be replaced during the procedure, but replacement may continue into the recovery period. In addition, if the gastrointestinal tract has been entered, the patient may not be permitted oral fluids or food on recovery. Therefore, both maintenance and ongoing losses must be provided parenterally in the postoperative period. Thus intravenous fluid therapy may continue well into the recovery period and beyond.

If oral food and fluid are contraindicated for more than 24 h, enteral feeding tubes (Table 10.1) may be used to provide the patient's nutritional requirements. The most commonly used feeding tubes, when the gastrointestinal tract is functioning normally, are naso-oesophageal tubes, pharyngostomy tubes and gastrostomy tubes. It is possible to feed patients through a jejunostomy tube in cases of pancreatitis or when gastric function is compromised, but these are not used routinely. In the recovery period, feeding tubes should be secured to the body with a dressing, to prevent interference by the patient and inadvertent removal. The skin around where the tube enters or exits should be

Table 10.1 Methods for use of enteral tubes.

Type of enteral tube	Exit site	Primary method of attachment of tube to patient	Secondary methods of attachment	Methods of preventing patient interference
Naso-oesophageal	Nostril	Cyanoacrylate glue Butterfly tapes Chinese finger-trap suture Friction suture	Attach to collar	Elizabethan collar In cats, run tube over the top of the head between the eyes, thus avoiding the whiskers
Pharyngostomy	Piriform recess	Chinese finger-trap suture Friction suture Butterfly tapes	Bandage	Bandage Stockinette Elizabethan collar
Gastrostomy	Left flank	Chinese finger-trap suture Friction suture Butterfly tapes Fixation device (Cook Veterinary Products)	Bandage	Bandage Stockinette Elizabethan collar
Jejunostomy	Right ventral abdomen	Chinese finger-trap suture Friction suture Butterfly tapes	Bandage	Bandage Stockinette Elizabethan collar

kept scrupulously clean, and disposable gloves should be worn when handling the tube.

Vomiting or regurgitation in the recovering patient is always a cause for concern. If this occurs, the head must be positioned lower than the stomach. If possible, pull the tongue forward gently out of the mouth and either suction or wipe the vomitus out of the mouth and pharynx. If any vomit or regurgitated material enters the respiratory tract the patient should be monitored closely for signs of dyspnoea. The acid contents of the stomach can cause severe bronchoconstriction in addition to aspiration pneumonia. It may be necessary to X-ray the patient to check for radiographic signs consistent with aspiration.

In patients with diarrhoea in the recovery period, it is important to ensure the surgical wound does not become contaminated. If this does happen, the wound must be thoroughly cleaned using surgical scrub and an aseptic technique.

Monitoring after urogenital procedures

Urine production
After most urogenital surgical procedures, it is of the utmost importance to ensure the patient is able to produce urine, and that the urine is free from bacterial

contamination. As with most patients recovering from a general anaesthetic, it may be some time before normal toilet habits can be adopted, so a means of measuring and collecting urine during this phase is useful. Monitoring urine production can be as simple as noting if and when the patient passes urine, and the appearance and smell of the urine. If it is important to know how much urine is being produced and what the biochemical parameters are, a more accurate and convenient means of measurement should be used. This is usually in the form of an indwelling catheter. The best method of collection is to use a closed urine collection system. This reduces the risk of bacteria tracking up the urethra and into the bladder. Urine collection bags can be purchased, or a system can be made from an empty fluid bag and a fluid giving set. When emptying the bag it is important not to disconnect the system, thus leaving it susceptible to ascending infection, but to remove the urine from the bag with a needle and syringe *via* the injection port in the fluid bag, after first swabbing the port with surgical spirit.

The intravenous fluid rate in these patients may be higher than normal in order to diurese the kidneys and flush out the bladder. An indwelling urinary catheter prevents excess pressure on the bladder wall that may have had a surgical procedure performed on it, giving the incision time to heal. However, extreme care must be taken not to introduce the urinary catheter too far into the bladder, causing direct trauma to the bladder wall wound. Most of these patients will require an Elizabethan collar to prevent premature removal of urinary catheters.

Monitoring after thoracic procedures

Thoracic drains
Management of thoracic drains is one of the most important duties of a recovery nurse. A patient with a thoracic drain in place must never be left unattended, because inadvertent removal of the drain, or any of the associated components, e.g. three-way stopcock, by the patient can have fatal consequences in a very short space of time (Fig. 10.3).

A sterile dressing should always cover the thoracic drain for reasons of asepsis and to prevent interference by the patient. The dressing must not restrict normal breathing efforts. To this end a simple dressing of sterile swabs and stockinette is usually sufficient without resorting to expensive and time-consuming thoracic bandages. However, a more elaborate dressing may be needed in certain situations, for example, following a median sternotomy when exudation from the wound may be expected.

Thoracic drainage may initially be required on a frequent basis. Sterile disposable gloves should always be worn when handling thoracic drains, and a sterile syringe used. Each time the chest is drained, the amount of air and fluid removed must be recorded. Fluid may need to be submitted to the laboratory

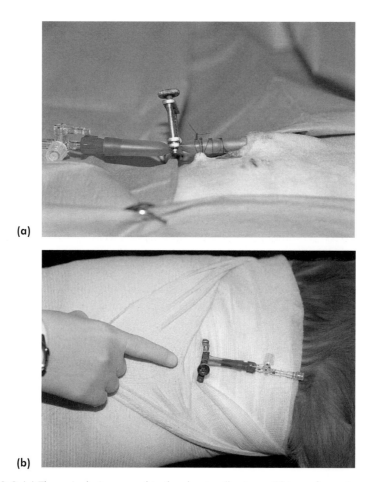

(a)

(b)

Fig. 10.3 (a) Thoracic drain secured to the chest wall using a Chinese finger-trap suture. A gate clamp provides additional security in the event that the three-way tap becomes dislodged. (b) A sterile dressing protects the thoracic drain and injection caps placed onto the three-way tap create a closed system.

for cytological or microbiological analysis and should be placed in appropriate containers.

Unfamiliar three-way stopcocks often present problems when draining chests, so it is essential that everyone involved with the nursing care of these patients understands how they work. Failure to do so can result in air being pushed into the thoracic cavity instead of being removed (iatrogenic pneumothorax), or large volumes of air may be appear to be withdrawn from the chest when in fact it is room air!

Analgesia

The normal movements required to breathe can produce intense pain in animals which have undergone thoracic surgery or suffered thoracic trauma. These patients take quick, shallow breaths, resulting in poor oxygenation of the tissues. Relieving this discomfort will encourage the patient to take deeper, more normal, breaths and will improve oxygenation. Although opioids are respiratory depressants and hence contraindicated in patients with poor oxygenation, the superior pain relief they provide allows the patient to breathe more efficiently and thus improve their oxygenation. Bladder and bowel movements, which cause the patient to strain, can induce quite severe pain. As well as using opioids in these patients, the use of a bowel regulator, and ensuring that the patient is given ample opportunity to empty the bladder voluntarily, can minimise these effects.

Oxygen

It may not be necessary to provide oxygen supplementation to all patients who have undergone thoracic surgery, but provision should be made in case the need arises. This may be as simple as having a mask and appropriate breathing system ready, or may involve the use of indwelling intranasal catheters. If using intranasal catheters, it is always a good idea to have them in place before you actually need them. Placing the catheter before the patient has fully recovered from the anaesthetic is the easiest option.

There are two types of catheter in common use. Paediatric feeding tubes are soft, flexible and inserted into the nares to the level of the medial canthus of the eye (Fig. 10.4). They are secured in a similar manner to naso-oesophageal tubes (see above). Disposable nasal cannulae have two short nasal prongs, which are inserted into the nostrils and fixed behind the head. This has the advantage of being easy to place in the conscious patient and twice as much oxygen can be delivered without causing high-pressure jetting injury and discomfort. Where possible, oxygen should always be humidified before being administered to the

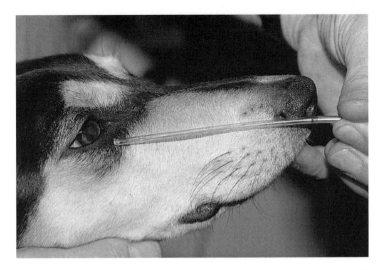

Fig. 10.4 Nasal oxygen tubing should not be advanced beyond the medial canthus of the eye.

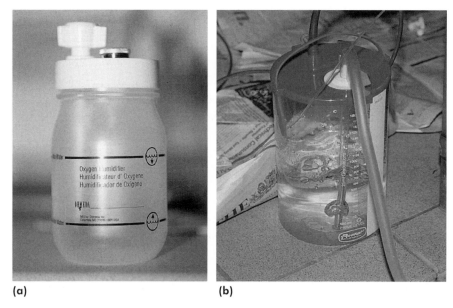

(a)   (b)

Fig. 10.5 (a) A commercial oxygen humidifier. (b) Oxygen may be humidified by bubbling the gas through distilled water.

patient (Fig. 10.5). It is contraindicated to give nasal oxygen to patients who have epistaxis, as the flow of oxygen may restart haemorrhage and could propel blood into the lungs, nor should it be given to patients who have undergone brain surgery, as any increase in cranial pressure should be avoided.

Monitoring after ear, nose and throat procedures
Protection
Following many of the surgical procedures that fall under this heading, wounds must be protected from interference by the patient, not only by licking but also by scratching. In the case of the ear and nose, this will probably mean an Elizabethan collar. Cervical neck wounds may be protected using bandages and/or vigilance on the part of the recovery nurse instead of an Elizabethan collar.

Due to the location of the facial nerve, many surgical procedures involving the ear are in danger of traumatising this nerve. This can cause paralysis of the facial muscles, characterised by a drooping lip and eyelid that is unable to blink. Often this is temporary, but in the recovery phase the surface of the eye should be kept moist and protected by the frequent application of an ophthalmic lubricant.

Tracheotomy
These patients are true intensive care cases. Whether the tracheotomy is temporary or permanent, these patients must be under 24-h watch in the early stages.

A temporary tracheotomy site allows patients to breathe directly through a tube placed in the trachea, until the normal airway is functional. Care and maintenance of these tubes requires vigilance by the recovery nurse. Soon after placement of a tracheotomy tube, the body begins to treat it like a foreign body. This results in large amounts of secretions forming around the tube. These must be suctioned out to prevent blocking of the tube (Fig. 10.6).

As the secretions are often thick and mucoid, it may be necessary to dilute them with some sterile saline prior to suctioning. Sterile saline (2–5 ml) is instilled into the tracheotomy tube following pre-oxygenation of the patient. Pre-oxygenation is required to avoid hypoxia during suctioning. Although a dog urinary catheter can be used to suction the secretions, these catheters are quite rigid and care must be taken not to traumatise the trachea. Tracheal suction catheters or infant feeding tubes are preferable. The longer the tracheotomy tube is in place, the fewer secretions will be produced. This means that in the early stages the tube should be suctioned every 20 min, but over time this can be reduced. Sometimes the tracheotomy tube may need to be changed if the secretions are building up on the inner surface and cannot be suctioned. Preplacement of stay sutures around the tracheal rings above and below the tracheotomy tube when it is inserted initially makes this an easier task. Double-lumen tracheotomy tubes make cleaning the tube much easier (Fig. 10.7). The inner cannula is simply removed, cleaned and replaced.

The skin around the tube must be kept clean and dry. The application of petroleum jelly around the tube will help to prevent excoriation of the surrounding tissue.

Many of the same principles regarding suction and attention to surrounding skin apply to patients with permanent tracheostomy sites. The only difference is that there is no plastic tube in place, just a permanent opening into the trachea.

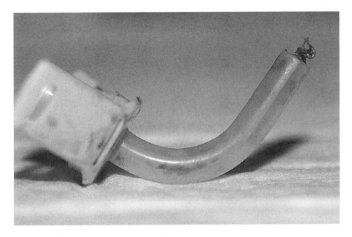

Fig. 10.6 A single-lumen tracheotomy tube blocked by secretions.

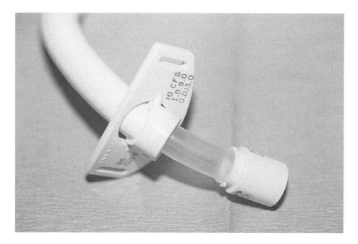

Fig. 10.7 A double-lumen tracheotomy tube. The inner tube is visible.

Patients with temporary or permanent tracheostomies bypass the nasal passages when breathing. Thus air is not humidified and warmed as it passes through the nasal chambers. These patients usually require intravenous fluid therapy in the postoperative period as they lose a lot of fluid through excess secretions and evaporation. Furthermore, bedding materials that do not shed lint that may be inhaled through the tube or stoma should be provided. In addition, excessive amounts of bedding should be avoided as this may cover the tube or stoma, and can quickly lead to suffocation.

Monitoring after orthopaedic procedures
Dressings
These are applied for support and/or protection and they come in many forms, from simple wound coverings to elaborate slings and casts. A newly applied dressing should be checked every 30 min for comfort and strikethrough and to ensure it is still doing the job it was applied to do. The materials used to apply a dressing should be noted on the patient's chart. This allows the recovery nurse to use the same materials if the dressing requires replacement.

Analgesics
All orthopaedic patients require analgesia. A well-applied dressing will help to ease discomfort, but most patients will require more than that. The practice of withholding analgesics to prevent orthopaedic patients moving around and disrupting the surgical repair is no longer acceptable on ethical grounds. A combination of non-steroidal anti-inflammatory drugs and opioids works well in these patients.

Assistance

Many of these patients may be temporarily para- or tetraparetic and will require assistance to move around the kennel, change position, reach food and water bowls, and empty bladders and bowels. The use of fleece-lined abdominal slings can be a great help to support these patients; however, a folded towel can be used. Any dog heavier than 25 kg will require at least two people to move and lift it.

Monitoring after neurological procedures

Position

Not all neurological patients will have had a surgical procedure. Many will have undergone investigations such as myelography, electromyography, computerised tomography (CT) or magnetic resonance imaging (MRI).

When performing myelography; dye can be injected into the subarachnoid space either in the lumbar or the cervical region. Following injection of dye into the cisterna magna, the patient should be positioned with the head raised on foam pads or blankets in the immediate postoperative period. This encourages dye to flow away from the brain, reducing the incidence of seizures. Other neurological investigations do not require any special positioning other than to ensure the patient's comfort.

If a surgical procedure has been performed it is important to ensure the patient is kept warm, as spinal surgery tends to be prolonged, with the potential for patients to become hypothermic.

Mental status

Rather than an absolute measurement, the important thing with mental status is noting changes and trends. Parameters that can be looked at include response to light and noise, and spatial awareness.

There may be changes in mental status before or after a seizure. These should all be noted and reported. The signs to look for include erratic movements, vocalisation, facial twitching, extension and rigidity of the limbs with hyperextension of the neck. If seizures are a possibility, the appropriate doses of suitable drugs should be drawn up and labelled, ready to administer should the need arise (see box). If seizures occur, help should be summoned and drugs should only be given on the instructions of a veterinary surgeon. Ensure that the intravenous catheter is patent. Dim the lights and reduce noise if possible. Before giving any drugs, check that a seizure has taken place, and not just postoperative excitement.

DRUGS USED IN THE POSTOPERATIVE PERIOD TO CONTROL SEIZURES

Diazepam

Dose: 0.5–1.0 mg/kg intravenously.

This can be repeated up to twice in 30 min and should be given slowly. This cannot be given as an infusion as it binds to the plastic in the giving set.

Midazolam

Dose: 0.2 mg/kg intravenously as a bolus, then 0.2 mg/kg/h as an infusion if desired.

Cannot be mixed with solutions containing calcium.

Assistance

The same restrictions apply to these patients as orthopaedic patients when moving them. Great care must be taken when moving patients with spinal fractures. The aim is to keep the spinal column completely supported and this is best achieved by the use of a rigid stretcher or board. It may be necessary to devise a means of securing the patient to the board, and this can be achieved with the use of broad nylon webbing which will secure the patient with comfort.

Patients who have undergone brain surgery should not receive nasal oxygen.

Monitoring patients with endocrine disease

Diabetes mellitus

Patients with diabetes mellitus are fasted overnight before surgery, following their normal evening feeding and insulin regime. On the morning of surgery they receive one half of the normal dose of insulin and food is withheld. It is important that these patients are scheduled for surgery early in the day to ensure that they have recovered fully from the procedure and are capable of eating their evening meal and receiving their evening medications as normal.

The stress of hospitalisation, anaesthesia and surgery can cause normally stable diabetic patients to decompensate, and so, in addition to the measures mentioned above, blood glucose levels should be checked every 30–60 min both intraoperatively and in the early stages of recovery. If hypoglycaemia occurs then 5% glucose solution should be infused intravenously at 10–15 ml/kg/h initially and the flow rate adjusted according to the blood glucose levels. Two catheters should be established, one for infusions and one for blood sampling to avoid falsely elevated blood glucose results being obtained.

Hypoadrenocorticism (Addison's disease)

These patients will usually have received glucocorticoids before the anaesthetic procedure, e.g. dexamethasone 1–2 mg/kg intravenously, to counteract the stress of the anaesthetic regime; it may be repeated in the postoperative period so venous access is important. In the recovery phase fluid therapy should be continued and the electrolytes, sodium and potassium, may be checked to ensure that the sodium is not too low and the potassium too high.

Monitoring patients with renal disease

Patients with renal dysfunction may take longer to recover following administration of anaesthetic drugs, as their kidneys may not be able to excrete these agents as efficiently as normal.

It is important to ensure that patients with any renal compromise are given fluids throughout the time of anaesthesia and surgery and well into the recovery period, and urine output should be measured. In addition, urine specific gravity should be measured using a refractometer each time the urine collection system is drained.

Severe hyperkalaemia is generally treated before patients are anaesthetised, but serum potassium levels may need to be monitored in the postoperative period. Electrocardiographic changes associated with hyperkalaemia, such as tall and/or peaked T-waves, and bradycardia, may alert the observant recovery nurse to impending problems.

Administration of non-steroidal anti-inflammatory drugs (NSAIDs) inhibits the production of prostaglandins. One of the functions of the prostaglandins is local vasodilation of renal vessels in conditions of hypovolaemia and hypotension to maintain renal blood flow and limit renal ischaemia. Thus, NSAIDs should be used with caution in patients with compromised renal function in the perioperative period, especially if they are hypovolaemic or hypotensive.

Monitoring patients with hepatic disease

Patients with any hepatic dysfunction may take longer to recover following administration of anaesthetic drugs, as their liver cannot metabolise these agents as efficiently as healthy livers. This effect may be compounded by hypoalbuminaemia as many anaesthetic drugs are carried round the body bound to this protein, and relative overdose of anaesthetic agents is possible.

Pre-anaesthetic measurement of serum albumin levels will indicate if the patient is hypoalbuminaemic. If this is the case then infusion of plasma or a colloid may be started during the anaesthetic and surgery, and may be continued into the postoperative period. If the patient has received crystalloids during the anaesthetic and surgery, then a blood sample to measure serum albumin levels in the recovery phase may be useful. This would indicate if the albumin levels had been further diluted by infusion of the crystalloid.

Disorders of coagulation may have been identified in patients with hepatic dysfunction prior to anaesthesia and surgery. In the postoperative period they should be observed closely for signs of unexpected bleeding and the veterinary surgeon alerted.

Many patients with hepatic disorders have a reduced capacity for gluconeo-genesis, combined with a tendency for prolonged recovery and thus a delay in return to enteral nutrition, so postoperative monitoring of blood glucose levels may be appropriate. This is especially true in patients with congenital disorders affecting hepatic function, such as portosystemic shunts.

Monitoring patients with gastrointestinal disease

If there is a history of vomiting then the endotracheal tube should be left in place as long as possible. Suction should be available and the patient should be placed with their head lowered in case vomiting should occur. Fluid therapy should be continued into the recovery phase. Disposable bedding may be used for patients with diarrhoea. These patients can also suffer from hypoalbuminaemia (see hepatic disease).

CONCLUSION

Ensuring the safe recovery of patients is a very important nursing skill to develop. Each recovery is different. Some may take minutes and be uneventful while others may be prolonged and take hours before the patient is stable enough to move. It need not be an expensive or difficult exercise to improve most recovery areas. Usually what is needed is just a little advance planning.

FURTHER READING

Moore, A.H. (1999) BSAVA *Manual of Advanced Veterinary Nursing.* British Small Animal Veterinary Association, Cheltenham.

Seymour, C. & Gleed, R. (1999) *BSAVA Manual of Small Animal Anaesthesia and Analgesia.* British Small Animal Veterinary Association, Cheltenham.

Moore, M. (1999) *BSAVA Manual of Veterinary Nursing.* British Small Animal Veterinary Association, Cheltenham.

Orpet, H. & Welsh, P. (2002) *Handbook of Veterinary Nursing.* Iowa State Press.

McKelvey, D. & Hollingshead, K.W. (2000) *Small Animal Anesthesia & Analgesia,* 2nd edition. Mosby, St Louis.

Cardiopulmonary Resuscitation and Other Emergencies

Kirstin Beard

Cardiopulmonary arrest (CPA) is defined as the sudden cessation of spontaneous and effective ventilation and systemic perfusion (circulation), which leads to inadequate oxygen delivery to tissues, shock and death. CPA may occur acutely due to a single devastating event or chronically from the cumulative effect of several factors. It is important to identify which patients are at risk for CPA (brachycephalic breeds during recovery, patients with respiratory compromise, hypotension, trauma, and so on) and anticipate potential problems, which can often be avoided by meticulous monitoring and observation. Prevention of a crisis is better than attempting a cure.

The goal of cardiopulmonary resuscitation (CPR) is to support ventilation and circulation until spontaneous functions can be restored and sustained. Cerebro-cardiopulmonary resuscitation (CCPR) is an alternative term which emphasises the importance of preserving cerebral function.

The long-term survival rates following CPR in dogs and cats are poor, with less than 5% of patients resuscitated being discharged from hospital. In view of this, there are several ways in which attempts can be made to improve patients' survival. It is essential to be well prepared for carrying out CPR, and a designated area should be assigned within the practice. Within this area, facilities and equipment required should be visible, organised and easily accessible. It is important to be familiar with the techniques necessary to perform effective CPR; therefore, practice training sessions can be carried out and a protocol developed which all members of staff understand. This leads to an efficient team that can respond rapidly to an emergency.

CARDIOPULMONARY ARREST

Early recognition of impending CPA is critical to successful CPR. The veterinary nurse is often in a position to detect changes in a patient's condition while monitoring anaesthesia, and to identify which animals are at risk of developing CPA. The anaesthetic record is vital to allow tracking of physiological parameters and to display sudden changes in trends. Signs indicative of deterioration include changes in respiratory rate, depth and pattern, changes in pulse quality or rhythm, unexplained changes in anaesthetic depth or abnormal ECG rhythms. If there is any doubt whether the patient is in CPA, resuscitation should be initiated immediately. A delay of 3–4 min before the onset of resuscitation can lead to irreversible and often fatal changes.

Causes of cardiopulmonary arrest
- Hypoxia and hypercapnia;
- Anaesthetic overdose (absolute or relative);
- Hypotension;
- Dysrhythmias;
- Pre-existing heart disease;
- Vagal stimulation;
- Electrolyte imbalances;
- Hypothermia;
- Toxaemia.

Signs of cardiopulmonary arrest
- No heart sounds on auscultation;
- Absence of palpable pulse;
- Fixed and dilated pupils (30–45 sec) and central eye position (Fig. 11.1);
- Apnoea or 'agonal' gasps;
- Grey or cyanotic mucous membranes;
- Dry cornea with loss of reflexes;
- Arrhythmia;
- Bleeding at surgical site stops or slows; blood becomes dark in colour;
- Loss of muscle tone and loss of cranial nerve reflexes.

The most common types of arrhythmia noted during CPA are electromechanical dissociation (EMD), asystole, and ventricular fibrillation. Additional rhythms encountered during CPA include sinus bradycardia, sinus tachycardia and ventricular tachycardia. Recognition of the cardiac rhythm will help to determine the type of therapy required. Do not assume that a normal ECG trace is indicative of effective cardiac output. Check for a palpable pulse, as in EMD the ECG can appear normal even though mechanical cardiac activity is lost.

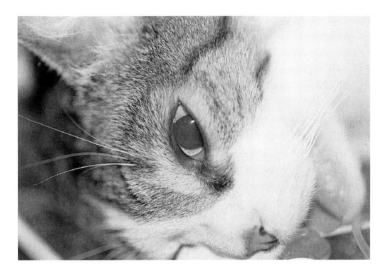

Fig. 11.1 Fixed dilated pupils and ashen mucous membranes in a cat that had suffered a cardiopulmonary arrest.

It is important to establish whether to perform CPR in patients with terminal disease, or those in which the likelihood of an arrest is anticipated and expected to be unsuccessful. Generally, CPR should only be performed when the arrest is unexpected, and the underlying cause of the CPA can be reversed. This will avoid inappropriate resuscitation and prevent undue suffering.

Cardiopulmonary resuscitation
Staff
A team approach to CPR is essential. One-person CPR is ineffective, and the ideal number of staff required in a resuscitation attempt is three to five. All staff within the practice should be trained in CPR techniques, and be capable of dealing with the initial management of CPA. An 'emergency plan' can be implemented which reflects individual practice facilities and staff. It is important for each member of the team to understand their role and responsibilities; this will avoid confusion and ensure an efficient, co-ordinated response.

Equipment
The facilities and supplies required to perform CPR should be readily available. The 'crash' box can be a simple small toolkit or an elaborate crash cart (Fig. 11.2). The cart has the advantage of additional storage space for equipment such as an ECG and defibrillator. Regardless of its form, the 'crash' box should be in a central location, fully equipped and regularly checked.

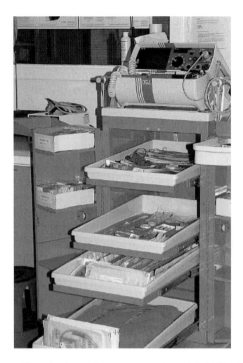

Fig. 11.2 A mobile, well stocked 'crash cart'. Note the ECG/defibrillator unit located on the top.

EMERGENCY EQUIPMENT CHECKLIST

Airway management

Endotracheal tubes (range 3–12 mm)
Laryngoscope
Stylet
Tracheostomy tubes
Large bore needles
ET tube ties

Vascular access

IV catheters (range of sizes)
Syringes
Needles
IV fluids set up – pressurised cuff
Scalpel blades
Intraosseus needle, spinal needles
Tape

(Continued)

Drugs

(see Table 11.1)

Emergency drug chart

Dosages in ml and defibrillator guidance

Additional facilities

Oxygen source
Ambu bag, breathing system, masks
Suction equipment: hand-held, suction pump
ECG: with pads attached to clips
Defibrillator: external and internal paddles, electrode gel
Stethoscope
Clock

Miscellaneous

Clippers
Scrub/spirit
Three-way taps, butterfly needles
Catheter bungs, extension sets
Urinary catheters: for IT drug administration
Surgical pack
Gloves
Suture material

The mnemonic ABCDEF is useful in remembering the elements of CPR. Each member of the team can then take responsibility for the treatment priorities of life support.

Airway (A)

Establish a patent airway. Intubate the patient with a well-fitting, cuffed endotracheal tube. Check that an existing tube is in the correct position and has not become blocked. In the event of upper airway obstruction, a long cannula can be passed to the tracheal bifurcation and oxygen insufflated until an emergency tracheostomy can be performed.

Breathing (B)

Perform intermittent positive pressure ventilation (IPPV) with 100% oxygen and an appropriate anaesthetic breathing system. Alternatively an Ambu bag (Fig. 11.3) can be used which will allow manual lung inflation with either air (21% oxygen) or 100% oxygen. Initially give the patient two breaths rapidly of 1–1.5 sec duration, and then ventilate once every 3–5 sec, interspersed with

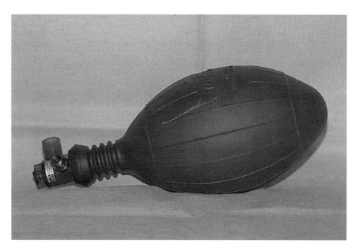

Fig. 11.3 An Ambu bag.

external chest compression. Inflation of the lungs should provide visible supranormal chest wall expansion. It is also important to allow the lungs to deflate fully after each ventilation to facilitate venous return.

Circulation (C)
Support of the circulation is essential to restore blood flow to vital organs and preserve cerebral function. It can be accomplished through external or internal cardiac compression. The breed of dog (size and shape) and chest wall compliance determine the effectiveness of the chosen method.

External cardiac compression
Blood flow during external cardiac compression is achieved by one of two mechanisms: the 'cardiac pump' and 'thoracic pump'.

- *Cardiac pump:* This is used in animals weighing less than 20 kg, or very narrow-chested dogs, e.g. greyhound. The aim is to squeeze the ventricles by compression of the ribcage over the cardiac area. This is performed with the patient positioned on a hard surface in right lateral recumbency with a slight head-down inclination. One or both hands are placed between the fourth to fifth intercostal space, at the costochondral junction, and the chest wall is compressed with the arms extended, force being applied by bending at the waist. The chest should be compressed by approximately one-third. A sandbag can be placed under the opposing chest wall for support. In cats, and patients weighing less than 5 kg, the thumb and forefingers can be used to compress the chest. The rate of compressions is approximately 90–120 per minute. The patient should be ventilated once every fifth or sixth compression.

- *Thoracic pump:* This technique is suited to larger dogs, or for those with 'barrel' chests. The chest is compressed at its widest part to increase intrathoracic pressure. This is transmitted to the intrathoracic vasculature, which leads to improved perfusion. Additional ways of improving venous return with this technique are:
  - Synchronous lung inflation with chest wall compression.
  - Abdominal binding of the hindlimbs and abdomen. This will direct blood flow from the abdomen towards the head.
  - Intermittent abdominal compression. The abdomen is slowly manually compressed as another means of improving blood flow.
  - Placing the patient in dorsal recumbency and compressing the sternum.

The effectiveness of CPR must be monitored within 3–4 min of onset. If the resuscitation efforts are not sufficient, the resuscitation technique must be changed. The following signs indicate generation of forward blood flow:

- palpation of a pulse during compression;
- constriction of pupil;
- improvement in mucous membrane colour;
- ECG changes.

Internal cardiac compression
Internal cardiac compression has been shown to be more effective than external chest compression in the artificial circulation of blood and perfusion of tissues during CPR. Internal cardiac compression is indicated in the following conditions:

- failed external cardiac compression;
- pneumothorax or haemothorax;
- pericardial tamponade;
- flail chest;
- diaphragmatic hernia;
- intra-operative thoracic or abdominal surgery.

The decision to perform a thoracotomy should be made after 5–10 min if the initial techniques employed are ineffective.

A rapid clip of the third to sixth intercostal space on the left side will remove the majority of long hair, and time should not be wasted in performing an aseptic surgical preparation of the site. The veterinary nurse should ensure that a surgical pack containing a loaded scalpel is prepared, and rib spreaders are available.

Internal compression allows visual and palpable assessment of ventricular filling, evaluation of the heart rhythm, accurate intraventricular injections, cross-clamping of the descending aorta, and assessment of lung inflation.

Disadvantages of internal compression include stopping cardiac compressions while performing a thoracotomy, potential damage to thoracic organs, unfamiliarity with the technique and postoperative sepsis.

Drugs (D)

Drug therapy during CPA is dependent on the situation and the type of cardiac rhythm; therefore ECG monitoring is generally required.

The principal drugs used in the treatment of CPA are adrenaline, atropine, and lignocaine. Additional drug therapy is based on the response to the initial stages of CPR. Some examples of the drugs that may be considered are shown in Table 11.1. There is considerable controversy regarding the value and place of many of the drugs suggested for use in CPR.

Table 11.1 Drugs commonly employed during and following cardiopulmonary resuscitation.

Drug	Indication	Dose rate
Adrenaline	Cardiac arrest	0.02–0.2 mg/kg IV
	Anaphylaxis	0.04–0.4 mg/kg IT
Atropine	Sinus bradycardia	0.02–0.04 mg/kg IV
	Atrioventricular block	0.4 mg/kg IT
	Ventricular asystole	
Lignocaine	Ventricular tachycardia	Dogs: 2–4 mg/kg IV
	Ventricular fibrillation	Cats: 0.5–1 mg/kg IV
Dobutamine	Myocardial failure	Dogs: 2–20 µg/kg/min CRI
	Low cardiac output	Cats: <4 µg/kg/min CRI
	Post CPR	
Dopamine	Hypotension	3–5 µg/kg/min CRI for
	Oliguria	increased renal perfusion
	Low cardiac output	5–10 µg/kg/min CRI for
		increased cardiac output
Frusemide	Cerebral/pulmonary oedema	Dogs: 2–4 mg/kg IV
	Oliguria	Cats: 1–2 mg/kg IV
	Congestive heart failure	
Methylprednisolone sodium succinate	Cerebral oedema post CPR	10–30 mg/kg IV
Naloxone	Opioid antagonist	0.04–1.0 mg/kg IV
	EMD	
Propranolol	Supraventricular tachycardia	0.02–0.06 mg/kg
Sodium bicarbonate	Severe metabolic acidosis	0.5–1 mEq/kg IV
	Prolonged CPR	
Bretylium tosylate	Ventricular fibrillation	5–10 mg/kg IV

Adrenaline

Adrenaline is an adrenergic agonist, which is considered to be the drug of choice in CPA. It produces an increase in heart rate, force of contraction and peripheral vasoconstriction, which increases arterial pressure and blood flow to vital organs.

Atropine

Atropine is a parasympatholytic agent that is used to treat arrhythmias arising from vagal stimulation. Its vagolytic action is indicated in the treatment of ventricular asystole and slow sinus or idioventricular rhythms.

Lignocaine

Lignocaine is an anti-arrhythmic agent. It is primarily used to treat ventricular arrhythmias. It may also be used to supplement treatment of ventricular fibrillation.

Routes of drug administration during CPR

Central venous route

This is the route of choice. Drugs are deposited near the heart, and provide high concentrations in a short period of time. Placement of a jugular catheter is required such that its tip lies within the cranial vena cava. This technique is useful in dogs and cats only when a central venous catheter has been preplaced.

Intraosseus route

This route is useful when vascular access is limited. There is rapid drug uptake from this site and large volumes can be administered. An intraosseus or spinal needle is inserted into the femur, humerus, wing of ileum or tibial crest.

Intratracheal route

Drugs may be administered into the trachea (IT route) by passing a urinary catheter through the endotracheal tube to the bifurcation of the trachea. Double the dose of the chosen drug is required and it should be diluted with saline to provide adequate volume to both distribute the drug and improve absorption. A limited number of drugs can be administered by this route. Drug uptake from this site may be slow and final blood concentrations reduced, but it is better than peripheral venous administration of drugs if there is poor forward flow of blood during CPR.

Peripheral venous route

This route is not ideal, but is often more convenient than others. Drugs take an excessive length of time to reach the heart, but following the drug with an intravenous bolus of sterile saline solution enhances response to peripheral venous injection.

Intracardiac route
This route of administration should be avoided unless open-chest CPR is being performed. Potential complications associated with this route of administration include coronary laceration, cardiac tamponade, myocardial trauma and refractory arrhythmias.

Fluid administration during CPR should be conservative unless hypovolaemia has been identified as an underlying cause of cardiac arrest because aggressive fluid therapy can rapidly lead to volume overload.

The veterinary nurse should ensure that drugs which are kept in the crash box remain within expiry dates. The practice of maintaining preloaded syringes with emergency drugs is not justified in veterinary practice. Unless the crash box is used on a routine basis, the drugs' life expectancy will be diminished; therefore the waste and costs involved do not make it practical. Additionally, the large range in animal body weights results in doses being variable.

An essential requirement of any crash box is a drug chart with dosages displayed in ml/kg. This allows rapid reference by a team member during CPR.

Electrical defibrillation (E)
The purpose of defibrillation is to convert the chaotic electrical activity of the fibrillating heart to sinus rhythm. The discharge of an electrical current through the myocardium aims to allow the pacemaker (sinoatrial node) to resume its normal rhythm. Defibrillation should be performed as soon as ventricular fibrillation is diagnosed, as success is inversely related to the elapsed time since fibrillation.

- *External defibrillation:* (See Fig. 11.4.) Conductive gel is applied to the defibrillator paddles, which are then placed firmly over the heart on each side of the chest. No personnel should be in contact with the patient at the time of discharge, therefore the operator should inform staff to 'clear'. Energy level = 1–5 J/kg.
- *Internal defibrillation:* (See Fig. 11.5.) The internal paddles should be covered in saline-soaked swabs to ensure good contact. The paddles cradle the heart opposite each other, and the procedure is carried out as above. Energy level = 0.1–0.5 J/kg.

When a defibrillator is not available a precordial thump may be effective. This involves delivering a sharp blow with a clenched fist over the precordium. Chemical defibrillation agents are of unknown value, but can be tried when a defibrillator is not available. Bretylium tosylate has been used at a dose of 5–10 mg/kg.

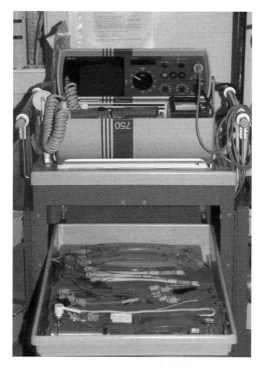

Fig. 11.4 A defibrillator with external paddles attached.

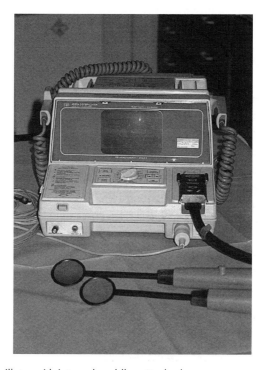

Fig. 11.5 A defibrillator with internal paddles attached.

Follow-up (F)

After successful CPR, continued support is required:

- Continue IPPV until the patient is breathing spontaneously. Provide a method of supplementing oxygen in the recovery period.
- Correct acidosis: Establish normal renal function or administer sodium bicarbonate if blood gas analysis is available.
- Cardiac support: Inotropes may be required to maintain cardiac output and improve renal blood flow.
- Fluid therapy: Fluids should be administered to maintain blood pressure and urine output.
- Minimise cerebral oedema: Position patient with head inclined upwards. Hyperventilate to reduce $PaCO_2$ and administer corticosteroids and/or mannitol if cerebral oedema is suspected.
- Assess neurological function.
- Monitor and maintain urinary output at 1–2 ml/kg/h.
- Maintain body temperature.

Intensive monitoring is very important in the post-resuscitative period. Special attention should be paid to monitoring the respiratory, cardiovascular, central nervous and urinary systems (see chapter 9). It is essential to monitor as many physiological variables as possible for each system to give an overview of the patient's status and prognosis.

OTHER EMERGENCIES AND ANAESTHETIC COMPLICATIONS

Good patient assessment and adequate preparation can prevent most anaesthetic emergencies and complications. Effective management of emergencies and complications requires continued vigilance, early detection and swift action. Remember, anaesthetic accidents can occur due to human error.

Respiratory emergencies

Apnoea and hypoventilation can result in severe hypoxia and hypercapnia, which can rapidly lead to cardiac arrest; therefore it is important to identify the cause and take immediate action. Often respiratory arrest is not detected before cardiac arrest, as they are almost simultaneous events.

Airway obstruction

This is most likely to occur in the pre-anaesthetic period or during recovery when the airway is unprotected and reflexes are diminished due to anaesthetic drugs. The exception is of course endotracheal tube and equipment-related problems during anaesthesia.

Causes of airway obstruction

- *Soft tissue entrapment (STE):* The tongue and soft palate are most commonly implicated. Brachycephalic breeds are susceptible to STE during recovery due to depression of oropharyngeal activity/reflexes (Fig. 11.6).
- *Foreign material:* Following upper airway, nasal, oral or dental surgery, blood, debris (e.g. calculus, tooth fragments), vomit, or saliva can lead to upper airway obstruction.
- *Mechanical obstruction:* Endotracheal tube problems such as kinking, over-inflation of the airway cuff, blockage or endobronchial intubation can cause obstruction.
- *Pathological:* For example, laryngeal paralysis, laryngospasm, tracheal collapse, bronchospasm.

Signs of airway obstruction

- Dyspnoea;
- Inspiratory snoring noises (stertor, stridor);
- Paradoxical thoracic wall movement;
- Cyanosis, reduced minute volume;
- Extreme respiratory efforts with no movement of reservoir bag.

Action

- If patient is vomiting or regurgitating, place in head-down position;
- Extend the head and neck and pull tongue forward;
- Insert mouth gag, clear oropharynx by swabbing or suction (Fig. 11.7);
- If intubated; check position and patency of tube and ventilate with 100% O_2;
- Consider the need for a tracheostomy if unable to relieve the obstruction.

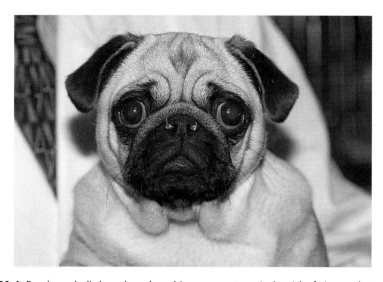

Fig. 11.6 Brachycephalic breeds such as this pug are at particular risk of airway obstruction.

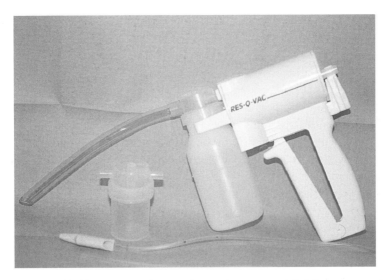

Fig. 11.7 A hand-held suction unit that may be used to remove debris from the oropharynx in an emergency.

Breathing

Transient apnoea is common following induction of anaesthesia with propofol and thiopentone. Assisted ventilation of the patient should be performed until spontaneous breathing resumes. Respiratory arrest can be obvious, but it is often preceded by hypoventilation that can be harder to assess.

Causes of respiratory depression or arrest
- *CNS depression:* e.g. anaesthetic overdose, increased intracranial pressure, severe head trauma, severe hypothermia, high dose opioids.
- *Chest wall fixation:* e.g. pneumothorax, neuromuscular blockade, restrictive bandages, pain following thoracotomy.
- *Pulmonary pathology:* e.g. pulmonary oedema, diaphragmatic hernia, restrictive lung lesions.
- *Tachypnoea:* e.g. inspired gas does not reach the alveoli. This may result from inadequate anaesthetic depth, pyrexia, hypoxia, or hypercapnia.

Signs of respiratory depression or arrest
- Reduced minute volume;
- Absence of ventilation;
- Cyanosis.

Action
- Establish a patent airway.
- Perform IPPV with 100% O_2 at a rate of 8–16 breaths per minute. Ensure good chest and lung compliance without the use of excessive pressure.

- Assess anaesthetic depth and stop administration of volatile, gaseous or intravenous agents if overdose suspected.
- Drug therapy may be required once the cause of respiratory arrest is diagnosed, e.g. opioid antagonists (naloxone), analeptics (doxapram), atipamezole.

Circulatory insufficiency

Failure of the circulation may be due to either inadequate circulatory volume (hypotension, hypovolaemia), or cardiac insufficiency (myopathy, arrhythmia). If left untreated, the decrease in effective circulating blood volume will lead to organ damage.

A patient is described as 'hypotensive' when the mean arterial blood pressure drops below 60 mmHg.

Causes of hypotension
- *Hypovolaemia:* e.g. absolute hypovolaemia due to volume deficit resulting from pre-existing fluid losses or severe haemorrhage or relative hypovolaemia following drug administration, the release of vasoactive substances, anaphylactic shock, and so on.
- *Decreased venous return to the heart:* This may occur with partial occlusion or compression of the caudal vena cava (large abdominal mass, gravid uterus). These effects are particularly marked when patients are placed in dorsal recumbency. Decreased venous return may also be caused by increased thoracic pressure during IPPV or if the expiratory valve of the breathing system is inadvertently closed.
- *Reduced systemic vascular resistance:* This is related to blood pressure and blood flow. It may be associated with vasodilation, excessive depth of anaesthesia, high doses of phenothiazines, endotoxaemia or anaphylaxis.
- *Myocardial depression:* This results in poor contractility of the heart. It can be associated with hypoxia, ischaemia, toxaemia, electrolyte disturbances, anaesthetic overdose or existing heart disease.
- *Inadequate cardiac output:* Tachycardia and/or inadequate stroke volume will affect cardiac output. Inadequate output may also occur with cardiac arrhythmias or disease, and hypovolaemia.

Signs of hypotension
- Weak peripheral pulses;
- Pale mucous membrane;
- Increased capillary refill time;
- Low measured blood pressure;
- Increased heart rate;
- Poor urinary output;
- Diminished bleeding.

Action

- Check that the expiratory valve is open.
- Assess depth of anaesthesia and reduce if necessary.
- Administer intravenous fluids rapidly, if hypovolaemia is present.
- Correct the inspiratory : expiratory ratio if using IPPV.
- If possible, reposition the patient from dorsal to lateral recumbency. Alternatively the table may be tilted to encourage abdominal structures to move caudally within the abdominal cavity.
- Control haemorrhage and relieve any factors reducing venous return.
- Inotropes may be considered, e.g. dobutamine, dopamine.

Tachycardia
Clinical tachycardia may be defined as heart rates above 180 beats per minute in the dog and 240 beats per minute in the cat. It is associated with decreased cardiac efficiency and increased cardiac workload. (See Table 11.2.)

Bradycardia
Clinical bradycardia may be defined as a heart rate below 60 beats per minute in the dog and 80 beats per minute in the cat. However, it is important to remember that there is marked variation between patients, and athletic dogs may normally have very low resting heart rates. Attention to possible causes is imperative to reduce the risk of CPA. (See Table 11.3.)

Miscellaneous
A number of other complications that may be encountered in the perianaesthetic period are detailed in Table 11.4.

Table 11.2 Causes of tachycardia and actions required.

Cause	Action
Inadequate anaesthesia, and pain	Check depth of anaesthesia
	Administer analgesics
Hypoxia	Ensure patent airway
	Check oxygen supply
	Remove nitrous oxide from inspired gases
	Ventilate with 100% oxygen
Hypercapnia	Ventilate with 100% oxygen
	Treat underlying cause (e.g. exhausted soda lime)
Hypotension	Administer fluids at rapid rates
	Treat underlying cause
Hyperthermia	Rapid cooling, e.g. ice-cold fluids, cold towels
Drugs	Parasympatholytic agents and β_1 agonists can cause tachycardia

Table 11.3 Causes of bradycardia and actions required.

Cause	Action
Anaesthetic overdose / Drugs	Check depth of anaesthesia and ventilate
Cardiovascular failure: hypoxaemia,	Ventilate with 100% oxygen
decreased venous return	Administer fluids
Hyperkalaemia	Ventilate with 100% oxygen
	Treat underlying cause
	Medical management
Vagal reflex: traction on viscera, ocular	Decrease surgical stimulation
pressure, laryngeal stimulation	Give atropine or glycopyrrolate
Hypothermia	Perform rewarming, supplementary heat

SUMMARY

Current survival rates for patients who experience cardiac arrest are low. The approach to CPR must be organised and a plan for CPA management must be made to attempt to improve success rates. It is very important to prevent the factors that contribute to arrest, therefore careful preparation and monitoring of patients is essential. Anticipation of potential problems in the high-risk patient and early recognition of changes in the physiological status of the anaesthetised patient will contribute to an efficient response and an improved outcome.

Several factors determine outcome in CPA: age of the patient, any concurrent disease, and current medical or surgical complications. The prognosis is improved in an acute, unexpected arrest where the animal is young and healthy, or in those who have had a drug overdose. Chronic arrests are more common, carry a poor prognosis and require aggressive management to be successful.

Knowledge of the owner's wishes with regard to CPR is advantageous. Prior discussion of the patient's prognosis and medical options will allow the owner time to become prepared and to make a decision, either to ask that everything possible should be done or to request a 'do not resuscitate' order if the likelihood of arrest is anticipated. This will prevent undue distress and inappropriate resuscitation.

When the cardiac resuscitative effort lasts in excess of 10–15 minutes, neurological outcome is worsened and long-term survival unlikely.

Most dogs and cats that show signs of recovery within 5 minutes of restoration of spontaneous circulation will recover with intact neurological function. However, following CPA patients are at risk of further arrests and so it is important that those animals that are successfully resuscitated receive continued intensive monitoring.

Table 11.4 Complications that may be encountered in the anaesthetic period.

Complication	Signs	Treatment	Comments
Drug overdose	Apnoea and/or hypoventilation Cardiac arrest	Discontinue anaesthetic drugs Administer IPPV Carry out CPR if required Fluid therapy Consider use of inotropes Drug antagonists when available, e.g. naloxone, atipamezole	Specific treatment will depend on the nature of the drug and relevant effects
Extravascular injections	Perivascular swelling around vein as drug is injected Pain on injection	Dilute with sterile saline by injecting 2–10 ml around affected vein, and massage well Lignocaine may be used as analgesia and to neutralise the alkalinity of the barbiturate	Barbiturates are irritant and can result in tissue sloughs following perivascular injection Avoid by venous catheterisation and adequate restraint
Haemorrhage	Increased blood at surgical site Tachycardia Pallor Weak pulse	Replace loss – blood, colloids, balanced electrolyte solution Estimate blood loss: weigh swabs, measure suction fluid	Blood loss leads to hypotension and hypovolaemic shock Clinical signs are evident when approx. 6–12 ml/kg lost
Vomiting or regurgitation	Presence of vomitus, oesophageal or gastric contents in oropharynx Dyspnoea	Protect patient airway – ensure airway cuff inflated if present Position patient head down Suction and clear oropharynx ± Irrigation of oropharynx Extubate with partially inflated cuff	This may occur because: Inadequate pre-anaesthetic fasting Prolonged gastric emptying Pressure from surgical manipulation or physiological state, e.g. pregnancy Disease or conditions associated with vomiting or regurgitation, e.g. mega-oesophagus
Hypothermia	Low core temperature Bradycardia Respiratory depression Prolonged recovery	Application of supplementary heat: heat pads, bubble wrap, blankets, hot water bottles, and wheat bags Avoid contact with cold surfaces Ensure warm ambient temperature Warm IV and lavage fluids Keep non-surgical areas of patient dry	Small animals are particularly susceptible Heat lost through evaporation, conduction, convection and radiation Avoid use of cold fluids Thermoregulation impaired by anaesthetics

FURTHER READING

Aeschbacher, G. & Webb, A.I. (1993) Intraosseous injection during cardiopulmonary resuscitation in dogs. *Journal of Small Animal Practice* **34**, 629–633.

Battaglia, A.M. (2001) Cardiopulmonary cerebrovascular resuscitation. In: *Small Animal Emergency and Critical Care*, WB Saunders.

Brodbelt, D.C. (1999) Anaesthesia and analgesia (eds D.R. Lane & B. Cooper). In: *Veterinary Nursing*, 2nd edition, Butterworth Heinemann.

Clutton, E. (1993) Management of perioperative cardiac arrest in companion animals, Part 1. *In Practice* **15**, 267.

Clutton, E. (1994) Management of perioperative cardiac arrest in companion animals, Part 2. *In Practice* **16**, 3.

Evans, A.T. (1999) New thoughts on cardiopulmonary resuscitation. *Veterinary Clinics of North America* **29**(3), 819.

Harvey, R.C. (1999) Anaesthetic emergencies and complications. In: *BSAVA Manual of Small Animal Anaesthesia and Analgesia* (eds C. Seymour & R. Gleed). British Small Animal Veterinary Association, Cheltenham.

Haskins, S.C. (1992) Internal cardiac compression. *Journal of the American Veterinary Medicine Association* **200**(12), 1945.

Kass, P.H. & Haskins, S.C. (1992) Survival following cardiopulmonary resuscitation in dogs and cats. *Journal of Veterinary Emergency and Critical Care* **2**, 57.

Marks, S.L. (1999) Cardiopulmonary resuscitation and oxygen therapy. *Veterinary Clinics of North America* **29**(4), 959.

Martin, M. & Corcoran, B. (1997) Cardiopulmonary resuscitation. In: *Cardiorespiratory Diseases of the Dog and Cat*. Blackwell Science, Oxford.

Muir, W.W. (1999) Cardiopulmonary-cerebral resuscitation in dogs and cats. In: *BSAVA Manual of Canine and Feline Emergency and Critical Care* (eds L. King & R. Hammond). British Small Animal Veterinary Association, Cheltenham.

Van Pelt, D.R. & Wingfield, W.E. (1992) Controversial issues in drug treatment during cardiopulmonary resuscitation. *Journal of the American Veterinary Medicine Association* **200**(12), 1938.

Rabbit, Ferret and Rodent Anaesthesia

12

Simon Girling

Sedation and anaesthesia (chemical restraint) may be required for a number of procedures in small mammals. However, there are some general broad common guidelines to follow before chemical restraint is attempted in order to safeguard the welfare of small mammal patients.

Aspects of chemical restraint

Chemical restraint may be necessary for a number of reasons in small mammals. It is often used to facilitate sample collection, such as blood testing or urine collection, and for procedures such as radiography, and oral examinations. Anaesthetic procedures are now becoming routine for most small mammals, and the improved levels of success in this area has been mainly due to the awareness of certain problems which frequently beset these patients, such as a high prevalence of low-grade respiratory infections, and the fine-tuning of the drugs used for individual species.

It is important to make an assessment as to whether or not the patient is fit for chemical restraint. To this end it is worthwhile noting the following points:

- *Respiratory infections:* Many members of the Rodentia and Lagomorpha families suffer from low-grade levels of respiratory infection all their lives. Many will cope with this on a day-to-day basis, but when anaesthetised, the respiratory rate slows, and respiratory secretions (already thickened or increased due to the chronic infections) become more tenacious and physical blockage of the airways can occur.
- *Upper airway anatomy:* The majority of the species considered are nose breathers, with their soft palates permanently locked around the epiglottis.

If the patient has a blocked nose, whether due to pus, blood, tumours or abscesses, then respiratory arrest is made much more likely under anaesthesia.

- *Hypothermia:* Due to their small size and large body surface areas to volume ratios, small mammals are prone to hypothermia during anaesthesia, from the cooling effect of the inhaled gases and from reduced muscular activity. It is therefore dangerous to place a patient that is already hypothermic through an anaesthetic without reversing this change.
- *Dehydration:* Respiratory fluid losses during the drying gaseous anaesthetic procedures are much greater than in cats, dogs or larger species. Hence placing a severely dehydrated small mammalian patient through an anaesthetic without prior fluid therapy is also dangerous.

If chemical immobilisation is then to take place, the following procedures should first be considered.

PRE-ANAESTHETIC PREPARATION

Weighing
It is vitally important that the animal be weighed accurately. A mistake of just 10 g in a hamster may lead to an under- or overdosage of 10%! The use of scales which will read accurately down to 1 g in weight is therefore essential.

Blood testing
Blood testing is now routine in cats and dogs prior to anaesthetic procedures if there is any doubt regarding the animal's overall health status. It is starting to become much more common in small mammals as well, and should be considered in every clinically unwell, or senior, patient where a large enough sample may be obtained.

Sites for venepuncture are as follows:

Lagomorphs (e.g. rabbits)
The lateral ear vein may be used with a 25–27 gauge needle. The prior application of a local anaesthetic cream to the site and the warming of the ear under a heat lamp or hot water bottle is advised to allow dilation of the vessel. Alternatively, the cephalic vein or the jugular vein may be used. The latter should be used with caution as it is the only source of blood drainage from the eyes and so, if a thrombus forms in this vessel, ocular oedema and permanent damage or even loss of the eye may occur.

Muridae (e.g. rats)

The lateral tail veins may be used in rats and mice. These run either side of the coccygeal vertebrae, and are best seen when the tail is warmed. As for the lateral ear vein in lagomorphs, a 25–27 gauge needle is required.

Mustelids (e.g. ferrets)

The jugular vein is probably the easiest to access, but may be difficult in a fractious animal. The positioning adopted for cats is used where one handler holds onto both forelimbs with one hand, clamping the body with forearm and elbow, the other hand placed under the chin and elevating the head. A towel may be used as a papoose to restrain a ferret. Cephalic veins may also be used, and 23–25 gauge needles suffice.

Hystricomorphs (e.g. chincillas)

The jugular veins are the most accessible. One handler holds both forelimbs with one hand and brings the patient to the edge of the table, raising the head with the other hand. The other operator may then take a jugular sample with a 23–25 gauge needle. Lateral saphenous veins may be used in guinea pigs, but chinchillas rarely have any other peripheral vessel large enough to sample.

Cricetidae (e.g. gerbils)

These are the most challenging, and blood sampling may not be possible. With care (particularly in gerbils) the lateral tail veins may be used. Frequently cardiac puncture under anaesthetic is the only way to get an adequate sample.

Scuiridae (e.g. chipmunks)

Jugular blood samples may be taken, but in nearly every case anaesthesia is required first.

Fasting

This again depends somewhat on the species.

Lagomorphs

These do not need to be fasted prior to anaesthesia, as they have a very tight cardiac sphincter preventing vomiting. Indeed starving may actually be deleterious to the patient's health as it causes a cessation in gut contractility and subsequent ileus. It is useful though to ensure that no food is present in the mouth at the time of induction, hence a period of 30–60 min starvation is used.

Muridae

Due to their high metabolic rate and likelihood of hypoglycaemia, rats and mice need only be starved a matter of 40–60 min (mice) to 45–90 min (rats) prior to induction of anaesthesia.

Mustelids
These may be starved for 2–4 hours. Any more than this will lead to hypoglycaemia as mustelids have a high metabolic rate and short gut transit times.

Hystricomorphs
Starvation may be performed for 3–6 hours prior to surgery to ensure a relatively empty stomach, and reduce pressure on the diaphragm. Again, prolonged starvation (> 4 h) will lead to hypoglycaemia, gut stasis and increase the risks of intra- or postoperative death.

Cricetidae
As for Muridae, a period of 45–90 min is usually sufficient. Fasting for longer than 2 hours is likely to result in postoperative hypoglycaemia.

Sciuridae
Periods of fasting of 2 hours have been reported as safe.

PRE-ANAESTHETIC MEDICATION

Pre-anaesthetics are used for a number of reasons: to provide a smooth induction; to aid a smooth recovery from anaesthesia; because they ensure a reduction of airway secretions, act as a respiratory stimulant, or prevent serious bradycardia.

Antimuscarinic drugs
Atropine is used in some species such as guinea pigs and chinchillas where oral secretions are high, and intubation difficult. Doses of 0.05 mg/kg (Mason 1997) have been used subcutaneously 30 min before induction. Atropine also acts to prevent excessive bradycardia that often occurs during the induction phase. It is not so useful in Lagomorphs as around 60% of rabbits have a serum atropinesterase that breaks down atropine before it has a chance to work. Glycopyrrolate, which functions in a similar manner, may also be used at doses of 0.01 mg/kg subcutaneously (Mason 1997).

Tranquillisers
Tranquillisers are frequently used to reduce the stress of induction, which plays a large part in the risks of anaesthetising Lagomorphs and Hystricomorphs. These species will hold their breath during gaseous induction, to the point where they go blue. In rabbits, the 'shock' organ is the lungs, and during intense stress the pulmonary circulation can go into spasm, worsening the hypoxia due to breath-holding, even to the point of collapse and cardiac arrest.

Acepromazine (ACP) can be used at doses of 0.2 mg/kg in ferrets, to 0.5 mg/kg in rabbits, and 0.5–1 mg/kg in rats, mice, hamsters, chinchillas and guinea pigs (Mason 1997). In general it is a very safe premedicant even in debilitated animals. However, it is advised not to use this in gerbils, as acepromazine reduces the seizure threshold, and many gerbils suffer from hereditary epilepsy.

Diazepam is useful as a premedicant in some species. In rodents doses of 3 mg/kg (Mason 1997) can be used even in gerbils. In rabbits, the benefits may be outweighed by the larger volumes required, as the intramuscular route is employed, which may be painful.

Neuroleptanalgesic drugs

Fentanyl–fluanisone combination (Hypnorm®) may be used at varying doses as either a premedicant, a sedative, or as part of an injectable general anaesthetic. As a premedicant doses of 0.1 ml/kg for rabbits, 0.08 ml/kg for rats and 0.2 ml/kg for guinea pigs (one-fifth the recommended sedation doses) can produce sufficient sedation to prevent breath-holding and allow gaseous induction. These doses are given intramuscularly 15–20 min before induction. Hypnorm® is an irritant and large doses at one site may cause postoperative lameness. It can be reversed with butorphanol at 0.2 mg/kg intravenously, or buprenorphine at 0.05 mg/kg (Mason 1997).

INDUCTION AND MAINTENANCE OF ANAESTHESIA

Induction agents are classified as injectable or volatile agents.

Injectable agents

The advantages of the injectable anaesthetics are that they are often easy to administer, they frequently involve minimal stress, and avoid the breath-holding problems associated with gaseous induction. Disadvantages include the problem of reversal for some agents, their often varying responses depending on the individual animal, and the frequent respiratory depression, hypoxia and hypotensive effects they produce.

Propofol

Propofol (Rapinovet® Schering-Plough) has some limited usage in small mammals. It may be used in ferrets at 10 mg/kg (Mason 1997) after the use of a premedicant such as acepromazine. However, in rabbits and hystricomorphs, the apnoea that ensues makes its use limited, and its need to be given intravenously limits its use in the smaller rodents.

Ketamine
Mustelids
Ketamine (Ketaset® Willows-Francis) may be used alone for chemical restraint in the ferret at doses of 10–20 mg/kg but, as with cats and dogs, muscle relaxation is poor, and salivation occurs. More often ketamine is combined with other

medicants such as the α_2 antagonists, xylazine and medetomidine. In ferrets 10–30 mg/kg ketamine may be used with 1–2 mg/kg xylazine, preferably giving the xylazine 5–10 min before the ketamine. (Information on dosage from Mason 1997.)

Lagomorphs

Ketamine is used at a dose of 20–35 mg/kg in conjunction with medetomidine at 0.3–0.5 mg/kg, or with xylazine at 5 mg/kg, using lower doses for debilitated animals. The advantages are a quick and stress-free anaesthetic, but the combination will cause blanching of the membranes, and make detection of hypoxia difficult. Respiratory depression during longer procedures may become a problem and intubation is often advised. The medetomidine may be reversed using atipamazole at 1 mg/kg. (Information on dosage from Mason 1997.)

Muridae and Cricetidae

Ketamine can be used at 90 mg/kg in combination with xylazine at 5 mg/kg intramuscularly or intraperitoneally in rats, with mice and hamsters requiring 100–150 mg/kg of ketamine and 5 mg/kg xylazine. (Information on dosage from Harkness & Wagner 1989.) These combinations provide 30 min or so of general anaesthesia (Mason 1997). In gerbils the dose of xylazine may be reduced to 2–3 mg/kg as they appear more sensitive to the hypovolaemic effects of the α_2 drugs, with ketamine doses at 50 mg/kg.

Ketamine may also be used in combination with medetomidine at doses of 0.5 mg/kg (Mason 1997). The advantages of the α_2 antagonists are that they produce good analgesia (which the ketamine does not) and that they may be quickly reversed with atipamazole at 1 mg/kg (Mason 1997). Their disadvantages include their severe hypotensive effects, and that once administered any injectable anaesthetic is always more difficult to control than a gaseous one. They also increase diuresis and may exacerbate renal dysfunction.

Hystricomorphs

Ketamine at 40 mg/kg may be used in conjunction with xylazine at 5 mg/kg in guinea pigs to produce a light plane of anaesthesia. Ketamine at 40 mg/kg may also be used with medetomidine at 0.5 mg/kg for guinea pigs, or ketamine at 30 mg/kg with medetomidine at 0.3 mg/kg for chinchillas. Reversal with 1 mg/kg atipamazole may be performed. Both of these may be improved after an acepromazine premedication of 0.25 mg/kg. (Information on dosage from Mason 1997.)

Alternatively for chinchillas a combination of ketamine (40 mg/kg) and acepromazine (0.5 mg/kg) can be used. Induction with these drugs takes 5–10 min and typically lasts for 45–60 min, but recovery may take 2–5 h for the non-reversible acepromazine combination, hence reducing this drug and using the reversible α_2 antagonists may be beneficial, but should be weighed against the greater hypotensive effects of the α_2 drugs.

Fentanyl–fluanisone (Hypnorm®)
This drug combination is a neuroleptanalgesic licensed for use in rats, mice, rabbits and guinea pigs. Fentanyl is an opioid, and fluanisone is a neuroleptic.

Lagomorphs
This may be used as sedation only on its own at a dose of 0.5 ml/kg intramuscularly. This produces sedation and immobilisation for 30–60 min according to the data sheets, but its analgesic effect due to the opioid derivative fentanyl will persist for some time after. It may be reversed with 0.5 mg/kg butorphanol intravenously, or 0.05 mg/kg buprenorphine, both of which will counteract the fentanyl and its analgesia and substitute their own pain relief.

Alternatively, to provide anaesthetic depth, fentanyl–fluanisone may be combined with diazepam (0.3 ml Hypnorm® to 2 mg/kg diazepam) intraperitoneally, or intravenously (but in separate syringes as they do not mix), or with midazolam (0.3 ml Hypnorm® to 2 mg/kg midazolam) intramuscularly or intraperitoneally in the same syringe.

Alternatively the Hypnorm® may be given intramuscularly first and then 15 min later the midazolam is given intravenously into the lateral ear vein. These two combinations provide good analgesia and muscle relaxation with duration of anaesthesia of 20–40 min. Again, the fentanyl may be reversed with buprenorphine or butorphanol given intravenously. In emergencies the drug naloxone at 0.1 mg/kg intramuscularly or intravenously may be given, but this provides no substitute analgesia.

Fentanyl–fluanisone combinations are well tolerated in most rabbits, but they can produce respiratory depression and hypoxia, which can lead to cardiac arrhythmias and even arrest.

Muridae
Hypnorm® may be used as sedation only on its own at a dose of 0.01 ml/30 g body weight in mice and 0.4 ml/kg in rats. Again this produces sedation and immobilisation for 30–60 min and may be reversed with buprenorphine or butorphanol as above.

Alternatively the drug may be combined with diazepam (mice 0.01 ml/30 g Hypnorm® with 5 mg/kg diazepam intraperitoneally; rats 0.3 ml/kg Hypnorm® with 2.5 mg/kg diazepam intraperitoneally) where the diazepam and Hypnorm® are given in separate syringes as they do not mix, or with midazolam. Midazolam is miscible with Hypnorm® and for rodents the recommendation is that each drug is mixed with an equal volume of sterile water first and then mixed together. Of this stock solution, mice receive 10 ml/kg and rats 2.7 ml/kg as a single intraperitoneal injection. These two combinations provide anaesthesia for a period of 20–40 min.

Hystricomorphs
Hypnorm® may be used for sedation only on its own at a dose of 1 ml/kg intramuscularly. This may be problematic in guinea pigs as large volumes are required and Hypnorm® is an irritant and may cause lameness when the whole dose is placed in one spot – multiple sites are therefore preferred. Alternatively the drug may be combined as above with diazepam (1 ml/kg Hypnorm® and 2.5 mg/kg diazepam) in separate syringes intraperitoneally, or with midazolam by making the stock solution as described for Muridae, and then administering 8 ml/kg of this solution intraperitoneally. Hypnorm® may be reversed with the partial opioid agonists, buprenorphine and butorphanol, or with the full antagonist naloxone.

Volatile agents
These have the advantage that it is relatively easy to change the depth of anaesthesia. The recovery times are often much shorter than with the injectable anaesthetics and frequently their side effects are less, particularly with isoflurane.

Their disadvantages include the fact that they have a drying effect on the airways of the patient, causing dehydration during long procedures. They also create problems if used as an induction agent, as many species will breath-hold during this procedure.

Halothane
This agent has been used in all small mammals; however, its margin of safety is less than that of isoflurane. Induction concentrations should not exceed 3%, and anaesthesia can be maintained with 1.5%. Disadvantages include possible induction of cardiac arrhythmias, particularly in lagomorphs, the main culprits of breath-holding. This may lead to apnoea and cardiac arrest. Halothane is best administered after premedication with acepromazine rather than Hypnorm® as Hypnorm® requires extensive hepatic metabolism, as does halothane.

Methoxyflurane
This anaesthetic gas has been oft quoted as the gas of choice for rodents and rabbits. However, the drug has now been withdrawn from the human anaesthetic market and is no longer available.

Isoflurane
This is now becoming the most widely used gas for maintenance and induction of anaesthesia. Usually a pre-anaesthetic medication is used with analgesia, as isoflurane's analgesic effects and rapidity of knockdown are less than those of methoxyflurane. Its main advantages are in its safety for the debilitated patient as < 1% of the gas is metabolised hepatically, the rest merely being exhaled for recovery to occur. Recovery is rapid. Induction levels vary at 2.5–4% and maintenance usually is 1.5–2.5%, assuming adequate analgesia. Breath-holding still occurs, but the practice of supplying 100% oxygen to the patient

for 2 min prior to anaesthetic administration helps minimise hypoxia. Then
gradually introduce the isoflurane, first 0.5% for 2 min, then, assuming regular breathing, increase to 1% for 2 min, and so on until anaesthetic levels are
reached, allowing a smooth induction.

Aspects of maintaining gaseous anaesthesia

As with all gaseous anaesthetics, after induction the placement of an endotracheal tube for maintenance is to be recommended whenever possible. This is
relatively straightforward in rabbits using a no. 1 Wisconsin flat-bladed paediatric laryngoscope and a 2–3 mm tube (Fig. 12.1). Ferrets are more easily
intubated. The aid of a rabbit mouth-gag helps visibility, however intubation
becomes a specialised procedure for rodents such as rats, mice and gerbils
where rigid guide tubes or guidewires and smaller scopes are used to guide the
tube into the larynx. In these species, therefore, face masks are more commonly
used (Fig. 12.2). In rabbits and ferrets the use of lignocaine spray on the larynx
is useful to reduce laryngospasm and aid intubation.

Intermittent positive pressure ventilation

This may be necessary in some individuals who breath-hold during induction.
If intubation is not possible then three options are available.

(1) A tight-fitting face mask and an Ayres T-piece or Mapleson C or modified
    Bain circuit with half-litre bag attached can be used to attempt ventila-
    tion.

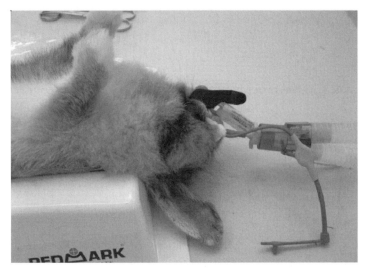

Fig. 12.1 Endotracheal intubation in a rabbit. Note the endotracheal tube cuff has not been
inflated and a pulse oximeter probe is attached to the tongue.

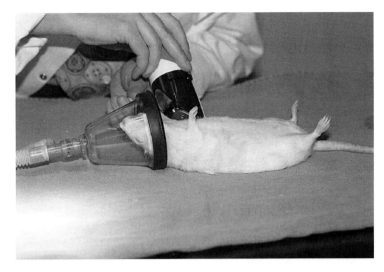

Fig. 12.2 Face masking of rodents such as this rat is often necessary owing to the increased difficulty of intubation.

(2) Place a nasopharygeal tube *via* the medial meatus of the nose into the pharyngeal area. Supply 4 litres or so of oxygen (to combat the resistance of the small diameter tubing of 1–2 mm) *via* this route.
(3) Perform an emergency tracheostomy with a 25–27 gauge needle attached to the oxygen outlet.

Anaesthetic breathing systems

Most of the small mammals described here are < 2 kg in weight. Thus, an Ayres T-piece, a modified Bain or Mapleson C circuit are preferred, minimising dead space. For larger rabbits, an Ayres T-piece is usually sufficient.

Additional supportive therapy

Positioning

During most surgical procedures positioning will be dependent upon the area being operated on. Frequently this necessitates the patient being placed in dorsal recumbency. This creates some problems with small herbivores. These species are differently proportioned from cats, dogs and carnivores in general. Most of the small herbivores have developed an enlarged hindgut because they rely on their gut flora to aid digestion. Therefore their abdomen to thorax ratio is 2 : 1 instead of 1 : 2 as with cats and dogs. More gut-fill therefore means when in dorsal recumbency more weight on the diaphragm, and so more resistance to inspiration. During lengthy surgical procedures this may lead to apnoea and hypoxia. The patient in dorsal recumbency should be positioned with the head elevated above the rest of the body.

Body temperature

Maintenance of core body temperature is vitally important in all patients to ensure successful recovery from anaesthesia, but is particularly important in small mammals. This is primarily due to their increased surface area in relation to their volume, so allowing more heat to escape per gram of animal. Anaesthetic gases have a rapidly cooling effect on the oral and respiratory membranes, and so patients maintained on gaseous anaesthetics will cool down more quickly than those on injectable agents. This effect worsens as the length of the anaesthetic increases. To help minimise this the following actions may be taken:

- Perform minimal surgical scrubbing of the site, and minimal clipping of fur from the area. Do not use surgical spirit as this rapidly cools the skin.
- Ensure adequate environmental room temperature.
- Place the patient on a water circulating heat pad, or place latex gloves or hot water bottles filled with warm water around the patient (making sure that the patient does not directly contact the containers as skin burns may ensue).
- Administer warmed isotonic fluids subcutaneously, intravenously, or intraperitoneally before and during surgery.

These actions will help prevent hypothermia. It is worth noting, however, that hyperthermia may be as bad as hypothermia. Small mammals generally have few or no sweat glands, and so heat cannot be lost *via* this route. In addition very few actually pant to lose heat so, if overwarmed, the core body temperature rises and irreversible hyperthermia will occur. A rectal thermometer is useful to monitor body temperature. Typical values are shown in Table 12.1.

Fluid therapy

Intra-, pre- and postoperative fluid therapy is very important in small mammals, even for routine surgery. Again, as with the issue of core body temperature, the small size and relatively large body surface area in relation to volume of these

Table 12.1 Normal body temperatures.

Species	Temperature (°C)
Rabbit	37–39.4
Rat	38 (av)
Mouse	37.5 (av)
Gerbil	37.4–39
Hamster	36.2–37.5
Guinea pig	37.2–39.5
Chinchilla	38–39
Ferret	37.8–40
Chipmunk	38 (av)

patients means that they will also dehydrate much faster, gram for gram, than a larger cat or dog. Studies have shown that the provision of maintenance levels of fluids to small mammals during and immediately after routine surgery improved anaesthetic safety levels by as much as 15% in some cases, with higher levels if the surgery was being performed on severely debilitated animals.

It is therefore strongly recommended that all small mammal patients receive fluids during and after all anaesthetics.

The volume of fluid to be administered can be calculated from Table 12.2.

These fluid rates are nearly double those for cats and dogs. The fluids administered will obviously depend on the health status of the small mammal patient, but a commonly used fluid for routine surgery is 0.18% saline–4% glucose. If dehydration is suspected or diagnosed then 0.9% saline–5% glucose should be used to replace the deficit. Fluid deficits should be replaced gradually, as for cats and dogs. A rough guide is as follows:

Day 1 – Replace 50% of fluid deficit + maintenance fluids
Day 2 – Replace 50% of fluid deficit + maintenance fluids
Day 3 – maintenance fluids.

Colloidal fluids should be contemplated if intravenous access can be achieved when haemorrhage occurs, and the use of lactated Ringer's solution for conditions where potassium loss and metabolic acidosis may occur (e.g. renal disease, chronic diarrhoea).

The routes by which these fluids may be administered will depend on the species and the degree of dehydration.

If the fluids are for routine intra- or postoperative requirements with minimal or no dehydration, then the subcutaneous route is satisfactory. The scruff region or the lateral thoracic wall may be utilised in any small mammal patient (Fig. 12.3). For more severe dehydration the intraperitoneal route or intravenous routes (in the larger patients) or intraosseous routes are required.

Intraperitoneal injections require the patient to be placed in dorsal recumbency with the head tilted downwards, so causing the abdominal viscera to

Table 12.2 Typical maintenance fluid levels.

Species	Maintenance fluid levels (ml/kg/day)
Rabbits	80–100
Ferrets	75–100
Rodents	90–100
Chinchillas	100
Guinea pigs	100
Chipmunks	100

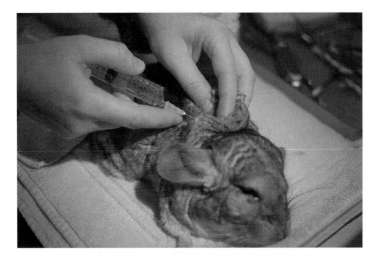

Fig. 12.3 Subcutaneous fluid therapy in the 'scruff' region should be performed after every routine minor sedation or anaesthetic, as in this chinchilla.

move cranially and away from the injection site, which is in the right lower quadrant of the ventral abdominal wall. The needle is angled between 20 and 40° in a cranial direction and advanced until it just pops through the peritoneum. The plunger is withdrawn on the syringe to ensure that bladder or gut puncture has not occurred and then the fluids may be administered.

In larger species such as rabbits, ferrets and even guinea pigs the intravenous route may be used. In rabbits use of the lateral ear vein is common, warming the ear to improve circulation, or using local anaesthetic cream to dilate the vessel. A 25–27 gauge butterfly catheter is the best method for this route, pre-flushed with heparin–saline, as it allows blood to flow back into the tubing, verifying access (Fig. 12.4). Conversely the lateral saphenous or cephalic veins may be used in rabbits, guinea pigs and ferrets (again, preferably, with 25–27 gauge butterfly catheters).

In guinea pigs, chinchillas and ferrets the jugular veins may also be used in a cut-down procedure which necessitates some form of sedation. The jugular vein can be used in rabbits but there is a danger that a thrombus will form in the vessel and in rabbits the external jugular veins are the sole drainage for the eyes and their orbits. Blockage therefore leads to ocular oedema and in severe cases loss of the eye.

In rats and mice the lateral tail veins may be used to administer small volumes of fluid; a 27 gauge needle or butterfly catheter will be required as well as warming the tail to improve vessel dilation.

For those species that have small or reduced peripheral circulation such as gerbils, hamsters or shocked patients, the intraosseous route can be used. In the majority of species the proximal femur is the site of choice (Fig. 12.5). Using

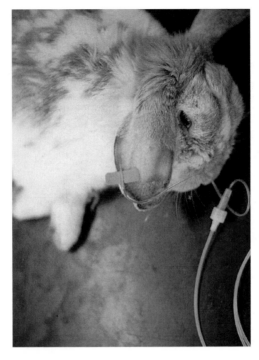

Fig. 12.4 The lateral ear vein may be catheterised using a pre-heparinised 25–27 gauge butterfly needle in rabbits for intravenous fluid therapy.

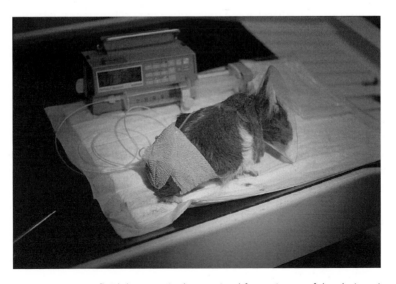

Fig. 12.5 Intraosseous fluid therapy via the proximal femur is a useful technique in small mammals which have collapsed peripheral circulation or difficult venous access such as this guinea-pig. Note the use of a syringe driver to increase accuracy of fluid administration.

a spinal needle or an ordinary hypodermic needle, the area over the femoral head is surgically prepared, and the needle advanced parallel to the long axis of the bone and inserted in the intertrochanteric fossa created between the hip joint and the greater trochanter. To perform this, sedation is often required, but the bone marrow cavity has direct access to the circulation. Because of the confining nature of the bone marrow cavity, only small boluses of fluid can be administered, and so an infusion device is important, such as a syringe driver. Asepsis must be strongly adhered to in the case of intraosseous catheters as osteomyelitis can easily ensue in debilitated patients.

MONITORING ANAESTHESIA

This becomes more and more difficult as the size of the patient decreases. No one factor (as with cats and dogs) will allow you to assess anaesthetic depth. Indeed in small mammals many of the useful techniques utilised in cats and dogs are not relevant. Eye position, for example, should not be used to assess depth of anaesthesia in small mammals. Instead a useful method is to assess depth by the response to noxious stimuli such as pain.

Initially the first reflex lost is usually the righting reflex; the animal is unable to return to ventral recumbency.

The next reflex to be lost in rabbits and guinea pigs is the swallow reflex; however, this may be difficult to assess. Palpebral reflexes are generally lost early in the course of anaesthetic, but rabbits may retain this reflex until well into the deeper planes of surgical anaesthesia. The palpebral reflex is also altered by the anaesthetic agent chosen, with most inhalant gaseous anaesthetics causing loss of the reflex early, but it is maintained with ketamine.

The pedal withdrawal reflex is useful in small mammals, with the leg being extended and the toe firmly pinched. Loss of this reflex suggests surgical planes of anaesthesia, but rabbits will retain the pedal reflex in the forelimbs until much deeper (and often dangerously deep!) planes of anaesthesia are reached. Other pain stimuli such as the ear pinch in the guinea pig and rabbit are useful; loss of this indicates a surgical plane, as does the loss of the tail pinch reflex in rats and mice.

Monitoring of the heart and circulation may be performed in a conventional manner with stethoscope and femoral pulse evaluation or, in larger species, using an oesophageal stethoscope. As with cats and dogs, increases in the respiratory and heart rates can be used to indicate lightening of the plane of anaesthesia. More sophisticated techniques may also be used with pulse oximetry to monitor heart rate and haemoglobin saturation. As with cats and dogs, the aim is to achieve 100% saturation, and levels below 90% would indicate hypoxaemia and the need for assisted ventilation. The ear is useful for this in rabbits using the clip-on probe; conversely the linear probes may be used successfully on the ventral aspect of the tail in most species. Other forms of cardiac monitoring include the ECG, which is frequently adapted to minimise trauma from the alligator forceps attachments by substituting fine needle probes, or by blunting the alligator teeth.

An extremely useful monitoring device is a Doppler probe that can detect blood flow in the smallest of vessels up to the heart itself. The Doppler probe converts blood flow into an audible sound through a speaker, which can then be assessed by the anaesthetist during surgery for changes in strength of the output and heart rates.

Respiratory monitors may be used if the patient is intubated and many pulse oximeters have outlets for these, allowing assessment of respiratory rates. Obviously these are not useful for patients that are being maintained on face masks or on injectable anaesthetics.

RECOVERY AND ANALGESIA

Recovery from anaesthesia is improved with the use of suitable reversal agents, if available. Examples include the use of atipamazole after medetomidine anaesthesia or sedation, and the use of naloxone, butorphanol or buprenorphine after opioid or Hypnorm® anaesthesia or sedation. Gaseous anaesthesia, particularly with isoflurane, tends to result in more rapid recovery than the injectable anaesthetics, but all forms of anaesthesia recovery are improved by ensuring adequate maintenance of body temperature during and after anaesthesia, as well as fluid balances.

Most small mammals will benefit from a quiet, darkened and warm recovery area allowing a controlled recovery; subsequent fluid administration the same day is frequently beneficial as many of these creatures will not be eating as normal for the first 12–24 h.

Analgesia is vitally important for a quick and smooth recovery process. Return to normal activity such as grooming, eating, drinking, and so on has been shown to be considerably shortened following adequate analgesia. Analgesics frequently used in small mammals include those listed in Table 12.3.

As with cats and dogs, and indeed humans, the administration of analgesia prior to the onset of pain makes for the most effective control of pain. Analgesics are therefore frequently used as part of premedication injections.

Table 12.3 Analgesics for use in small mammals. Dosages given in mg/kg body weight.

Drug	Ferret	Rabbit	Rodent	Chinchilla	Guinea pig	Chipmunk
Butorphanol*	0.3	0.3	1–5	2	2	1–5
Buprenorphine†	0.02	0.03	0.07	0.05	0.05	0.05
Carprofen‡	4	4	5	5	5	4
Flunixin‡	1	1.5	2.5	2.5	2.5	2.5

*Every 4 hours, †every 8 hours, ‡every 24 hours
Source: Mason (1997)

Choice of analgesic depends on the level of pain and other factors such as
concurrent disease processes. Flunixin (Finadyne® Schering-Plough), for example, is not a good analgesic to use in dehydrated animals or those with renal
disease; opioids act to depress respiration and so may be contraindicated in
severe respiratory disease cases. Buprenorphine (Vetergesic® Animalcare) is
effective as twice daily administration, and carprofen (Rimadyl® Pfizer) has
been shown to be useful on a once-a-day basis.

REFERENCES AND FURTHER READING

Beynon, P.H. & Cooper, J.E. (1991) *Manual of Exotic Pets*. British Small Animal Vet-
erinary Association, Cheltenham.
Flecknall, P.A. (1998) Analgesia in small mammals. In: *Seminars in Avian and Exotic
Pet Medicine*, 7(1), 41–47. WB Saunders, Philadelphia.
Flecknall, P. (2000) *Manual of Rabbits*. British Small Animal Veterinary Association,
Cheltenham.
Harkness, J.E. & Wagner, J.E. (1989) Anaesthesia. *The Biology and Medicine of Rab-
bits and Rodents*, 3rd edition, pp 61–67. Lea & Febiger, Philadelphia.
Mason, D.E. (1997) Anaesthesia, analgesia, and sedation for small mammals. In: *Fer-
rets, Rabbits and Rodents* (eds E.V. Hillyer & K.E. Quesenberry), pp 378–391. WB
Saunders, Philadelphia.
Meredith, A. & Redrobe, S. (2001) *Manual of Exotic Pets*, 4th edition. British Small
Animal Veterinary Association, Cheltenham.

Avian Anaesthesia

Simon Girling

Firstly a decision must be made as to whether anaesthesia is actually safe in the avian patient. If the answers to the questions below suggest that anaesthesia may be detrimental to the avian patient's health, or even risk a fatality, then anaesthesia should obviously be postponed until such times as it is safe to proceed.

The first requirement before anaesthesia is induced is to ensure that the bird can be successfully physically restrained for anaesthesia to be induced. The pros and cons of physical restraint will therefore also have to be considered at this stage.

Requirements for restraint

This may seem a basic point but it is sometimes necessary to be sure that restraint is required. The veterinary nurse needs to make a value decision on whether the bird in question is safe to restrain – not only from a danger to his/her own welfare (in the case of an aggressive or potentially dangerous bird of prey) but also from a medical aspect regarding the patient's health.

Points to consider include:

- Is the bird in respiratory distress, and therefore is the stress of handling going to exacerbate this?
- Is the bird easily accessible, allowing quick, stress-free and safe capture?
- Is the avian patient a potentially dangerous species such as a large eagle or swan, and is the correct equipment available to ensure safe restraint?

It is worthwhile remembering that many avian patients are highly stressed individuals and any restraint should therefore involve minimal periods of handling and capture.

HANDLING AVIAN PATIENTS

It is helpful to remember that the majority of avian patients seen in practice (with the exception of the owl family, Strigiformae) are diurnal and so reduced or dimmed lighting in general has a calming effect. Dimming the lights may be adequate or, for birds of prey, there may well be access to the bird's own 'hood'. This is a leather cap which slots over the head, covering the eyes but leaving the beak free, used to calm the bird when on the wrist or during handling or transporting.

Reducing noise levels when handling birds is also advisable as their sense of hearing is their best sense, after sight. With these two initial approaches, stress and time for capture can be greatly reduced.

Handling birds of prey

Falconiformes is the order of birds of prey, containing the following families – falcons, hawks, vultures and eagles. These birds are mainly diurnal and make up the most commonly seen group of birds of prey in practice.

Strigiformes is the order containing the owl species. They are generally nocturnal, so the use of hoods and darkening the room will not quieten these birds. However, as an order, they tend to be docile, and short periods of bright light may be used to temporarily pacify them.

The use of a hood in Falconiformes has already been mentioned, and many of these birds will also have jesses on their legs. These are the leather straps attached to their 'ankles' (lower tarso-metatarsal area) *via* a leather loop known as an 'aylmeri', and allow the falcon to be restrained while on the owner's fist.

Leather gauntlets are necessary for handling all raptors as their talons and power of grasp of each foot can be extremely strong. The feet of raptors, not the beak, represent the major danger to the handler. It is important to note that, when the bird of prey is positioned on the gauntletted hand, the wrist of this hand (traditionally the left hand in European falconers) is kept *above* the height of the elbow. If not, the bird has a tendency to walk up the arm of the handler, with serious and painful results!

The gauntletted hand is placed into the cage or box or beside the bird's perch, and grasps the jesses with the thumb and forefinger to encourage the bird to step up onto the glove. Once on the hand, the hood is slipped over the bird's head. The raptor may then be safely examined 'on the hand' and frequently is docile enough to allow manipulation of wings and beak and for small injections to be administered.

Casting a raptor

If the diurnal raptor does not have jesses attached but is trained to perch on the hand, it may well step up onto the gauntlet of its own accord. If not, then the room should be darkened (a blue or red light source could also be used, allowing the handler to see the bird but preventing the bird of prey seeing normally), and the bird grasped from behind in a thick towel, ensuring that the handler is aware of where the bird's head is. The bird is grasped across the shoulder area with the forefingers pushing forward underneath the beak to extend the head away from the hands. The hood can then be applied. The middle finger and fourth finger of each hand are looped, respectively, in front of and behind the upper legs, and the legs are presented away from the handler's body. This helps prevent the raptor from grasping one taloned foot with the other, which may cause significant self-trauma. This technique is known as **casting** the bird of prey. In this position general anaesthesia may be induced, or the raptor medicated.

Handling parrots and other cage birds

Psittaciformes is the order of birds within which the entire parrot group of birds is contained. Passeriformes is an enormous order containing over half of all living species of birds, the 'perching' birds. In both groups the use of subdued or blue or red light will aid in calming the bird and allow it to be restrained with minimal fuss.

In Psittaciformes the main weapon is the beak, with a powerful bite possible. The hyacinth macaw, the largest in the family, can produce 330 pounds per square inch of pressure with its beak, allowing it to easily crack the largest Brazil nuts, and enough to badly damage or even sever a finger.

In Passeriformes the main weapon may again be the beak; this is less damaging as a biting weapon, but may still be a sharp stabbing weapon in the case of starlings and mynahs.

It is advised that heavy gauntlets are not used, as they do not allow easy judgement of the strength of the handler's grip on the bird and may lead to significant restriction of breathing. Instead, dish towels or bath towels for the larger species and paper towels for the smaller ones provide some protection from being bitten without masking the true strength of the handler's grip.

The towel and hand are introduced to the cage and the bird is firmly but gently grasped from the back, ensuring the head is located first to allow the thumb and forefingers to be positioned underneath the lower beak, pushing it upwards and preventing the bird from biting. The rest of the towel is used to wrap around the bird to gently restrain wing movements to avoid excessive struggling and wing trauma (Fig. 13.1).

Handling other avian species

Toucans/Hornbills

These have an extremely impressive beak with a serrated edge to the upper bill. Providing the head is initially controlled using the towel technique previously described for parrots, an elastic band or tape may be applied around the bill, preventing biting; however, the handler still needs to be careful of stabbing manoeuvres and a second handler may be needed. Otherwise this group of birds may be restrained in much the same way as one would cast a raptor.

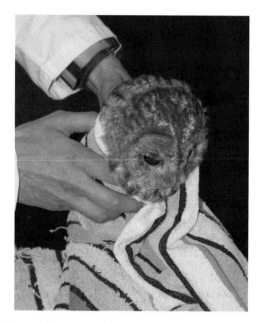

Fig. 13.1 Method of restraining an owl using a towel.

Waterfowl

Restraint of these species may become hazardous with the larger swan and goose family. Control of the head is important, by grasping the waterfowl around the upper neck from behind, ensuring the fingers curl around the neck and under the bill whilst the thumb supports the back of the neck and the potentially weak area of the atlanto-occipital joint (which in birds has only one condyle, unlike mammals).

Alternatively a shepherd's crook or other such adapted smooth metal, or wooden pole with an attached hook can be used to catch the neck, high up under the bill.

The wings should be rapidly controlled before the bird has a chance to damage itself or you! This is achieved by using a towel, thrown or draped over the patient's back and loosely wrapped under the sternum. Some practices may have access to more specialised goose/swan cradle bags that wrap around the body, containing the wings but allowing the feet, head and neck to remain free.

CHEMICAL RESTRAINT

Due to the highly stressed nature of many avian patients, the use of chemical restraint, whether full general anaesthesia, or less commonly, sedation, is being used more and more in avian practice.

Naturally all methods of chemical restraint require that the patient be restrained manually, before the medication can be administered. The advantage therefore does not lie so much in avoiding manual restraint but in minimising the period of manual restraint in order to reduce stress.

Before any form of chemical immobilisation can be used, an assessment of the patient's status has to be made. Is the procedure necessary for life-saving medication or treatment, and is the patient's condition likely to be worsened by the drugs used?

Next, the avian patient's natural respiratory physiology must be considered and appreciated.

Overview of avian respiratory anatomy and physiology

For an overview of the respiratory cycle of the avian patient see chapter 2.

The avian respiratory system differs in a number of ways from the mammalian system, namely (starting cranially):

(1) Vestigial larynx. The bird has a glottis, but no vocal cords or epiglottis. All sound comes from an area known as the syrinx, lying at the bifurcation of the trachea into the bronchi deep within the 'chest'.

(2) Complete cartilaginous rings to the trachea (Fig. 13.2). This is important for two reasons. First, it is relatively difficult (although not impossible!) to throttle a bird around the neck. Second, there is no 'give' to the trachea and so inflatable cuffs on endotracheal tubes should not be over-inflated as this will cause pressure necrosis to the lining of the trachea. Instead it may be better to use a snug-fitting uncuffed tube. In some cases, such as flushing the crop of a bird, it may be necessary to use and inflate a cuffed tube to prevent inhalation pneumonia. Extreme care should then be used.

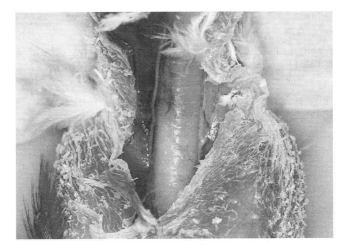

Fig. 13.2 The avian trachea has complete cartilaginous rings.

(3) The avian respiratory cycle is such that the bird may gain oxygen from air on inspiration and expiration (see chapter 2). A series of balloon-like air sacs exist inside the body of the bird, which in combination with the movement of the avian ribcage and sternum act to push air backwards and forwards through a rigid lung structure, enabling oxygen to be extracted from the air on both inspiration and expiration. This makes birds very efficient at gaseous exchange and allows the clinician to utilise this to advantage should the upper airway or trachea become blocked. In this instance the caudally located air sacs may be cannulated with a cut-down endotracheal tube and the patient ventilated *via* this route (see below).

Pre-anaesthetic preparation

Blood testing

It is useful to run biochemical and haemocytological tests on avian patients before administering anaesthetics. Blood can be taken from the right jugular vein in all species, from the brachial vein (in the larger species) running cranially on the ventral aspect of the humerus, and from the medial metatarsal vein in many waterfowl. The minimum tests include an assessment of the haematocrit, the total blood proteins, blood calcium, uric acid levels for kidney function and if possible both aspartamine transaminase (AST) and bile acid levels to assess liver function. More comprehensive tests in the case of seriously ill patients should of course be performed if required.

Fasting

Because of the high metabolic rate of avian patients, extended fasting may be detrimental to health, as hepatic glycogen stores can be quickly depleted. Birds larger than 300 g body weight are slightly less likely to become hypoglycaemic.

Fasting ensures emptying of the crop (the sac-like structure which acts as a storage chamber for food and sits at the inlet of the bird's neck), and so stops passive reflux of fluid or food material during the anaesthetic. Some species do not have a crop (most ducks and geese, penguins, seagulls and toucans), but they have a more distensible oesophagus that acts as a storage chamber.

Most birds are fasted 1–3 h before anaesthesia, depending on body size – the smallest having the shortest period of fasting (e.g. canaries, budgerigars). Birds > 300 g may be able to tolerate an overnight fast of 8–10 h, assuming good health and body condition, and this may be necessary if surgery on the gastrointestinal system or crop is intended.

Whatever the period of fasting, water should only be withheld for 1 h before anaesthesia.

Local anaesthesia

This may be combined with a sedative/tranquilliser such as midazolam (see below) for minor procedures where general anaesthesia is not required, such as minor skin wound repairs and reduction of cloacal prolapse. The local anaesthetic of choice is lignocaine hydrochloride with adrenaline. The adrenaline component is necessary to prevent rapid absorption of the lignocaine, which may induce fatal arrhythmias. It is advised that the stock solution, generally 2% concentration, be diluted with three parts sterile water to create a 0.5% solution, particularly if dealing with smaller species. Even then, parrots below 200 g should be given small doses (average 0.1–0.15 ml per 100 g of a 0.5% solution).

Pre-anaesthetic medication
These are used in cats and dogs to provide cardiopulmonary and central nervous system stabilisation, a smooth anaesthetic induction, muscle relaxation, analgesia and a degree of sedation.

Pre-anaesthetic medications are used infrequently in birds. However, fluid therapy is important as it can make the difference between successful surgery or failure.

Atropine and glycopyrrolate will reduce vagally induced bradycardia and oral secretions that may block endotracheal tubes. Both, however, may have unwanted side effects, the main ones being an unacceptably high heart rate, increasing myocardial oxygen demand, and making oral/respiratory secretions so tenacious that endotracheal tube blockage is even more likely.

Diazepam or midazolam may be used as premedicants in waterfowl, as these species may exhibit periods of apnoea during mask induction of anaesthesia. This is due to a stress response (often referred to, inaccurately, as a 'diving response') mediated by the trigeminal receptors in the beak and nares, whereby the breath is held and blood flow is preferentially diverted to the kidneys, heart and brain.

Induction using injectable agents
The advantages of injectable anaesthetics include the ease of administration, rapid induction, low cost and availability. Disadvantages include the fact that recovery is often dependent on organ metabolism, potentially difficult reversal of medications in emergency situations, prolonged and sometimes traumatic recovery periods, muscle necrosis at injection sites, and lack of adequate muscle relaxation with some drugs.

Propofol
This must be used intravenously, and hence a jugular, medial metatarsal or brachial vein catheter needs to be placed. It produces profound apnoea and is rarely used as an induction or anaesthetic agent in birds.

Ketamine and ketamine combinations
When used alone ketamine produces inadequate anaesthesia and recoveries are often traumatic with the patient flapping wildly (doses of 20–50 mg/kg are quoted) (Beynon 1996). In addition due to the high doses required, the

duration of anaesthesia may be prolonged, leading to potential hypothermia and hypoglycaemia, with poor recovery rates.

However combining ketamine with other injectable anaesthetic agents allows a reduction of the dose and therefore allows faster recovery times.

Diazepam at a dose of 0.5–2 mg/kg allows the ketamine to be reduced to 10–20 mg/kg or midazolam (Hypnovel®) at a dose of 0.5–1.5 mg/kg (Curro 1998) allows the ketamine dose to be reduced to 10 mg/kg. These two tranquillisers help with muscle relaxation and sedation, and reduce flapping on recovery as well as shortening recovery time.

Ketamine may also be combined with xylazine (Rompun® Bayer) at 1–2.2 mg/kg (Beynon 1996) which can reduce the dose of ketamine to 5–10 mg/kg. Coles (1997) has recommended a dosage of 20 mg/kg ketamine and 4 mg/kg xylazine, intramuscularly, and finds that this gives 10–20 min of anaesthesia with full recovery in 1–2 h. However, this combination should be avoided for pigeons and doves, and for all wading birds.

Use of medetomidine (Domitor® Pfizer Ltd) at 60–85 µg/kg (Beynon 1996) can reduce the ketamine dose to 5 mg/kg. However, slightly higher doses of 10 mg/kg ketamine and 100–150 µg/kg medetomidine may be required for full surgical anaesthesia in some species such as waterfowl and owls.

The use of α_2 agonist drugs reduces the ketamine dosage appreciably and so improves recovery rates, while enhancing sedation levels and analgesia. Xylazine has the side effect of inducing respiratory and cardiac suppression and so has become less popular and should be used with caution in debilitated patients. It may be reversed with the drug yohimbine at 0.1 mg/kg intravenously, but this may not fully reverse its effects. Medetomidine may be reversed fully with atipamizole (same volume as medetomidine given) and does not seem to produce such profound side effects, making this α_2 agonist a very useful injectable anaesthetic. It can still have cardiopulmonary depressive effects and may compromise blood flow to the kidneys, risking renal damage. Sun conures have been noted to be particularly intolerant of ketamine–α_2 combinations (Rosskopf et al. 1989).

The above combined medications are given intramuscularly generally and induction will take on average 5–10 min. Complete recovery may take 2–4 h or more unless reversible agents are used.

Midazolam
Midazolam (Hypnovel®) may be used on its own as a sedative in many species, and of course as an anti-convulsant. Doses for sedation in geese and swans have been quoted as 2 mg/kg (Valverde et al. 1990).

Extending and maintaining anaesthesia
It is always advisable, if using injectable anaesthetics, that the avian patient is intubated and oxygen is supplied, or at least is on standby. This also allows the above-noted injectable anaesthetic combinations to be extended beyond

15–20 min, by introducing low levels of isoflurane (0.5–1%) if the surgical procedure is likely to be prolonged.

Alternatively, anaesthesia may be induced directly using an inhalational agent.

Induction using inhalation agents
Nitrous oxide
This has been used in avian anaesthesia. It has good analgesic properties, but accumulates in large hollow viscous organs. There is some thought that it may therefore accumulate in the air sacs and may prolong anaesthetic recovery times. Recent evidence disputes this but it cannot be used on its own for anaesthesia, and halothane or isoflurane are required to allow a surgical plane to be reached. It should not exceed 50% of the anaesthetic gas supplied, and should not be used if respiratory disease is suspected. As with mammalian anaesthesia, the nitrous oxide supply must be discontinued some 5–10 min prior to the end of anaesthesia to minimise diffusion hypoxia.

Halothane
Induction is with 3–4% halothane *via* a face mask. Halothane may be reduced to 2–3% and delivered either *via* a face mask or preferably *via* an endotracheal tube to maintain anaesthesia. Halothane is partly metabolised by the liver and, as many sick avian patients have some degree of hepatic function impairment, this can place the patient at some risk. Recovery is often extended and cardiac arrest often occurs at the same time as respiratory arrest, giving little response time in an emergency. Halothane also depresses the responsiveness of the bird's intrapulmonary chemoreceptors (IPC) to carbon dioxide. This is important as the IPCs only respond to increasing carbon dioxide levels in the unanaesthetised bird, and not to hypoxia. Hence birds anaesthetised with halothane are less able to adjust ventilation in response to changes in carbon dioxide levels.

Isoflurane
This is the anaesthetic gas (and anaesthetic in general) of choice for the avian patient. Induction may be achieved by face mask on 4–5% concentration, being turned down to 1.25–2% for maintenance, preferably *via* an endotracheal tube – face masks requiring a 25–30% increase in gas concentration.

Its advantages include low blood solubility with minimal metabolism of the drug by the bird (< 0.2%) allowing rapid changes in anaesthetic depth. At sedative or light anaesthesia levels the adverse cardiopulmonary effects are minimal. The drug does not require hepatic metabolism for recovery to occur. Hence it is a useful anaesthetic for sick birds. Cardiovascular arrest does not occur at the same time as respiratory arrest, which tends to be the case with halothane, so giving some time for resuscitation.

Sevoflurane

This is a newer anaesthetic gas now being used in avian patients. It produces a quicker recovery time than isoflurane, but seems to have the same safety margins and anaesthetic effects. It often requires higher induction doses than isoflurane (5–6% as compared with 3–4%). This is due to its much lower blood solubility (blood : gas coefficient 0.68), which leads to rapid recovery rates once supply of the anaesthetic is discontinued. Maintenance levels average at 3%. It is minimally metabolised in the body (< 1%) and like isoflurane seems not to produce cardiac dysrhythmias. Its current restricted use is mainly due to its high cost. However its rapid recovery rate may make it the future gaseous anaesthetic of choice in avian patients.

Maintaining anaesthesia

For prolonged anaesthetic procedures, gaseous general anaesthesia is required, with isoflurane being the agent of choice.

For avian patients larger than 100 g it is advisable to intubate the bird for this period, as more effective control of rate and depth of anaesthesia can be achieved. Also isoflurane causes dose-dependent respiratory depressive effects, hence with prolonged procedures, the patient may become apnoeic and require positive pressure ventilation.

Intubation

Intubation is easily achieved once general anaesthesia is induced *via* a face mask. Once resistance is reduced the beak may be opened using an avian gag, or simply by attaching one piece of bandage material to the lower beak and one to the upper, while a second operator places the endotracheal tube through the glottis, which is easily visible *per os* at the base of the tongue. Visibility is improved with a directional light source and by grasping the tongue, in those species with a mobile tongue, with a pair of atraumatic forceps and pulling it and the attached glottis rostrally. It is better not to inflate the cuff on endotracheal tubes due to the risk of causing severe damage to the lining of the rigid avian trachea. A good-fitting tube is thus necessary or, if positive pressure ventilation is required or if performing a stomach wash to remove foreign bodies, gentle inflation of the cuff may be used – only enough to prevent air escaping when ventilated and refluxed fluid being aspirated.

Anaesthetic breathing systems

Anaesthetic circuits used must minimise dead space and be non-rebreathing as many avian patients are much smaller than cats and dogs. Modified Bain circuits are useful, as are the more exotic Mapleson C circuits (Fig. 13.3) for these reasons; even the Ayres T-piece may be used for larger parrots and waterfowl. In any instance a 0.5 litre rebreathing bag is frequently necessary.

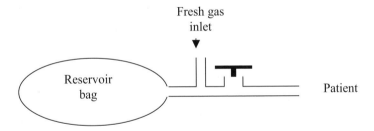

Fig. 13.3 A Mapleson C circuit may be used for avian patients.

Air sac catheterisation

In the event of an airway obstruction, or if head or oral cavity surgery is required, it may be necessary to deliver anaesthetic gases *via* a tube placed directly into one of the air sacs. This is possible due to the close proximity of many of the air sacs to the skin surface, and the fact that they take no part in gaseous exchange, but simply shunt the air back and forth through the rigid lung structure.

The clavicular and the abdominal/caudal thoracic air sacs may be catheterised. A small stab incision is made in the skin over the air sac, and the underlying muscle bluntly dissected with a pair of mosquito haemostats. The endotracheal tube is then inserted to a depth of 4–5 mm and sutured in place.

The clavicular air sacs lie at the thoracic inlet, just dorsal to the clavicles; the caudal thoracic air sacs may be entered between the sixth and seventh ribs; the abdominal air sacs may be entered by raising the leg cranially and incising just caudal to the stifle through the lateral body wall.

ADDITIONAL SUPPORTIVE THERAPY

Positioning

Due to the unique anatomy of the avian patient's respiratory system, it is vitally important that the ribcage can move freely, otherwise hypoxia will develop. Common positions include lateral or dorsal recumbency. Dorsal recumbency may be a problem in larger species where the bulkier abdominal contents may press on the air sacs when in this position, so increasing respiratory effort. However, smaller species generally do not suffer from this problem and may be positioned according to need.

Intermittent positive pressure ventilation

If the respiratory rate becomes depressed for periods > 15–20 sec, respiratory assistance should be provided. The usual anaesthetic checklist should be run through – checking flow rates, patency of any endotracheal tubes, anaesthetic gas levels, and so on, and the anaesthetic turned down.

If the bird is still breathing sporadically, then positive pressure ventilation 2–3 times a minute should be started. If possible a mechanical ventilator unit should be used, providing a maximum inspiratory pressure of 10–15 cmH$_2$O. If manual ventilation is used, then the gentlest of touches on the bag, enough just to allow the bird's ribcage to rise, should be used. If the bird is apnoeic, then a rate of 10–15 breaths per minute should be used. The cardiorespiratory stimulant doxapram (Dopram –V® Willows Francis) may be administered intravenously, or intramuscularly at 5–10 mg/kg once only if severe respiratory depression is observed.

If the bird is on a face mask rather than intubated, the uppermost wing may be grasped at the carpus, and gently but firmly moved in and out at 90° to the chest wall. This will stimulate movement of the ribcage, and so allow air to move back and forth through the air sacs and lungs. Alternatively the sternum may be pushed from the ventral aspect, dorsally, which can be useful for cardiac massage in cases of cardiac arrest. Frequently apnoea is quickly followed by cardiac arrest, from which the avian patient is difficult to revive. Adrenaline may be given at 1000 units/kg body weight *via* endotracheal tube, or intravenously *via* the right jugular vein, or the brachial wing vein, but generally has a poor success rate.

The type of anaesthetic used will influence the likelihood of apnoea occurring. Xylazine is a notorious respiratory depressant (Curro 1998). Isoflurane in African grey parrots will also produce respiratory depression, even at the lowest surgical levels (Taylor 1988).

Body temperature

Hypothermia is a problem in most of the avian patients seen as they are generally small in size and therefore have a large body surface area to volume ratio, leading to a much faster rate of heat loss than in larger species. In addition most avian species have a core body temperature between 40 and 44°C, and anaesthetic gases are cooling in their effect, causing a potential for hypothermia.

To minimise hypothermia the surgical field should be plucked minimally of feathers, with minimal soaking with surgical antiseptic solutions (avian skin is relatively poorly populated with contaminant bacteria and fungi anyway in comparison to cats and dogs). The patient can be covered with surgical drapes, with clear drapes being preferred for ease of observation. The patient may be placed onto a circulating warm water blanket, the room temperature should be raised, an angle-adjustable lamp may also be used to increase the environmental temperature. Warm water blankets or filled latex gloves may be placed close to the patient, although care should be taken not to allow them to directly contact the bird, as when too hot they may scald, and as they cool they may actually draw heat away from the patient.

During the procedure the cloacal temperature can be measured directly using an electronic probe.

Fluid therapy

It should be noted that, as with small mammals, postoperative fluid therapy may enhance the recovery rate and improve the return to normal function of the patient.

Healthy, anaesthetised birds should receive replacement fluids at 10 ml/kg/h for the first 2 h, and then at 5–8 ml/kg/h thereafter to prevent overhydration (Curro 1998). If blood loss should occur during surgery then the replacement volume of crystalloid fluid should be three times the blood loss volume. If the volume of blood lost is > 30% of the normal total blood volume, then a blood transfusion should be considered. Other indicators for blood transfusions are a total plasma protein level below 25 g/l and a PCV below 15%. Blood donors should at least be of the same avian group (e.g. parrot to parrot), and preferably the same species (e.g. from one budgerigar to another). One drop of blood is roughly equivalent to 0.05 ml, and the estimated blood volume of an avian patient is 10% body weight in grams. Therefore a 500 g African grey parrot will have roughly 50 ml of blood circulating in its body. Note that a 40 g budgerigar will have only 4 ml of blood and the loss of just 20 drops (1 ml) will represent 25% of its blood volume.

Routes of fluid administration will depend on the procedure and health status of the patient. Subcutaneous routes are used for healthy birds undergoing minor or routine surgery. Areas used include the interscapular area, the axillae, the propatagium (wing web between the shoulder and carpus), and the inguinal skin fold which lies cranial to each leg.

Advanced dehydration requires that intraosseous or intravenous routes should be used. Intraosseous routes include the proximal tibia and distal ulna; intravenous routes include the right jugular vein, the medial metatarsal vein and the brachial veins. The right jugular vein is usually larger than the left and may be catheterised relatively easily in most species, a 25 gauge catheter being sufficient in birds down to 100 g. The brachial vein runs caudal to the humerus and is visible on the underside of the wing. It tends to be smaller, but is still relatively easily catheterised in birds over 100–200 g. The medial metatarsal vein runs along the medial aspect of the lower leg, distal to the intertarsal ('hock') joint and is particularly useful in waterfowl and many raptors as it is less mobile and less fragile than the previously mentioned veins.

The most commonly used fluid is lactated Ringer's solution, but dextrose solutions may be used to treat hypoglycaemia in malnourished cases. All fluids should be warmed to 39–40°C before being administered.

Monitoring anaesthesia

During the initial stages of anaesthesia (planes 1 and 2), the respiratory rate will be shallow and erratic. The patient will be lethargic, have drooping eyelids, a lowered head and ruffled feathers. As anaesthetic depth increases, palpebral, corneal, pedal and cere reflexes will remain, but all voluntary movement ceases.

As stage 3 is reached, the respiration rate becomes regular, and depth of breathing is increased and corneal and pedal reflexes are slow but the palpebral reflex disappears. If anaesthesia is allowed to progress, respiratory rate and tidal volume will continue to decrease, until respiratory arrest occurs. Therefore monitoring the rebreathing bag, for rate and depth of respiration, can provide valuable information to the anaesthetist.

Heart rates can be monitored directly using a stethoscope, and ECG leads may be attached to allow monitoring of electrical output. The attachment of the leads is modified in avian cases by using adhesive pads or fine needles to attach to the skin, rather than traumatic alligator clips. These may be applied to the wing web (propatagium) or the fold of skin in front of the legs. The avian ECG differs somewhat from its mammalian counterpart in that the wave appears to be inverted in most species on lead II as the RS wave is the most developed part of the QRS complex as a norm (Fig. 13.4). Heart rates in smaller birds may be too fast (> 300 beats per minute) for an ECG to accurately trace.

The use of Doppler flow apparatus is extremely useful. These detect movement of fluid, in this case blood flow through a superficial blood vessel, and convert this to an audible sound or visual trace. It provides information therefore on the strength of the pulse, pulse rate and perfusion of tissues, and can often cope better than the ECG with higher pulse rates.

Respiratory flow monitors can be used if endotracheal tubes are used, although the very low flow rates of some smaller avian species may not register.

Pulse oximeters may also be used, to measure the relative saturation of the haemoglobin with oxygen. Reflector probe attachments are the best, and may be used cloacally, or orally; however, many oximeters will not be able to cope with the high heart rates of smaller birds. The Heska® oximeter will allow detection of heart rates in the 300 beats per minute range.

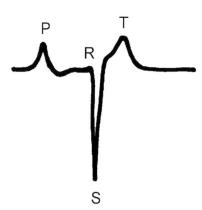

Fig. 13.4 The avian ECG differs somewhat from its mammalian counterpart in that the wave appears to be inverted in most species on lead II as the RS wave is normally the most developed part of the QRS complex.

RECOVERY AND ANALGESIA

Recovery involves ventilation with 100% oxygen. The endotracheal tube is removed once the bird starts to object to its presence. Regardless of the anaesthetic used, practically all patients will appear disorientated and will attempt to flap their wings during recovery. Every attempt should be made to gently constrain them (without restricting respiration) to ensure that they do not damage their wings or feathers. This can be best achieved by lightly wrapping them in a towel. Usually with isoflurane anaesthesia, recovery is over in 5–10 min; however, if ketamine is used, recovery may take much longer. During any recovery period the environmental temperature should be kept in the 25–30°C range to prevent hypothermia. Keep the recovery area quiet and dimly lit to ensure minimal adverse stimulation.

The patient should be encouraged to take food as soon as it is able; this will minimise the deleterious effects of hypoglycaemia seen in these high metabolic rate species.

Analgesia

Analgesia has been shown to reduce the time taken for birds to return to normal eating and preening behaviour, to reduce induction doses of anaesthetic required if administered preoperatively, and to result in less wound breakdowns due to self-trauma.

Opioids such as butorphanol (Torbugesic® Fort Dodge) at 3–4 mg/kg (Bauck 1990) have been used in cockatoos and African grey parrots. Doses may need to be repeated three times daily due to the drug's relatively short-acting duration. It does however have some respiratory suppression side effects, and requires liver metabolism for excretion. Other opioids used include buprenorphine (Vetergesic® Animalcare) at doses of 0.1 mg/kg intravenously or intramuscularly twice daily.

Non-steroidal anti-inflammatory drugs (NSAIDs) such as carprofen (Rimadyl® Pfizer Ltd) at 4–5 mg/kg once daily have been used. Others include meloxicam (Metacam® oral drops Boehringer Ingelheim Ltd) at 1–2 drops/kg body weight once daily, ketoprofen (Ketofen® 1% Merial) at 2 mg/kg intramuscularly once daily or flunixin meglumine (Finadyne Injection® for dogs Schering Plough) at 1–10 mg/kg once daily (Curro 1998). As these are all NSAIDs, particular care should be taken in patients with gastrointestinal or renal disease; avian patients due to their kidney structure are more sensitive to some of these side effects. Concurrent fluid therapy is therefore often advised when using NSAIDs, with or without gastrointestinal protectants such as sucralfate and cimetidine.

REFERENCES AND FURTHER READING

Bauck, L. (1990) Analgesics in avian medicine. In: *Proceedings of the Association of Avian Vets*, pp 239–244.

Beynon, P.H. (1996) Formulary. In: *Manual of Psittacine Birds* (eds P.H. Beynon, N.A. Forbes & M.P.C. Lawton). British Small Animal Veterinary Association, Cheltenham.

Beynon, P.H., Forbes, N.A. & Harcourt-Brown, N.H. (1996) *Manual of Raptors, Pigeons and Waterfowl*. British Small Animal Veterinary Association, Cheltenham.

Beynon, P.H., Forbes, N.A. & Lawton, M.P.C. (1996) *Manual of Psittacine Birds*. British Small Animal Veterinary Association, Cheltenham.

Coles, B.H. (1997) *Avian Medicine and Surgery*, 2nd edition. Blackwell Science, Oxford.

Curro, T.G. (1998) Anaesthesia of pet birds. *Seminars in Avian and Exotic Pet Medicine*, Jan, pp 10–21.

Ritchie, B.W., Harrison, G.J. & Harrison, L.R. (1994) *Avian Medicine: Principles and Applications*. Wingers Publishing, Lake Worth, FL.

Rosskopf, W.J., Woerpel, R.W. & Reed, S. (1989) Avian anaesthesia administration. *Proceedings of the American Animal Hospital Association*, pp 449–457.

Taylor, M. (1988) General cautions with isoflurane. *Assoc Avian Vet Today*, **2**, 96–97.

Valverde, A., Honeyman, V.L. & Dyson, D.H. Determination of a sedative dose and influence of midazolam on cardiopulmonary function in Canada geese. *American Journal of Veterinary Research*, **51**, 1071–1074.

Reptile Anaesthesia

Simon Girling

Reptiles tend to be less easily stressed than their avian cousins, and so restraint may be performed without as much risk in the case of the debilitated animal. It is still worthwhile considering how to successfully and safely restrain the reptile patient for it to be anaesthetised, as well as some tips that may make restraint less dangerous to animal and handler alike.

Initial restraint of the reptile patient

Points to consider include:

- Is the patient suffering from disease? Examples include patients with pneumonia, where mouth breathing and excessive oral mucus may be seen. Vigorous manual manipulation can exacerbate the condition.
- What is the species? Day geckos are extremely delicate and very prone to shedding their tails when handled. Similarly, species such as green iguanas are prone to conditions such as metabolic bone disease whereby their skeleton becomes fragile and spontaneous fractures are common. Some reptiles are naturally aggressive, for example, snapping turtles, Tokay geckos, and rock pythons. Other species are potentially dangerous, such as venomous species of snake, or lizard (e.g. rattlesnakes, cobras, Gila monsters and beaded lizards).

The need for restraint therefore needs to be considered carefully before physical attempts are made.

Restraint techniques and equipment
Order Sauria

This includes members of the lizard family such as geckos, iguanas, chameleons and agamas.

Lizards come in many different shapes and sizes, from the 4-foot long adult green iguana to the 4-inch long green anole. They all have roughly the same structural format with four limbs (although these may become vestigial, for example, the slow-worm) and a tail. Their main danger areas therefore include their claws, teeth and, in some species such as iguanas, their tails which can lash out in a whip-like fashion.

Restraint is best performed by grasping the pectoral girdle with one hand from the ventral aspect, so controlling one forelimb with the thumb and the other between index and middle finger. The other hand is used to grasp the pelvic girdle from the dorsal aspect, controlling one limb with the thumb and the other again between index and middle finger (Fig. 14.1). The lizard may then be held in a vertical manner with head uppermost to put the tail out of harm's way. The handler should allow some flexibility in this method as the lizard may wriggle, and overly rigid restraint could damage the spine.

The use of a thick towel to control the tail and claws is often very useful for aggressive lizards. Occasionally gauntlets are necessary for very large liz-

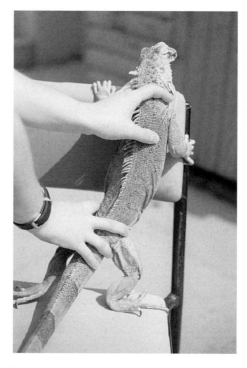

Fig. 14.1 Method of approaching the restraint of a large lizard such as a green iguana by controlling both the pectoral and pelvic limbs from the dorsal aspect.

ards, and for those which may have a poisonous bite (the Gila monster and the beaded lizard). It is important to ensure that the lizard is not restrained with too much force, as those with skeletal problems such as metabolic bone disease may be seriously injured. In addition lizards, like other reptiles, do not have a diaphragm and so overzealous restraint will lead to the digestive system pushing onto the lungs and increasing inspiratory effort.

Geckos can be extremely fragile and the day gecko may be best anaesthetised in a clear plastic container rather than physically restraining it. Other geckos have easily damaged skin and so latex gloves and soft cloths should be used.

Small lizards may have their heads controlled between the index finger and thumb to prevent biting. *Under no circumstances should lizards be restrained by their tail*. Many will shed their tails at this time, but not all of them will regrow: green iguanas, for example, will only regrow their tails as juveniles, < 2.5–3 years of age. After this they will be left tail-less.

Vago-vagal reflex

There is a procedure that can be used to place members of the lizard family into a trance-like state. It involves closing the eyelids and placing firm but gentle digital pressure onto both eyeballs. This stimulates the parasympathetic autonomic nervous system that results in a reduction in heart rate, blood pressure and respiration rate. Providing no loud noises are made, the lizard after 1–2 min of this may be placed on its side, front and back so allowing radiography to be performed without further physical or chemical restraint. A loud noise or physical stimulation will immediately revert the lizard to its normal wakeful state.

Order Serpentes

This is the snake family. Examples encompass a wide range of sizes from the enormous anacondas and Burmese pythons, which may achieve lengths up to 30 feet or more, down to the thread-snake family that may be a few tens of centimetres long. They are all characterised by their elongated form with an absence of limbs. Their danger areas are their teeth (and in the case of the more poisonous species such as the viper family their fang teeth) and in the case of the constrictor and python family their ability to asphyxiate their prey by winding themselves around the victim's chest or neck.

Non-venomous snakes can be restrained by initially controlling the head. This is done by placing the thumb over the occiput and curling the fingers under the chin. Reptiles, like birds, have only the one occipital condyle so it is important to stabilise the neck occipital–atlantal joint. It is also important to support the rest of the snake's body so that not all of the weight of the snake is suspended from the head (Fig. 13.2). This is best achieved by allowing the smaller species to coil around the handler's arm, so the snake is supporting itself. In larger species it is necessary to support the body length at regular intervals – hence the help of several people may be necessary. Above all it is important not to grip

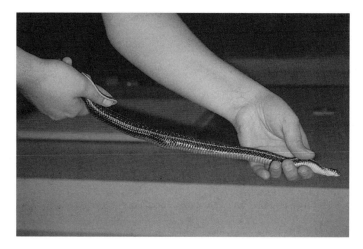

Fig. 14.2 It is important to provide support at regular intervals along the body of a snake such as this garter snake, to avoid undue pressure or dependent weight on any one part of the spine.

the snake too hard as this will cause bruising and the release of myoglobin from muscle cells that will damage the kidney filtration membranes.

Poisonous species (such as the viper family, rattlesnakes, and so on) or very aggressive species (such as anacondas, reticulated and rock pythons) may be restrained using snake hooks. These are 1.5–2 foot steel rods with a blunt-ended shepherd's hook on the end and are used to loop under the body of a snake to move it at arm's length into a container. The hook may also be used to trap the head flat to the floor before grasping it with the hand. Once the head is controlled safely the snake is rendered harmless, unless it is a member of the spitting cobra family. These are unlikely to be encountered in general practice, but if they are, plastic goggles should be worn, as the poison is spat into the prey or assailant's eyes, causing blindness.

Order Chelonia

This includes all land tortoises, terrapins and aquatic turtles, varying in size from the small Egyptian tortoise weighing a few grams to Galapagos species weighing several hundred kilograms. The majority are harmless, although surprisingly strong. Exceptions include the snapping turtle and the alligator snapping turtle, both of which can give a serious bite, as do most of the soft-shelled terrapins. They also have mobile necks. Even red-eared terrapins may give a nasty nip!

The mild-tempered Mediterranean species of tortoise may be held with both hands, one on either side of the main part of the shell, behind the front legs. To keep the tortoise still for examination it may be placed onto a cylinder or stack of tins which ensure that its legs are raised clear of the table, balancing on the centre of the underside of the shell (plastron).

For aggressive species it is essential to hold the shell on both sides behind and above the rear legs, to avoid being bitten. For examination of the head region in these species it is necessary to chemically restrain them.

For soft-shelled and aquatic species, soft cloths and latex gloves may be necessary to avoid marking the shell.

Order Crocodylia
This family is rarely seen in general practice and includes the crocodiles, both fresh and saltwater, the alligators, the fish-eating gharials, and the caimans. Their dangers lie in their impressively arrayed jaws and their sheer size – an adult bull Nile crocodile may weigh many hundreds of kilograms and may live for up to 50 years or more. Readers are advised to consult standard texts for further information.

CHEMICAL RESTRAINT

Chemical restraint is often necessary in reptile medicine to facilitate procedures, from extracting the head of a leopard tortoise or box turtle simply to enable a jugular blood sample to be obtained, to coeliotomy procedures such as surgical correction of egg binding.

Before any anaesthetic or sedative is administered, an assessment of the reptile patient's health is necessary. Is sedation or anaesthesia necessary for the procedure required? Is the reptile suffering from respiratory disease, or septicaemia, hence is the reptile's health likely to be made worse by sedation or anaesthesia?

Before any attempt to administer chemical restraint the reptilian respiratory system should be understood.

Overview of reptilian respiratory anatomy and physiology
The reptilian respiratory system differs in a number of ways from the basic mammalian system, namely (starting cranially):

(1) Reduced larynx. Like the avian patient the reptile patient has a glottis, which lies at the base of the tongue, more rostrally in snakes and lizards and more caudally in Chelonia. At rest the glottis is permanently closed, opening briefly during inspiration and expiration. In crocodiles the glottis is obscured by the basihyal valve that is a fold of the epiglottis, which has to be deflected before they can be intubated (Bennet 1998).
(2) The trachea varies between orders. The Chelonia and Crocodylia have complete cartilaginous rings similar to the avian patient, with the Chelonia patient having a very short trachea, bifurcating into two bronchi in the neck in some species. Serpentes and Sauria have incomplete rings, such as are found in the cat and dog, with Serpentes having a very long trachea.

(3) The lungs of Serpentes and saurian species are simple and elastic in nature. The left lung of most Serpentes is absent or vestigial but may be present in the case of members of the Boid family (e.g. boa constrictors). The right lung of Serpentes ends in an air sac. Chelonia species have a more complicated lung structure, and the paired lungs sit dorsally inside the carapace of the shell. Crocodylia have lungs not dissimilar to mammalian ones and are paired.

(4) No reptile has a diaphragm, although Crocodylia species have a pseudo-diaphragm that changes position with the movements of the liver and gut, so pushing air in and out of the lungs.

(5) Most reptiles use intercostal muscles to move the ribcage in and out, as with birds, the exception being the Chelonia. These species require movement of their limbs and head into and out of the shell in order to bring air into and out of the lungs. This is important when they are anaesthetised as such movements and therefore breathing ceases.

(6) Some species can survive in oxygen-deprived atmospheres for prolonged periods. Chelonia species may survive for 24 h or more, and green iguanas may even survive for 4–5 h, making inhalation induction of anaesthesia almost impossible in these animals.

Pre-anaesthetic preparation
Blood testing
It is useful to test biochemical and haemocytological parameters before administering anaesthetic drugs. Blood samples may be taken from the jugular vein or dorsal tail vein in Chelonia, the ventral tail vein, palatine vein or cardiac puncture in Serpentes, and the ventral tail vein in Crocodylia and Sauria. The minimum tests advised are haematocrit, blood calcium levels, blood total protein levels, aspartamine transaminase (AST) levels for hepatic function and uric acid levels for renal function.

Fasting
This is necessary in Serpentes for a period of 2 days before anaesthesia to prevent regurgitation and pressure on the lungs and/or heart. Chelonia rarely regurgitate and so do not need much fasting. It is important not to feed live prey to insectivores (e.g. leopard geckos) 24 h before anaesthesia, as the prey may still be alive when the reptile is anaesthetised!

Pre-anaesthetic medications
Antimuscarinic drugs
Atropine (0.01–0.04 mg/kg intramuscularly) or glycopyrrolate (0.01 mg/kg intramuscularly) can reduce oral secretions, and prevent bradycardia. However, these problems are rarely of concern in reptile patients.

Tranquillisers

Acepromazine (0.1–0.5 mg/kg intramuscularly) may be given 1 h before induction of anaesthesia to reduce the dose of anaesthetic required. Diazepam (0.22–0.62 mg/kg intramuscularly in alligators) and midazolam (2 mg/kg intramuscularly in turtles) are also useful.

Alpha$_2$ adrenoceptor agonists

Xylazine (Rompun® Bayer) can be used 30 min before ketamine at 1 mg/kg in Crocodylia to reduce the dose of ketamine. Medetomidine (Domitor® Pfizer) may be used at doses of 100–150 µg/kg, so reducing the dose required of ketamine in Chelonia, and has the advantage of being reversible with atipamezole (Antisedan® Pfizer) at 500–750 µg/kg.

Opioids

Butorphanol (Torbugesic® Fort Dodge) at 0.4 mg/kg intramuscularly can be administered 20 min before anaesthesia, providing analgesia and reducing the anaesthetic dose required. It may be combined with midazolam (Hypnovel®) at 2 mg/kg.

Induction using injectable agents

Advantages of injectable anaesthetics include ease of administration, avoiding breath-holding and prolonged induction, low cost and availability. Disadvantages include a recovery often dependent on organ metabolism, potential difficulty reversing medications in emergency situations, and prolonged recovery periods, as well as necrosis of muscle cells at injection sites. Also, due to the renal portal system, drugs injected into the caudal half of a reptile may either be excreted by the kidneys before they take effect, or increase renal damage if potentially nephrotoxic (see chapter 2). Injectable medications should therefore be administered in the cranial half of the body.

Ketamine (Ketaset® Fort Dodge)

The effects of ketamine are species and dosage dependent. Recommended levels range from 22–44 mg/kg intramuscularly for sedation to 55–88 mg/kg intramuscularly for surgical anaesthesia, lower levels being needed if combined with a premedicant such as midazolam or medetomidine.

Effects occur in 10–30 min but may take up to 4 days to wear off, particularly at low environmental temperatures. It is mainly used therefore at the lower dose range to allow sedation and facilitate intubation and maintenance of anaesthesia by a gaseous means in species such as Chelonia which may breath-hold.

Disadvantages are that it is frequently painful to administer; effects are prolonged and ketamine is excreted *via* the kidneys; administration of ketamine in the cranial half of the body is recommended.

Alphaxalone–alphadolone (Saffan® Schering-Plough)

Saffan® can allow intubation within 3–5 min when administered intravenously. It may be administered intramuscularly but induction will take longer (25–40 min). If used alone it will provide anaesthesia for 15–35 min at a dose of 6–9 mg/kg for intravenous administration, or 9–15 mg/kg if given intramuscularly. Recovery is quicker than with ketamine, although full recovery may still take 1–4 h.

Propofol

Propofol produces rapid induction and recovery, and is becoming the induction agent of choice. Its advantages include a short elimination half-life and minimal organ metabolism, making it safer in debilitated reptiles. The disadvantage is that it requires intravenous access, although use of the intraosseous route has been shown to be successful in green iguanas at a dose of 10 mg/kg. Propofol produces transient apnoea and cardiac depression, often necessitating positive pressure ventilation.

Doses of 10–15 mg/kg in Chelonia given *via* the dorsal coccygeal (tail) vein have successfully induced anaesthesia in under 1 min, allowing intubation and maintenance on a gaseous anaesthetic if required. Used alone it provides general anaesthesia for 20–30 min.

Succinylcholine

This is a neuromuscular blocking agent, and produces immobilisation without analgesia. It should be used to aid the administration of another form of anaesthetic, or to aid in transportation, and not as a sole method of anaesthesia.

It can be used in large Chelonia at doses of 0.5–1 mg/kg intramuscularly and will allow intubation and conversion to gaseous anaesthesia. Crocodilians can be immobilised with 3–5 mg/kg intramuscularly, with immobilisation occurring within 4 min and recovery in 7–9 h. Respiration usually continues without assistance at these doses, but it is important to have assisted ventilation facilities to hand as paralysis of the muscles of respiration can easily occur.

Reversal of succinylcholine can be effected with neostigmine (an acetylcholinesterase inhibitor) at doses of 0.03–0.07 mg/kg intramuscularly.

Induction using gaseous agents

The usual gaseous agents (see below) may be used to induce anaesthesia, either in an induction chamber or *via* face masks. Face masks may be bought or, for snakes, syringe cases may be modified to form elongated masks for induction.

Maintenance of anaesthesia with injectable agents

Ketamine

This may be used on its own for anaesthesia at doses of 55–88 mg/kg intramuscularly. As the dosages increase the recovery time also increases, in some instances to several days, and doses above 110 mg/kg will cause respiratory arrest and bradycardia.

Ketamine may be combined with other injectable agents to provide surgical anaesthesia. These include midazolam at 2 mg/kg intramuscularly with 40 mg/kg ketamine in turtles (Bennet 1998); xylazine at 1 mg/kg intramuscularly, given 30 min before 20 mg/kg ketamine in large crocodiles (Page 1993); and meditomidine at 100 µg/kg intramuscularly with 50 mg/kg ketamine in kingsnakes (Malley 1997).

Propofol
Propofol may be used to give 20–30 min of anaesthesia, which allows minor procedures. It may be 'topped-up' at 1 mg/kg/min intravenously or intraosseously. Apnoea is extremely common and intubation and ventilation with 100% oxygen is advised.

Alphaxalone–alphadolone
Saffan® can be used for induction and for short periods of anaesthesia (average 25 min) at 6–9 mg/kg intravenously. Intramuscular doses may be given but onset of anaesthesia may take 20–30 min.

Disadvantages include prolonged recovery time of 1–4 h, the relatively large doses of this medication required *via* an intravenous route, and the need to intubate many reptiles due to relaxation of the muscles which keep the glottis open to allow breathing.

Maintenance of anaesthesia with gaseous agents
Halothane
Halothane can be used for both maintenance and induction in reptiles. Face masks or induction chambers can be used for induction at levels of 4–5%, although certain species such as Chelonia can breath-hold for long periods, negating its use for induction. Maintenance can be achieved at 1–2.5%.

Disadvantages are that it can induce myocardial hypoxia and dysrhythmias. For recovery 15–20% metabolism by the liver will occur. As many diseased reptiles have damaged livers, this makes its use limited. Cardiac arrest and apnoea frequently occur simultaneously, reducing resuscitation response times. It can also induce a period of excitement in reptiles during the induction phase.

Isoflurane
This is the gaseous maintenance anaesthetic of choice. Although more expensive than halothane, it scores over it in several areas. It is minimally metabolised in the body (<1%), and has a very low blood gas partition coefficient (1.5 compared with 2.5 for halothane in human trials). Hence it has a very low solubility in blood, so as soon as isoflurane administration is stopped the reptile starts to recover. It also has lower fat solubility than halothane and so excretion from

the body is quicker still. Finally, it has excellent muscle relaxing properties and is a good analgesic, and apnoea precedes cardiac arrest.

Induction of anaesthesia is by face mask, or induction chamber in those species not exhibiting breath-holding, 4–5%. Maintenance of anaesthesia, preferably *via* endotracheal tube, is at levels of 2–3% depending on the procedure.

Nitrous oxide
This can be used in conjunction with halothane or isoflurane, so reducing the percentage of the gaseous anaesthetic required for induction and maintenance of anaesthesia. Its other advantages include good muscle relaxation and analgesic properties, making it useful in orthopaedic procedures.

Maintaining anaesthesia
Inhalant gaseous anaesthesia is becoming the main method of anaesthetising reptiles for prolonged procedures and as described above offers many benefits. These are enhanced still further if the reptile is intubated, allowing the inhalant anaesthetic to be delivered in a controlled manner.

Intubation
The glottis, which acts as the entrance to the trachea, is relatively cranial in many species. It is kept closed at rest, so the operator must wait for inspiration to occur to allow intubation. Reptiles produce little or no saliva when not eating, so blockage of the endotracheal tube is uncommon.

In Serpentes, the glottis sits rostrally on the floor of the mouth, caudal to the tongue sheath. Intubation may be performed while the reptile is conscious, if necessary, as they do not have a cough reflex; the mouth is opened with a wooden or plastic tongue depressor and the endotracheal tube inserted during inspiration. Alternatively, an induction agent may be given and then intubation attempted.

In Chelonia the glottis sits caudally at the base of the tongue. The trachea is very short and the endotracheal tube should only be inserted a few centimetres, otherwise there is a risk one or other bronchus will be intubated, leading to only one lung receiving the anaesthetic. As mentioned, an induction agent such as ketamine or propofol is advised for Chelonia prior to intubation due to breath-holding and difficulty in extracting the head from the shell.

Sauria vary depending on the species, most having just a glottis guarding the entrance to the trachea, but some species (e.g. geckos) possess vocal folds. Some may be intubated while conscious; most are better induced with an injectable preparation, or following gaseous induction by face mask. Some species may be too small for intubation.

Crocodylia have a basihyal fold (Bennet 1998)that acts like an epiglottis and needs to be depressed prior to intubation. These species require some form of chemical injectable sedation or induction prior to intubation for operator safety.

Intermittent positive pressure ventilation

If intubation is performed on a fully conscious patient, anaesthesia may be induced, even in breath-holding species, by using positive pressure ventilation, in a matter of 5–10 min. This has some advantages as avoiding injectable induction agents leads to rapid postoperative recovery.

Many species require positive pressure ventilation during anaesthesia. Chelonia, for example, are frequently placed in dorsal recumbency during intracoelomic surgery (the absence of a diaphragm leads to one body cavity – the coelomic cavity). As they have no diaphragm, and the lungs are situated dorsally, the weight of the digestive contents pressing on the lungs will depress inspiration and lead to hypoxia. In addition most inspiratory effort is induced by movement of the chelonian's limbs, which are (one hopes!) immobile during anaesthesia. If a neuromuscular blocking agent such as succinylcholine has been used, positive pressure ventilation may be needed as respiratory muscle paralysis may occur.

The aims of intermittent positive pressure ventilation (IPPV) are to just inflate the lungs for an adequately oxygenated state to be maintained, and for the animal to remain anaesthetised. Most reptiles require 2–6 breaths a minute, at a maximum inflation pressure of 10–15 cmH$_2$O. A ventilator unit is useful (Fig. 14.3) but, with experience, manual ventilation with enough pressure to

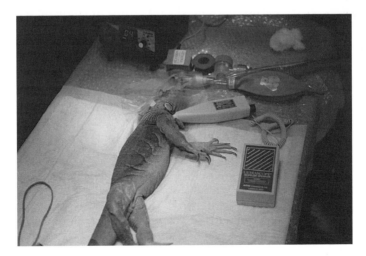

Fig. 14.3 Ventilator units such as this Vetronic® small animal ventilator (top left of picture) are extremely useful when performing IPPV in reptiles. Note also the use of a Doppler probe at the thoracic inlet (the heart of green iguanas is relatively cranial) to monitor cardiac output during anaesthesia.

just inflate the lungs and no more can be achieved. A rough guide is to inflate the first two-fifths of the reptile's body at each cycle (Malley 1997).

Anaesthetic breathing systems
For species less than 5 kg a non-rebreathing system with oxygen flow at twice the minute volume (which approximates to 300–500 ml/kg/min for most species) is suggested (Bennet 1998). Ayres T-pieces, modified Bain circuits or Mapleson C circuits may all be used.

ADDITIONAL SUPPORTIVE THERAPY

Positioning
Many chelonians will be placed in dorsal recumbency for intracoelomic surgery. Other groups of reptiles may be placed in this position for similar techniques. Therefore foam wedges, or positional polystyrene-filled vacuum bags, are essential to maintain stability.

Snakes become extremely flaccid during surgery and may be strapped to a long board, or wedged in place with foam or vacuum bags.

Body temperature
Reptiles should be maintained as near to their optimal environmental body temperature as possible (22–30°C for most species). The reptile may be placed onto a circulating water heating pad during anaesthesia; environmental room temperatures should be kept up to reduce losses. Warmed subcutaneous or intracoelomic fluids can be used. Alternatively hot water bottles, or hot water-filled latex gloves may be used (wrapped in towelling to prevent direct contact with the reptile) to group around the patient. Care should be taken when these cool down as they may then draw heat away from the patient rather than provide it.

Clear drapes will also help to preserve heat, and light sources for surgery will radiate heat.

During the procedure a cloacal probe attached to a digital thermometer may be used to monitor body temperature.

Fluid therapy
Postoperative fluid therapy enhances the recovery rate and improves the return to normal function of the patient.

Fluids may be administered *via* intravenous, intraosseous or intracoelomic routes. Serpentes may have fluids administered intravenously in larger species *via* the palatine vein that runs either side of midline in the roof of the mouth;

catheters must be removed prior to recovery. The alternative is to do a cut-down procedure and catheterise the jugular vein 5–10 cm caudal to the angle of the jaw, or intra-operatively to administer bolus fluids intracardially. Anaesthesia or sedation is therefore needed. While the reptile is conscious, fluids are given intracoelomically. To avoid organ puncture this is performed in the caudal third of the snake, two rows of scales dorsal from the ventral body scales on the side of the snake. The needle is pushed just through the body wall, between the ribs.

Chelonians may have a catheter placed in the jugular vein, this again may require a cut-down procedure in some species. Fluids and drugs may also be given *via* the dorsal tail vein, but this is more a sinus or collection of small vessels rather than one discrete vessel and so long-term therapy is difficult. In-traosseous fluids in Chelonia can be *via* the pillars – the part of the shell which connects the carapace to the plastron. Access is in a caudal to cranial direction from in front of the hindlimb, screwing a hypodermic or spinal needle into the marrow cavity, keeping the direction parallel to the outer shell wall (Fig. 14.4). The proximal tibia may also be used. Intracoelomic fluids may be given either

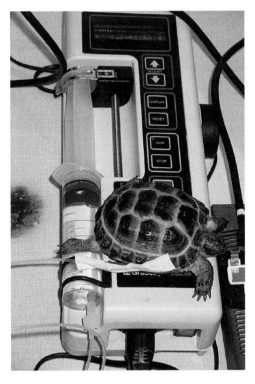

Fig. 14.4 Intraosseous fluid therapy in a Horsfield's tortoise via the caudal pillar of the shell. The use of syringe drivers is invaluable when administering small volumes of fluids over a 24-hour period.

side of the neck inlet, in a cranial-caudal direction keeping close to the floor of the plastron, or cranial to either hindlimb. Care should be taken to avoid puncturing the urinary bladder *via* the latter route.

Sauria may have intravenous fluids administered *via* the cephalic vein in larger species. A cut-down procedure is required across the humerus in a line perpendicular to its long axis. The ventral abdominal vein, running just beneath the skin on ventral midline, may also be used. Intraosseous fluids can be given into the proximal end of the femur, or into the proximal end of the tibia, using a hypodermic or spinal needle. Intracoelomic fluids may be administered in the right lower quadrant of the lizard after placing it on its back with its head down to allow the gut to fall away from the injection site.

Fluid volumes are recommended at 20–25 ml/kg every 24 h, and certainly should not exceed 2–3% body weight in chelonians (Bennet 1998).

Most reptiles should receive lactated Ringer's and glucose saline fluid mixes; a common combination is lactated Ringer's 33%, 0.9% saline–5% glucose 33% and sterile water 33%. This is to reduce the isotonicity, as most terrestrial reptiles have a plasma concentration of 0.8% saline rather than the mammalian 0.9%.

Monitoring anaesthesia

Reptiles will pass through similar definable stages of anaesthesia to mammals.

Stage 1

This is marked by a reduction in the rate of movement, although the reptile maintains the ability to right itself after being turned on its back. In addition tongue withdrawal reflexes and palpebral reflexes are present.

Stage 2

In this stage the righting reflex often disappears, and the reptile ceases to respond to mildly noxious stimuli. The palpebral and vent reflexes are diminished, and movement ceases.

Stage 3

This is the stage of surgical anaesthesia classically. The tongue withdrawal reflex disappears, and the muscles are totally relaxed. In snakes the Bauchstreich reflex (where stroking the ventral scutes produces normal movement of the body wall) ceases. There is no response to noxious stimuli, and the vent reflex is much reduced, although total loss of this response indicates the reptile may be too deeply anaesthetised. Chelonia still possess a corneal reflex at this stage

Stage 4

This stage precedes death. Respiratory movements cease or slow markedly, Chelonia lose their corneal reflexes, and all reptiles lose their vent reflexes.

Monitoring the heart rate and rhythm can be extremely difficult with a conventional stethoscope, due to the rough scales of the reptile interfering with sound transmission and the three-chambered heart of reptiles that reduces the clarity of the heart beat. Some of this can be overcome by placing a damp towel over the area to be auscultated, so deadening the sound of the scales, but in many cases the best solution is to resort to using a Doppler probe which produces an audible response to movement of blood through a superficial vessel or heart (Fig. 14.5).

ECG leads may be attached to the patient to give an electrical trace of heart activity. The alligator clips on the leads may be attached to hypodermic needles that can then be attached to the patient to minimise the crushing effects of the forceps on small fragile patients. In snakes these can still be used, even in the absence of limbs; the leads are placed two heart lengths cranial and caudal to the heart. In some Sauria such as iguanas, skinks, chameleons and water dragons the heart is situated far cranially and hence the forelimb leads are better placed cervically.

Respiratory flow monitors are not so useful due to the need for IPPV in most reptile species. Pulse oximeters are useful, with reflector probes being used per cloaca, or orally, to measure the percentage saturation of the haemoglobin with oxygen.

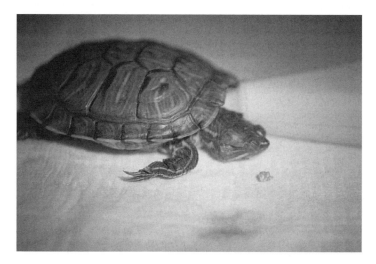

Fig. 14.5 Cardiac output monitoring with a Doppler ultrasound probe in a red-eared terrapin. The area of skin between the neck and forelimb provides a useful point for anaesthetic monitoring, allowing the rate and quality of blood flow to be assessed.

RECOVERY AND ANALGESIA

Reptiles often will recover rapidly from isoflurane anaesthesia. But if other injectable drugs are used such as alphadalone–alphaxolone or ketamine, recovery may be prolonged. It is thus essential to keep the reptile patient calm, stress-free and at its optimum preferred body temperature. It may be necessary to keep the patient intubated and on IPPV with oxygen if high doses of the above agents have been used, until the reptile is once again breathing for itself. Care should be taken though as high levels of oxygen actually suppress the stimulus for a reptile to breathe, as this is induced by a low level of PaO_2 rather than high $PaCO_2$ as in mammals. The use of doxapram (Dopram®) at a dose of 5 mg/kg intramuscularly or intravenously helps stimulate respiration.

Fluid therapy also helps to speed recovery, especially with agents such as ketamine which are cleared through the kidneys. Once recovery occurs, patients should be encouraged to eat, or if anorexic then assisted feeding or stomach-tube feeding should be initiated.

Analgesia is, as with other animal groups, an important aspect of postoperative recovery. Reptiles provided with analgesia have been shown to return to normal behaviour, eating, and so on, more quickly than those who do not receive analgesia.

Opioids have been shown to have some effect; butorphanol at 0.4 mg/kg by the intramuscular, intravenous or subcutaneous route, and buprenorphine at 0.01 mg/kg intramuscularly have been recommended (Malley 1997; Bennet 1998).

NSAIDs also seem to be beneficial with carprofen (Rimadyl®) at doses of 2–4 mg/kg intramuscularly initially, and then 1–2 mg/kg every 24–72 h thereafter (Malley 1997), meloxicam (Metacam®) at 0.1–0.2 mg/kg orally every 24 h (Malley 1997), ketoprofen (Ketofen®) at 2 mg/kg intramuscularly every 24 h (Bennet 1998) and flunixin meglumine (Finadyne®) at 0.1–0.5 mg/kg intramuscularly every 24 h (Malley 1997), all recommended. It should be noted that all these drugs are potentially nephrotoxic and have gastrointestinal side effects, and hence fluid therapy and close monitoring should be performed.

REFERENCES AND FURTHER READING

Bennet, R.A. (1996) Anaesthesia. In: *Reptile Medicine and Surgery* (ed. R. Mader), pp 241–247. WB Saunders, London.
Bennet, R.A. (1998) Reptile anaesthesia. *Seminars in Avian and Exotic Pet Medicine*, Jan, pp 30–40. WB Saunders, Philadelphia, PA.
Beynon, P.H., Lawton, M.P.C. & Cooper, J.E. (1992) *Manual of Reptiles*. British Small Animal Veterinary Association, Cheltenham.
Fryer, F. (1994) *Biomedical and Surgical Aspects of Captive Reptile Husbandry*. Krieger Publishing, Malabar, FL.

Lawton, M.P.C. (1992) Anaesthesia. In: *Manual of Reptiles*. British Small Animal Veterinary Asociation, Cheltenham.

Mader, D. (1996) *Reptile Medicine and Surgery*. WB Saunders, Philadelphia.

Malley, D. (1997) Reptile anaesthesia and the practising veterinarian. *In Practice*, July/August, 351–368.

Page, C.D. (1993) Current reptilian anaesthesia procedures. In: *Zoo and Wildlife Medicine: Current Therapy*, 3 (ed. M. Fowler). pp 140–143. WB Saunders Philadelphia, PA.

Porter, K.R. (1972) *Herpetology*. WB Saunders, Philadelphia, PA.

Large Animal Anaesthesia

Elizabeth Welsh

The basic principles of good anaesthetic practice apply regardless of the size and species of the animal to be anaesthetised. It is equally important to obtain a complete history, perform a thorough physical examination, undertake pre-anaesthetic tests (as indicated) and obtain informed consent from owners prior to anaesthetising large animals such as horses, ponies, cattle, sheep and goats. Many horses, ponies and valuable breeding or showing animals will be insured. If feasible, the insurance company should be informed of the need for general anaesthesia, although in many emergency situations this will not be possible.

Many of the problems encountered in anaesthetising large animals arise from the sheer size and weight of the patient, and the safety of the personnel involved must be considered. This is particularly important if the animals are not familiar with being restrained, or become excited when handled.

EQUINE ANAESTHESIA

Both local and general anaesthetic techniques are used in horses although some procedures may be performed under standing surgical anaesthesia (standing chemical restraint or standing sedation). Many tranquillisers, sedatives and general anaesthetic agents may not be used in animals intended for human consumption and, although most horses and ponies in the UK are kept for pleasure or sporting purposes, this should be borne in mind.

Unlike small animals, horses and ponies are often anaesthetised 'in-the-field', i.e. on the premises (in a loose box or field) where they are stabled rather than in a veterinary clinic (Fig. 15.1). In this environment it is particularly important to ensure the safety of the people involved and to have a source of

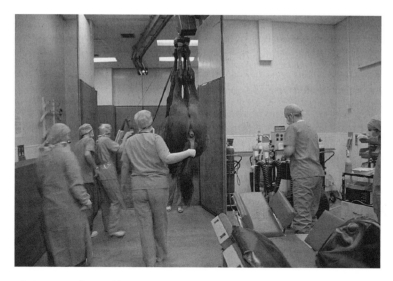

Fig. 15.1 An anaesthetised horse is moved to the recovery box using a hoist following anaesthesia. Note the padding on the surgical table and the endotracheal tubes on the wall. Photograph courtesy of Louise Clark.

oxygen available if required e.g. an oxygen cylinder with a Hudson demand valve attached.

Pre-anaesthetic considerations

Horse shoes

It is important to remove all horse shoes prior to general anaesthesia for the safety of the patient, the anaesthetist and surgical personnel and to protect the padding of the induction and recovery area. If the shoes cannot be removed, clenches and shoes should be well padded or covered with adhesive tape.

The hooves of horses must be cleaned thoroughly before anaesthesia to remove organic matter and reduce the risk of postoperative infection originating from the microbial population present on the hooves. A recent study compared two different methods for presurgical disinfection of the hoof and found that, regardless of the disinfection protocol used, the bacterial load remained high (Hennig *et al.* 2001). Thus water-impermeable coverings should be placed on the hooves during the surgical procedure when possible.

Pre-anaesthetic fasting

Patients should be fasted overnight for 12–18 h prior to general anaesthesia. This may be achieved by placing the patient in a stall with wood shavings or a similar material rather than straw for bedding. In emergencies this may not be possible. Access to fresh water should be denied from the time of pre-anaesthetic medication.

Fasting reduces the volume and weight of gastrointestinal contents and increases functional residual capacity by reducing pressure on the diaphragm.

It is often difficult to maintain an acceptable level of general anaesthesia in physically fit horses and they may be prone to the development of intra- and postoperative complications such as hypotension and myopathy. Consequently, elective surgical procedures in fit performance horses may be delayed for a period of time during which the dietary protein and carbohydrate levels are decreased.

Intravenous catheterisation

In horses and ponies the jugular vein is catheterised using a 13–16 gauge catheter. Aseptic technique is observed during placement of the catheter. Jugular catheters are secured using sutures rather than tape. Most general anaesthetic techniques use intravenous induction agents. Sedatives, fluids and other drugs also may be administered *via* the catheter. Furthermore, it provides rapid intravenous access in the event of an emergency.

If scales are not available to provide an accurate weight for a horse before anaesthesia, the following equation may be used:

$$\text{Horse's weight} (\pm 25 \text{ kg}) = \frac{\text{Girth (inches)}^2 \times \text{Length (inches)}}{660}$$

Pre-anaesthetic medication

Many of the same sedatives, tranquillisers and analgesics used in small animals are also used in equine anaesthesia.

Acetylpromazine

Acetylpromazine (ACP) has the same pharmacological effects in horses following parenteral administration as those found in small animals and it may be administered by the same routes (including orally as a paste). Although it is rarely used in isolation for pre-anaesthetic medication due to its unreliable sedative properties, ACP is useful for the sedation of young, nervous horses and ponies prior to further pre-anaesthetic medication and induction of anaesthesia.

Acetylpromazine is specifically contraindicated for use in breeding stallions because of the risk of priapism and paraphimosis. If used in other male horses the lowest dose recommended to produce the desired effect should be administered. Horses and ponies should not be ridden within 36 h of administration of ACP due to the prolonged duration of action in this species.

Unlike the solution for injection in dogs and cats (0.2% solution; 2 mg/ml) the solution available for horses is 1% (10 mg/ml).

Alpha-2 adrenoceptor agonists

Xylazine, romifidine and detomidine are used in horses. These drugs cause profound standing sedation following administration and are used either as sedatives in their own right or as part of a general anaesthetic protocol. Donkeys and mules are less sensitive to the effects of α_2 adrenoceptor agonists than horses and ponies.

The α_2 adrenoceptor agonists are the main agents used in standing sedation when they are combined with analgesic agents such as butorphanol (agonist–antagonist) or morphine (agonist). Standing sedation avoids many of the problems encountered under general anaesthesia and an increasing number of procedures are performed safely using this technique. However, horses may become ataxic, increasing the risks to all involved.

Atipamezole, an α_2 adrenoceptor antagonist, may be used to reverse the sedative effects of medetomidine in small animals, but in the UK there is no specific antagonist licensed to reverse the effects of α_2 agonists in horses. However, atipamezole exerts similar effects in horses.

Analgesics

Peripheral nerve blocks using local analgesia techniques are used in the diagnosis of lameness. In addition local analgesic techniques, including extradural injection, are particularly valuable in horses as part of a balanced anaesthetic technique. Opioids, local anaesthetics and α_2 adrenoceptor agonists are all suitable extradural analgesic agents. The sacrococcygeal or first intercoccygeal space is used to inject drugs extradurally in horses.

Opioid and non-steroidal anti-inflammatory drugs are used routinely to provide pain relief. As in small animals, pethidine is the only full agonist licensed for use in horses, and similarly should not be injected intravenously when excitement may be observed.

Other agents

Large Animal Immobilon® (ACP and etorphine) a reversible neuroleptanalgesic, is available for restraint and minor surgical intervention in horses. Large Animal Immobilon® is a Schedule 2 controlled drug. Extreme care must be taken when handling this drug, as etorphine can be life-threatening to humans if absorbed by any route. When this agent is being used, an assistant must be present who is capable of giving an intravenous injection of the reversing agent (Large Animal Revivon®, diprenorphine) to the individual administering Large Animal Immobilon. In addition to Large Animal Revivon® a stock of naloxone (Narcan®) must always be available. Following accidental injection of humans, antagonism of the effects of etorphine with naloxone is preferred to diprenorphine. Enterohepatic recycling of etorphine can cause excitement, walking and head-pressing 6–8 h following administration of Large Animal Revivon® to horses.

Benzodiazepines (diazepam and midazolam) may also be used in horses and are commonly given with ketamine to produce a smooth anaesthetic induction following pre-anaesthetic medication with an α_2 adrenoceptor agonist.

Atropine and glycopyrrolate are not used for pre-anaesthetic medication unless specifically indicated (e.g. vagally induced bradycardia), because of their side effects on gut motility, visual disturbance, and so on.

Induction of general anaesthesia
Induction of anaesthesia using inhalation of volatile anaesthetic agents in oxygen *via* face mask or nasotracheal intubation is limited to foals. This induction technique may increase anaesthetic risk.

In adult horses and ponies, induction of general anaesthesia is accomplished using injectable anaesthetic agents such as ketamine or thiopentone. To limit the volume required for injection, solutions of thiopentone are more concentrated than those used in small animals (5–10%). Consequently perivascular injection of this irritant drug must be treated promptly and aggressively to avoid tissue necrosis and skin sloughing.

Endotracheal intubation
Cuffed endotracheal tubes are considerably larger than those used in dogs and cats, e.g. 30 mm tube for 500 kg horse. Direct visualisation of the rima glottidis in horses and ponies is not possible. Gags are used to hold the incisors apart before the tube is inserted blind to the level of the larynx and passed down the trachea.

Anaesthetic breathing systems
Rebreathing systems (circle and to-and-fro) are used to deliver anaesthetic gases to equine patients. Non-rebreathing systems would require extremely high fresh gas flow rates (outwith the specifications of most flowmeters), resulting in considerable expense.

Maintenance of general anaesthesia
Both halothane and isoflurane may be administered *via* calibrated out-of-circuit vaporisers to horses and ponies. The use of rebreathing anaesthetic gas delivery systems can slow the rate of change of anaesthetic depth in response to increasing or decreasing the concentration of the volatile agent if the system is used with low fresh gas flows. Unexpected decreases in the depth of anaesthesia may be managed by intravenous injection of low doses of ketamine, ketamine and midazolam or thiopentone.

Nitrous oxide may be used as a carrier gas in equine anaesthesia but reduces the inspired oxygen concentration and functional residual capacity. This may exacerbate hypoxia, and monitoring PaO_2 by arterial blood gas analysis is essential.

Total intravenous anaesthetic techniques are also possible using a combination of ketamine, an α_2 adrenoceptor agonist and guaiphenesin (sometimes referred to as GGE). Guaiphenesin is a centrally acting muscle relaxant. Propofol used both as a sole agent and in combination with ketamine also has been described for total intravenous anaesthesia in horses and ponies. Currently combinations including propofol are prohibitively expensive.

Intra-operative monitoring

Monitoring of physiological responses under general anaesthesia is of equal importance in horses as in small animals. It is preferable to monitor the electrical activity of the heart continuously using an ECG and also direct arterial blood pressure (see complications of general anaesthesia, below).

Recovery of consciousness and postoperative monitoring

Once the endotracheal tube has been removed following recovery of laryngeal reflexes, the anaesthetic personnel should observe the patient until it is standing and no longer ataxic. In specialist clinics, horses and ponies generally recover from general anaesthesia in a padded room to limit self-inflicted trauma. It is extremely important to avoid unnecessary visual or auditory stimulation during the recovery period. Dimmer switches allowing modulation of the light levels in the recovery box are useful.

Occasionally the nasal mucous membranes of horses and ponies become oedematous following prolonged periods of recumbency, which leads to snoring during recovery. If this causes obstruction to free air flow through the nasal passages, a nasotracheal or orotracheal tube should be placed to maintain the airway and oxygen may be insufflated through these tubes. Such tubes may be taped into position and removed once the horse is standing.

Complications of general anaesthesia

The mortality rate following general anaesthesia in horses is tenfold greater than that in dogs and cats (1.0% versus 0.1%) with cardiac arrest, perioperative fractures and postoperative myopathy the most commonly cited factors.

Hypotension

Suppression of the central nervous system during general anaesthesia is accompanied by depression of the cardiovascular and respiratory systems. Horses in particular are prone to hypotension. A mean arterial blood pressure > 60–70 mmHg is thought to ensure adequate blood flow to organs, and simple measures such as intra-operative administration of intravenous fluids (crystalloids and or colloids) and refining anaesthetic technique to limit administration of hypotensive agents (such as halothane which significantly decreases myocardial contractility in horses) helps to maintain blood pressure within acceptable limits. However, administration of inotropic agents such as dobutamine or dopamine by infusion may be required to maintain blood pressure within acceptable limits.

Hypoxia

In a healthy, conscious, standing horse breathing air, both lung fields are well ventilated and receive adequate blood flow. The PaO_2 is normal. In healthy, unconscious recumbent horses the dependent lung fields (the lower lung field in lateral recumbency and the dorsal lung fields in dorsal recumbency) are no longer normally ventilated but continue to be normally perfused. This occurs because of the combination of the weight of the abdominal viscera pressing on the diaphragm in addition to drug-induced depression of respiration. This effect is compounded if the perfusion of the upper lung is compromised because of hypotension. This phenomenon is referred to as ventilation/perfusion mismatch and can cause hypoxia even when the horse is breathing 100% oxygen. Uncorrected hypoxia and hypercarbia have deleterious effects on the myocardium and may lead to cardiac arrhythmias and ultimately arrest.

The severity of ventilation/perfusion mismatching may be limited by:

- Maximising functional residual capacity (e.g. pre-anaesthetic fasting, treatment of respiratory disease prior to anaesthesia, delaying elective procedures in pregnant mares).
- Allowing horses positioned in dorsal recumbency to recover in left lateral recumbency to ensure the greatest lung mass is uppermost. (*Note:* Do not place horses that have been in right lateral recumbency during a prolonged procedure onto the contralateral side during recovery. This is because there will be atelectasis and hypostatic congestion present in the right lung following right lateral recumbency, obliterating the usual beneficial effects of having this lung field uppermost.)
- Allowing horses to breathe oxygen during anaesthesia (connect endotracheal tube to anaesthetic breathing system or Hudson Demand Valve. Alternatively, insufflate oxygen intranasally or via endotracheal tube at 10–15 litres per minute.)
- Ventilating horse to lower $PaCO_2$ if hypercapnia is severe.
- Using standing restraint. If this is not possible it is best to position horses in left lateral recumbency > right lateral recumbency > dorsal recumbency.

Size

The size and weight of horses and ponies present problems in manoeuvring them when they are anaesthetised. In the field it is important to select a safe environment to induce general anaesthesia. This may be in a grassed field or a well-padded loose box. Careful restraint using experienced handlers and smooth induction of general anaesthesia allows some manipulation of the horse during the transition from standing to lateral recumbency. In specially equipped veterinary clinics, tilting tables, hoists, overhead tracks and floor partitions in the induction/recovery box that also serve as the operating table facilitate the movement of the anaesthetised patient.

Mypopathy

Postanaesthetic myopathy is a distressing condition causing a range of clinical signs from temporary lameness to prolonged recumbency, inability to rise necessitating euthanasia, or incoordination resulting in limb fractures. The pathogenesis of the condition is not completely understood but a number of factors have been implicated including reduced muscle perfusion, duration of recumbency, hypotension, hypoxia, anaesthesia of physically fit horses, high carbohydrate diets, size of horse and poor positioning.

To limit development of this condition, anaesthetised horses are positioned in such a way as to maintain blood supply to limbs. In lateral recumbency the uppermost legs are supported to avoid pressure on the lower legs that may compromise blood circulation of the lower limbs. Padding is important to distribute weight evenly and alleviate pressure points such as the edge of the table. In addition hypoxia, hypotension and prolonged duration of anaesthesia should be avoided.

Neuropraxia

The facial nerve, which courses over the edge of the mandible, is prone to damage during general anaesthesia. Care should be taken to avoid trauma to this area during induction of general anaesthesia, and head collars should be removed for the duration of the general anaesthetic. Damage to other nerves can also occur, e.g. brachial plexus, femoral, peroneal nerves and so on.

Other complications

A number of other complications may be encountered following general anaesthesia in horses and ponies. These include myelomalacia (spinal cord necrosis); tympany (gas accumulation within the gastrointestinal tract); 'excited' recoveries causing self-inflicted trauma that can range from simple abrasions and cuts to disruption of the surgical wound, fractured limbs or pelvis.

RUMINANT ANAESTHESIA

Sheep, goats and cattle are ruminants. Ruminants regurgitate and remasticate solid food and unlike cats, dogs and horses, ruminants have four stomachs. These stomachs are called the reticulum, rumen, omasum and abomasum.

During and following general anaesthesia ruminants are prone to regurgitation with possible aspiration of rumenal contents, bloating (tympany) and excess salivation. In addition, many of the problems encountered in horses and ponies are also encountered in ruminants, e.g. hypotension, myositis and neuropraxia (see above).

Pre-anaesthetic considerations

Many ruminants will not be accustomed to physical restraint, and experienced assistance when handling the larger species is imperative. Preoperative fasting is particularly important to reduce the risk, not only of regurgitation but also of bloat, as ruminants produce large amounts of gas (carbon dioxide and methane) during their normal digestive processes. Food deprivation for 24 h prior to anaesthesia is normal.

Pre-anaesthetic and anaesthetic drugs

Many anaesthetics are not approved for use in food-producing animals, and due consideration must be made to the final fate of ruminants undergoing general anaesthetic procedures, i.e. whether or not they will enter the human food chain. Even when licensed drugs are used (Table 15.1), withdrawal periods for milk and meat must be observed. Withdrawal periods can vary considerably and must always be checked according to manufacturer's instructions.

Because of these limitations, in addition to the complications that may occur under general anaesthesia, local anaesthetic techniques are commonly used in ruminants for a wide variety of procedures including caesarean operation, claw surgery, rumenotomy, dehorning, and so on. Nevertheless a large number of unlicensed pre-anaesthetic and general anaesthetic drugs are used in ruminants (Tables 15.1, 15.2, and 15.3).

Table 15.1 Pre-anaesthetic and anaesthetic drugs licensed for use in ruminants in the UK.

Drug	Animal
Xylazine*	Cattle
Atropine	Cattle, sheep
NSAIDs: Flunixin, carprofen, meloxicam, ketoprofen, tolfenamic acid	Cattle
Halothane	Cattle, sheep
Local anaesthetics: Prilocaine, Procaine	Cattle

*Ruminants are very sensitive to the effects of α_2 adrenoceptor agonists and the dose is approximately one-tenth that used in horses.

Table 15.2 Drugs used for pre-anaesthetic medication in ruminants.

Drug	Comments	Species
Acetylpromazine	Tendency to increase regurgitation	Bovine, ovine, caprine
Alpha-2 adrenoceptor agonists	Only xylazine licensed in cattle; increase salivation	Bovine, ovine, caprine
Benzodiazepines	Intravenous or intramuscular injection; may be administered by mouth to aid restraint of aggressive sheep and goats	Bovine, ovine, caprine

Table 15.3 Drugs used to induce and maintain general anaesthesia in ruminants.

Drug	Comments	Species
Ketamine	Intravenous injection	Bovine, ovine,
	Frequently used in combination with α_2 adrenoceptor	caprine
	agonists to reduce the likelihood of regurgitation on	
	induction	
	May be used by infusion with guaiphenesin	
Thiopentone (Fig. 15.2)	May be used by infusion with guaiphenesin	Bovine, ovine, caprine
Pentobarbitone	May be used for sedation at reduced doses	Bovine, ovine, caprine
Alphaxalone–alphadolone	Expensive	Ovine, caprine
Propofol	Expensive	Ovine, caprine
Halothane	Delivered in oxygen	Bovine, ovine,
	Kids, lambs and calves are amenable to mask induction	caprine
Isoflurane	Delivered in oxygen	Bovine, ovine,
	Kids, lambs and calves are amenable to mask induction	caprine

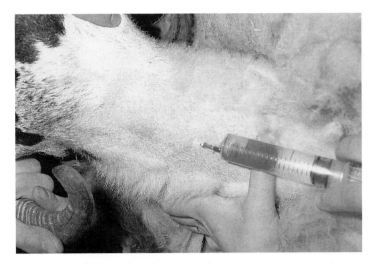

Fig. 15.2 Induction of general anaesthesia in a sheep by intravenous injection of 2.5% thiopentone.

Complications of general anaesthesia

Regurgitation

A number of factors are thought to predispose to regurgitation including choice of induction agent, light general anaesthesia, relaxation of the sphincter mechanisms between the pharynx and oesophagus and the oesophagus and the reticulum (the first of the four stomachs) under deeper general anaesthetic levels, and increased pressure on the rumen during recumbency. In anaesthetised ruminants the protective reflexes of the larynx are suppressed or abolished and aspiration of regurgitated food and fluid may occur. This can cause broncho-constriction or aspiration pneumonia.

There are a number of ways to limit regurgitation or minimise the complications following regurgitation.

Pre-anaesthetic fasting

Mature ruminants should be fasted for up to 24 h. Periods up to 48 h have been suggested but cause the rumen contents to become more fluid. Access to water is removed at least 12 h pre-induction. Ruminants under 1 month of age should not be fasted prior to anaesthesia.

Endotracheal intubation

Cuffed endotracheal tubes help to protect the lower airways from aspiration. Intubation of ruminants is less straightforward than in small animals. Adult cattle tend to be intubated manually by direct palpation with the aid of a gag (e.g. Drinkwater gag). A laryngoscope with a suitably long, compact blade is useful for sheep, goats and calves. The tube is removed only when the patient is in sternal recumbency or can definitely eructate and swallow. The cuff of the tube may be only partially deflated before removal, helping to clear any regurgitated material from the oropharynx (Fig. 15.3).

Recovery

Ruminants should be moved into sternal recumbency as soon as possible during recovery to aid eructation and limit regurgitation.

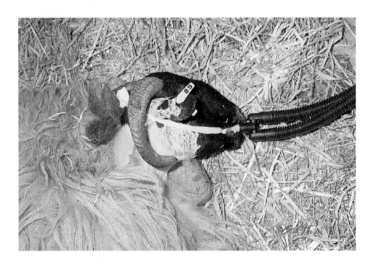

Fig. 15.3 Endotracheal intubation in ruminants protects the lower airways in the event of regurgitation. Note also the sandbag under the neck to incline the nose downwards, allowing saliva to drain from the mouth.

Bloat (tympany)

During normal digestive processes, ruminants, which are herbivores, naturally produce a large amount of gas within the gastrointestinal tract. Much of this is passed out of the gastrointestinal tract during the process of eructation where gas is passed back up the oesophagus to the oropharynx. Eructation normally occurs once per minute. Under general anaesthesia ruminants are no longer able to eructate, which in association with reduced ruminal motility causes gas build-up within the bowel (bloat). This in turn can lead to a reduction in functional residual capacity because of increased pressure on the diaphragm, and also decreases venous return, reducing cardiac output and mean arterial blood pressure. Ruminants are prone to ventilation/perfusion mismatching under general anaesthesia and this effect is compounded by the development of bloat. Appropriate pre-anaesthetic fasting will help to minimise bloat, but a stomach tube may be passed or rumenal trocharisation performed to relieve any excessive build-up of gas that occurs.

Salivation

Ruminants normally produce large volumes of alkaline (bicarbonate-rich) saliva and production continues under general anaesthesia. However because swallowing is not present the saliva either remains within the mouth (from where it may be aspirated) or drains from the mouth. Antisialogogues such as atropine do not reduce the volume of saliva produced but increase the viscosity and are not used. The most efficient method of dealing with saliva under general anaesthesia is to allow it to drain by gravity from the mouth (Fig. 15.3). This may be achieved by positioning the animal in a nose down, tail down position i.e. with the top of the head higher than the rest of the body. This position also aids drainage of regurgitated material from the mouth.

SUMMARY

Many of the basic anaesthetic principles and anaesthetic drugs for large animals are similar to those for small animals. However, the sheer size of many large animal patients, in addition to the different anatomical and physiological considerations between large and small animal species, mean that veterinary nurses involved in anaesthetising horses and ruminants must be familiar with the particular challenges these animals present.

REFERENCES AND FURTHER READING

Clutton, E. (1997) Remote intramuscular injection in unmanageable horses. *In Practice*, **19**, 316–319.

Hall, L.W., Clarke, K.W. & Trim, C.M. (eds) (2001) *Veterinary Anaesthesia*, 10th edition. WB Saunders, Philadelphia.

Hennig, G.E., Kraus, B.H., Fister, R., *et al.* (2001) Comparison of two methods for presurgical disinfection of the equine hoof. *Veterinary Surgery*, 30, 366–373.

Muir, W.W. III & Hubbell, J.A.E. (1992) *Equine Anesthesia Monitoring and Emergency Care*. Mosby Year Book, St Louis, MO.

Webb, A.I. (1984) Nasal intubation in the foal. *Journal of the American Veterinary Medical Association*, 185, 48–51.

White, K. & Taylor, P. (2000) Anaesthesia in sheep. *In Practice*, 22, 126–135.

Index